An Introduction to

VETERINARY IMMUNOLOGY

IAN TIZARD, PhD., B.Sc., B.V.M.S., M.R.C.V.S.

Professor and Head, Department of Veterinary Microbiology and Parasitology
College of Veterinary Medicine, Texas A & M University
College Station, Texas 77843

Second Edition

W. B. SAUNDERS COMPANY

PHILADELPHIA • LONDON • TORONTO

MEXICO CITY • RIO DE JANEIRO • SYDNEY • TOKYO

W. B. Saunders Company: West Washington Square
Philadelphia, Pa. 19105

1 St. Anne's Road
Eastbourne, East Sussex BN21 3UN, England

1 Goldthorne Avenue
Toronto, Ontario M8Z 5T9, Canada

Apartado 26370—Cedro 512
Mexico 4, D.F., Mexico

Rua Coronel Cabrita, 8
Sao Cristovao Caixa Postal 21176
Rio de Janeiro, Brazil

9 Waltham Street
Artarmon, N.S.W. 2064, Australia

Ichibancho, Central Bldg., 22-1 Ichibancho
Chiyoda-Ku, Tokyo 102, Japan

Library of Congress Cataloging in Publication Data

Tizard, Ian R.
  An introduction to veterinary immunology.
  Includes bibliographies and index.
  1. Veterinary immunology. I. Title. [DNLM: 1. Animals—Immunology. 2. Animal diseases—Immunology. 3. Immunologic diseases—Veterinary. SF 757.2 T625i]
SF757.2.T59 1982   636.089'6079   81-40517
ISBN 0-7216-8882-9   ACCR2

Spanish (*1st Edition*)—Nueva Editorial Interamericana

German (*1st Edition*)—Verlag Paul Parey

An Introduction to Veterinary Immunology   ISBN 0-7216-8882-9

Last digit is the print number: 9 8 7 6 5 4

To Claire, Robert and Fiona

Preface to
the Second Edition

The discerning reader, wishing to know whether to invest in a copy of this book, will be interested to note the changes between this and the first edition.

No chapter has entirely escaped revision. The major changes and additions will be found in the descriptions of phagocytic cells, the genetics of immunoglobulin synthesis, the cellular interactions in immune responses and the regulation of immune responses through the activities of genes found in the major histocompatibility complex. Recent advances in our knowledge of resistance to infectious diseases have been less dramatic, but much new information has become available on interferon as well as on immunity to virus-induced tumors and to helminths. There has also been significant growth in information on autoimmune and immunodeficiency diseases of domestic animals.

The quantity of new data presents severe problems to a textbook author. On one hand, the text must expand in order to accommodate the new information. On the other hand, both veterinary students and practicing veterinarians have many demands on their time and rarely have an opportunity to study a comprehensive textbook at leisure. An author must therefore seek to balance these conflicting requirements and at the same time convey a sense of the fascination of this rapidly advancing area of veterinary science. The revisions in this edition have been undertaken with these considerations in mind, and I hope that it will continue to serve a useful role in the teaching of veterinary immunology.

This book could not have been revised without the generous assistance and sound advice of my colleagues Drs. J. B. Derbyshire, T. T. Kramer, P. Eyre and S. Yamashiro. I would like to express my gratitude to Dr. A. Mellors, in whose laboratory most of the revision was undertaken. I would especially like to thank Mr. R. Kersey and the staff of W.B. Saunders Company for their advice and professional skill in nurturing this book through the publishing process. Finally, I must thank my wife Claire, not only for her help and encouragement, but also for her tolerance while the manuscript was in preparation and usually widely scattered across the floor.

IAN TIZARD

Guelph, 1981

Contents

Glossary

ADCC Antibody-dependent cellular cytotoxicity. Lysis of target cells through the actions of antibody and neutrophils, macrophages or null cells.

Adjuvant Material that enhances the normal immune response.

Affinity A measure of the binding strength between an antibody-combining site and an antigenic determinant. It is derived through the law of mass action and is expressed in liters per mole.

Agglutinaton The bringing together of particulate antigens such as bacteria or erythrocytes by antibody.

Allergen An antigen that stimulates the production of reaginic antibodies.

Allergy A term that now encompasses any immunologically mediated adverse consequences of exposure to antigens, but which should be restricted to describing immediate (Type I) hypersensitivity.

Allogeneic Genetically dissimilar but of the same species.

Allograft A graft between allogeneic animals. (The term homograft was once employed in this respect.)

Allotype Genetically controlled antigenic determinants found on protein molecules from some individuals of a species.

Anamnestic response A secondary immune response. The term is generally applied to a secondary response occurring some considerable time after first exposure to antigen.

Anaphylactoid reaction A shock syndrome that superficially resembles anaphylaxis but is not immunologically mediated.

Anaphylaxis A form of immediate (Type I) hypersensitivity mediated by reaginic antibodies and resulting from the acute release of pharmacologically active agents from mast cells or basophils. It may be local or systemic.

Anergy An absence of a cell-mediated immunity (usually a delayed hypersensitivity reaction) in an animal that has been sensitized.

Antibody Immunoglobulins formed in response to the introduction of material into the body that is recognized by the body as foreign. Their characteristic property is to combine under physiological conditions with the inducing material (antigen).

Antigen Material that can bring about an immune response.

Antiglobulin test A test that employs an antibody directed against immunoglobulins to agglutinate particles carrying nonagglutinating antibody on their surface. This is also called the Coombs' test, after the veterinarian who developed it.

Arthus reaction A local immune complex–mediated (Type III hypersensitivity) inflammatory reaction in the skin.

Atopy A term used to describe the inherited tendency to develop immediate (Type I) hypersensitivity found in some humans and dogs.

Autoantibody Antibody directed against antigenic determinants on an animal's own body constituents.

1

Autogenous vaccine   A vaccine prepared from the organisms causing disease in an individual or herd and subsequently used in that same individual or herd in order to stimulate immunity with the intention of assisting recovery. This may be useful when immunity is highly strain-specific.

Autoimmune disease   Disease caused by an immune response directed against an animal's own tissues.

Avidity   A confusing term used by some to describe a property of antibody that determines the rate at which the antibody reacts with antigen, but used by others to refer to the strength of combination of an antiserum with an antigen.

Bacterin   A preparation of killed bacteria used for immunization.

Bence Jones proteins   Proteins found in the urine of individuals with a myeloma. They coagulate on heating the urine to about 60° C and redissolve at higher temperatures. Bence Jones proteins are usually immunoglobulin light chains.

Blastogenesis   The production of dividing cells.

Blocking antibody.   A noncytotoxic, noncomplement-fixing antibody that, by coating cells, can protect them against cell-mediated destruction.

Capping   The aggregation of cell-membrane molecules at a restricted region of a cell surface.

Carrier   An immunogenic molecule to which a hapten is bound.

Chemotaxis   The movement of cells or organisms under the influence of an external chemical stimulus. It may be either positive or negative.

Chimera   An animal that has been successfully populated either naturally or artificially by allogeneic cells.

Clone   A population of identical cells or organisms derived from a single precursor cell or organism.

Complement   A rather complex linked-enzyme and self-aggregating protein system that is activated by a number of factors, particularly antigen-antibody interaction, and that results in a wide variety of biological consequences such as cell membrane lysis and opsonization.

Conglutinin   A constituent of bovine serum, unrelated to immunoglobulins, that combines with fixed third component of complement. If this fixed C3 is attached to a particle such as an erythrocyte, then conglutinin will cause the erythrocyte to aggregate in a reaction known as conglutination.

Coombs' test   See *Antiglobulin test*.

Cytophilic antibodies   Immunoglobulins that are able to bind to cell receptors by virtue of a specific site on their Fc region.

Delayed hypersensitivity   A cell-mediated skin reaction to injected antigen. So-called because the reaction does not reach maximal intensity until 24 to 48 hours after administration of antigen. An example of this is the tuberculin reaction.

Effector cell   A cell performing a specific function.

Endotoxin   A lipopolysaccharide component of gram-negative bacterial cell walls that possesses nonspecific toxic activity.

Enhancement   The prolongation of allograft survival or enhancement of tumor growth brought about by blocking antibodies.

Exotoxin   Soluble proteins, either secreted by living bacteria or released from the cytoplasm of dead organisms, that have a specifc toxic effect. They are usually produced by gram-positive organisms.

Flocculation   A form of precipitation reaction seen when horse serum is used as a source of antibody, in which the precipitate appears as floccules and in which the ratio of antigen-antibody mixtures that give a precipitate is relatively restricted.

Gamma globulins   The group of plasma proteins that have the slowest electrophoretic mobility. It is within this group that antibodies (immunoglobulins) are found.

Globulins   Proteins precipitated by the addition of an equal volume of a saturated solution of ammonium sulfate to serum.

Gnotobiotic animal   An animal that is either germ-free or contaminated with a known bacterial population.

Hapten   A nonprotein molecule that can combine with specific antibody-combining sites but cannot, by itself, initiate an immune response.

Hemadsorption   The attachment of red blood cells to the surface of cultured animal cells following infection with certain viruses.

Hemagglutination   The bringing together of red blood cells by antibody or virus.

Hemagglutination-inhibition   Inhibition of viral hemagglutination mediated by specific antibody against the virus.

Heterophile antigens   Antigenic determinants found widely distributed in nature, e.g., on bacteria, plants and several species of animal.

Histocompatibility antigens   Antigens found on the surface of nucleated cells, which are characteristic of an individual and which provoke allograft rejection, and regulate immune reactions.

Homocytotropic antibodies   A term that includes cytophilic antibodies and all antibodies that attach specifically to cells in the same species as that in which they are made. By convention, use of this term is confined to those antibodies that bind to mast cells or basophils and mediate type I hypersensitivity—i.e., reaginic antibodies.

Hybridoma   A cultured cell line formed by fusion of myeloma cells with antibody-producing B cells.

Idiotype   Antigenic variability of a population of protein molecules within an individual animal. This type of variation is seen in immunoglobulins and is associated with the different amino acid sequences of the antibody-combining sites.

Immediate hypersensitivity   Reaginic antibody-mediated hypersensitivity in which the administration of antigen produces a detectable response within seconds or minutes.

Immunization   Strictly speaking, the administration of antigen to an animal with the intention of producing protective immunity. However, it is now commonly used to describe the procedure for inducing an immune response.

Immunoconglutinins   Autoantibodies directed against fixed third or fourth components of complement. When these complement components are fixed to particles, the presence of immunoconglutinins may cause them to clump. This is called immunoconglutination.

Immunogen   A substance that is able to elicit an immune response.

Immunoglobulins   The class of proteins that have antibody activity.

Immunological tolerance   A form of immune response in which an animal becomes specifically unresponsive to an antigen and in which neither antibodies nor effector lymphocytes are produced.

Incomplete antibodies   Antibodies that, although they may bind to antigenic particles, are unable to link them together to cause agglutination. A preferable term is nonagglutinating antibodies. They may be detected by means of an antiglobulin test.

Interferons   A group of low molecular weight proteins that possess the ability to interfere with viral replication and regulate immune reactivity.

Isogeneic   See *Syngeneic*.

Isotype   Antigenic variability between related proteins found in all animals of the same species. For example, the antigenic differences between immunoglobulin subclasses are isotypic.

K cells   Non-T, non-B lymphocytes that can destroy target cells by ADCC.

Lectins   Proteins, usually of plant origin, that bind to specific monosaccharides. Most lectins used in immunology stimulate lymphocyte proliferation when they bind to cell membrane sugars.

Lymphokines   Lymphocyte-derived glycoproteins that control the activities of other cells. In this way they serve to regulate many aspects of the immune responses.

Mitogen   A substance that stimulates cells to proliferate.

Mixed vaccine   A vaccine containing a mixture of different antigens. Used with the intention of promoting immunity against a number of microorganisms or toxins by a single injection. For instance, canine distemper, infectious hepatitis, and Leptospira vaccines may be satisfactorily combined as a mixed vaccine.

Monokines   Protein products of mononuclear phagocytes that influence the activities of other cell populations.

Myeloma   A tumor of plasma cells.

Null cells   Lymphocytes that lack recognizable T or B cell surface markers.

Natural killer (NK) cell   An ill-defined lymphoid cell found in normal animals and capable of destroying tumor- or virus-infected cells.

Opsonin   A substance that binds to particles and facilitates their phagocytosis.

Passive hemagglutination test   A hemagglutination test brought about by antibody directed against an antigen artificially bound to the surface of erythrocytes. This may also be called indirect hemagglutination.

Pathogenic microorganism   A microorganism that has the ability to cause disease in susceptible animals.

Phagocytosis   Eating by cells. The term encompasses a number of processes, including chemotaxis, adherence, ingestion and digestion of particles.

Pinocytosis   Literally, drinking by cells. A term used to indicate the engulfing of fluid droplets at the cell surface.

Precipitation   The bringing together of soluble antigen molecules by antibody to produce a visible precipitate. The visible precipitate will contain both antigen and antibody.

Premunition   A form of immunity seen in protozoan and some helminth infections that is dependent upon the continued presence of the parasite. Superinfection is prevented as long as parasites persist in the host, but the immunity disappears rapidly after parasite elimination.

Prozone   The absence of detectable immunological reaction in a test system in the presence of low dilutions of high-titered antiserum. This may be due to gross antibody excess or to inhibition of agglutination by complement or nonagglutinating antibody.

Pyroninophilic   Stained by the pink dye pyronin. Pyronin has an affinity for RNA and thus detects ribosomes in cell cytoplasm. Since ribosomes are associated with protein synthesis, a cell with a pyroninophilic cytoplasm is a protein-synthesizing cell.

Reaginic antibody   Antibody that mediates type I hypersensitivity, i.e., IgE and some IgG subclasses.

Rheumatoid factor   An autoantibody directed against normal immunoglobulin. It is found in many autoimmune diseases, especially rheumatoid arthritis and systemic lupus erythematosus.

Serotype   A subtype within a group of organisms that can be identified only by serological techniques.

Serum   The clear yellow fluid expressed when blood has clotted and the clot has been permitted to contract.

Shwartzman reactions   Toxic reactions to bacterial endotoxins in which either a local or a systemic intravascular coagulation occurs. The reaction is precipitated by activation of the alternate pathway of complement.

Syngeneic   Genetically identical.

Titer   A measure of the number of antibody units per unit volume of serum. It is usually expressed as the reciprocal of the dilution of serum in the last tube in a series of increasing dilutions that shows the desired effect.

Tolerance   The failure of the immune system to respond to specific antigen.

Toxoid   The modification of a toxin in such a way that its toxicity but not its immunogenicity is destroyed. This is usually done by treating the toxin with formaldehyde.

Vaccination   The administration of antigen (vaccine) to an animal with the intention of stimulating a protective immune response.

Viral hemagglutination   The clumping of red blood cells that occurs in the presence of certain viruses as a result of attachment of virus to the red cells.

Virulence   This term is used to quantitate the disease-producing power of a particular pathogenic microorganism.

Xenograft   A graft between xenogeneic individuals (i.e., individuals of different species).

1

General Features of the Immune Responses

Humoral Immune Response
Cell-Mediated Immune Response
Tolerance
Mechanism of the Immune Responses

If a piece of living tissue is surgically removed from one animal and grafted onto another of the same species, it usually survives only for a few days before being destroyed by the recipient. This process is significant, not so much for the difficulties it presents to the transplantation surgeon but because it is a reflection of the capacity of the animal body to recognize and then destroy material regarded as foreign. This process is known as an immune response, and the study of immune responses, their mechanisms and consequences, is known as immunology.

The rejection of foreign tissue grafts is but one form of the immune response. Nevertheless, it is of importance as an indication of the existence of a mechanism whereby cells, differing only slightly from an animal's own normal cells, are recognized and promptly eliminated. In general, aged and dying cells are removed from the body by nonimmunological processes. However, cells with minor structural abnormalities may be recognized as "foreign" by the "immune system" and eliminated even though they are otherwise apparently healthy. The immune response to foreign cells as shown by graft rejection may therefore be considered to be an indication of the existence of some form of "surveillance system" that identifies and removes abnormal cells. This system could thus function to prevent the development of tumor cells. In addition, the ability to distinguish between normal body constituents and foreign material is also essential if the body is to maintain itself free from invasion by microorganisms or parasites. In the absence of an effective immune system, massive infections leading to death are inevitable.

The identification of the defensive functions of the immune system long preceded the suggestion that surveillance for abnormal cells might also be necessary. Thus, in the eleventh century the Chinese observed that individuals fortunate enough to recover from smallpox were resistant to further attacks of this disease. Being practical people, they introduced the custom of deliberately infecting infants with smallpox in order to protect them from this disease in later life. The great risks inherent in this procedure were acceptable in an era of high infant mortality, and on gaining experience with the technique they found that the least severe reactions were obtained by selecting the smallpox scabs used in this process from the mildest cases available. The technique gradually spread westward to Europe, where "variolation," as it was called, came to be widely employed in the latter half of the eighteenth century. As a consequence, there occurred a dramatic drop in mortality due to smallpox, resulting in a population explosion that served both to provide soldiers for the Napoleonic wars and to hasten significantly the development of industrial society in Europe.

In 1798, Edward Jenner, an English physician, confirmed the suggestion of one of his patients, a dairy maid, that cowpox could substitute for smallpox in variolation. Since cowpox does not cause severe disease in humans, its use effectively reduced to insignificant levels the risks incurred in protecting against smallpox; the effectiveness of this technique is such that smallpox has become the first major infectious disease to be eradicated from the world.

The general implications of Jenner's observations on smallpox were not realized until 1879, when Louis Pasteur in France made some experimental observations on the resistance of chickens to the causal agent of fowl cholera (*Pasteurella multocida*) (Fig. 1–1). Pasteur possessed a culture of this organism that was accidentally allowed to "age" for several days on a laboratory bench. Nevertheless, he tried to infect chickens with this culture but without success. Being economically inclined, Pasteur kept these chickens for a second experiment, in which they were challenged again, this time with a fresh culture of *P. multocida* known to be capable of killing chickens. To his surprise these chickens still did not die. On investigating the problem further, Pasteur realized that this phenomenon was similar in principle to Jenner's use of cowpox. He therefore called the process vaccination (*vacca* is Latin for "cow"). In vaccination, exposure of an animal to a strain of an organism that will not cause disease (an avirulent strain) can provide protection against a subsequent infection by a disease-producing (virulent) strain of the same, or closely related, organism. (It is of interest to note at this point that vaccination of poultry against fowl cholera is still relatively unsatisfactory, despite Pasteur's initial successes.) Having established the general principle of vaccination, Pasteur applied it to anthrax, rendering the organisms avirulent by growing them at an unusually high temperature. He also developed a successful rabies vaccine by allowing

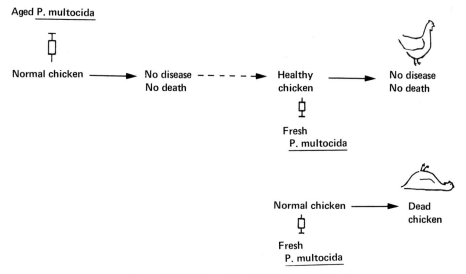

Figure 1–1 Pasteur's fowl cholera experiment.

spinal cords taken from rabies-infected rabbits to dry, and then using the dried cords as his vaccine material, since the drying process effectively rendered the rabies virus avirulent. While Jenner and Pasteur both used avirulent but living organisms in their vaccines, it was not long before other investigators demonstrated that killed organisms, or even some filtrates taken from bacterial cultures, could also give effective protection in other diseases.

HUMORAL IMMUNE RESPONSE

After Pasteur had discovered that it was possible to produce resistance to infectious agents by vaccination, it was soon recognized that the substances that provided this resistance could be found in blood serum. It was shown, for instance, that serum from a vaccinated animal could be used to transfer immunity to a nonvaccinated one. For example, if serum is obtained from a horse made resistant to tetanus toxin by vaccination and this serum is injected into a normal horse in appropriate quantities, then that normal horse will become temporarily resistant to tetanus. The serum from the immune horse is known as tetanus antitoxin and is widely used for the prevention of this disease.

The factors found in serum that confer resistance in this way are known as antibodies. Antibodies to tetanus toxin are not found in normal horse serum but are produced as a result of vaccination. Tetanus toxin is just one example of a foreign substance that stimulates antibody production. The general term for such a substance is antigen. If an antigen is injected into an animal, then antibodies that can combine with that antigen are produced. Antibodies usually only combine specifically with the antigen that stimulates their production so that, for example, the antibodies produced by exposure to tetanus toxin react only with tetanus toxin. If serum containing these antibodies is mixed in a test tube with a solution of tetanus toxin, then a visible precipitate develops as a result of the combination of antibody with the toxin. In addition, the antibody serves to "neutralize" the toxin so that it is no longer toxic. It is by means of this neutralization process that antibodies protect animals against the lethal effects of tetanus toxin.

The time course of the immune response of a horse to tetanus toxin can be followed by bleeding it at intervals after vaccination (Fig. 1–2). The amount of antibody in the serum may be estimated either by measuring the amount of precipitate formed on adding toxin or, alternatively, by measuring the ability of the serum to neutralize a fixed amount of toxin. Both methods yield approximately the same results. Following a single injection of toxin (or its chemically neutralized derivative, tetanus toxoid) into a horse that has never been exposed to it previously, no response is detectable for several days. This is known as the lag period. Antibodies become detectable about one week after the first injection, and the amount present in serum then climbs to reach its highest level by 10 to 14 days before declining rapidly. In general, the amount of antibody formed, and hence the amount of protection conferred, during this first or "primary" response is relatively small. If, some time after the first, a second dose of toxin is given to the same horse and the antibody response again followed, then the lag period lasts for no more than two or three days. The amount of detectable antibody then rises rapidly to a high level before declining slowly. A third dose of toxin given to the same animal results in an immune response characterized by an even shorter lag period and a still higher and more prolonged antibody response. The stimulation of resistance to disease through the use of multiple

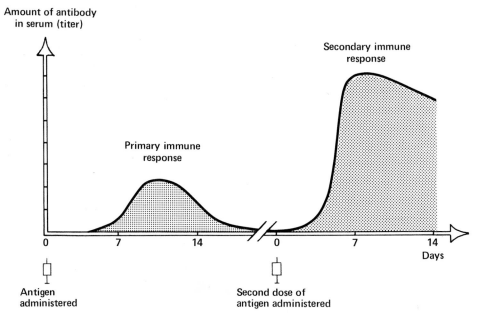

Amount of antibody
in serum (titer)

Secondary immune
response

Primary immune
response

0   7   14   0   7   14

Days

Antigen
administered

Second dose of
antigen administered

Figure 1–2 The time course of the immune response to an antigen as measured by serum antibody levels.

injections of antigen in this way forms the basis of current vaccination techniques employed against infectious diseases.

As we have seen, the response of an animal to a second dose of antigen is very different from the first in that it occurs much more quickly and antibodies reach very much higher levels. This "secondary" response is specific in that it can be induced only by an antigen identical to the first. A secondary response may be invoked many months or years after the first injection of antigen, although its magnitude does tend to decline as time passes. A secondary response can also be induced even though the response of the animal to the first injection of antigen was so weak as to be undetectable. Thus, the antibody forming system possesses the ability to "remember" previous exposure to an antigen. For this reason, the secondary immune response is sometimes known as an anamnestic response (*anamnesko* is Greek for "recollection").

If a second dose of antigen is given to an animal still possessing serum antibodies remaining after its primary immune response, then the level of these antibodies may drop for a few days before the secondary immune response gets under way. This so-called negative phase occurs as a result of the injected antigen binding and removing antibodies from the circulation. It should also be noted that repeated injections of antigen do not lead to greater and greater immune responses indefinitely. The total level of antibodies in serum is relatively well controlled, so that they tend to "plateau," or reach a constant level, even after multiple doses of antigen or exposure to many different antigens.

CELL-MEDIATED IMMUNE RESPONSE

If a skin graft is transplanted from one dog to a second, unrelated dog, it will survive for about 10 days; the graft will initially appear to be healthy, and vascular connections will be established between the graft and its host. By about one week, however, these new blood vessels will begin to degenerate, as a consequence of which the blood supply to the graft will be cut off so that the graft will die and be shed. This slow rejection process is known as a "first-set reaction" (Fig. 1–3). If a second graft is taken from the original donor and placed on the same recipient, then that second graft will survive no longer than one or two days before being rejected. This rapid rejection process is known as a "second-set reaction." Thus, in the process of graft rejection we see that the response to a first graft is relatively weak and slow and analogous to the primary antibody response, whereas a second graft stimulates a very rapid and powerful second-set reaction similar in many ways to the secondary antibody response. Graft rejection, like antibody formation, is specific, in that a second-set reaction occurs only if the second graft is from the same donor as the first. Like antibody formation, the graft rejection process also possesses a "memory," since a second graft may be rapidly rejected many months or years after loss of the first.

However, the graft rejection process is not entirely identical to the process involved in protection against tetanus toxin, since it cannot be transferred from a sensitized to a normal animal by means of serum antibodies. The ability to mount a second-set reaction to a graft can only be transferred between animals by means of living cells. The cells that perform this function are known as lymphocytes and are usually derived from the spleen, lymph nodes or peripheral blood. Because of this, we must conclude that the process of graft rejection is mediated primarily by lymphocytes and not by serum antibodies.

TOLERANCE

We have already discussed how it is essential for the immune system to be able to identify antigens, such as tetanus toxin, or grafts from other animals as foreign. It is an absolute corollary to this that the immune system must be able to recognize antigens on its own cells as being "not-foreign," and it must not mount an immune

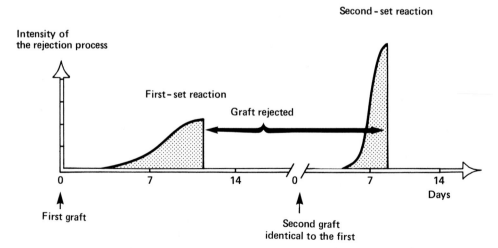

Figure 1–3 The time course of the immune response to a foreign skin graft. Notice how similar this diagram is to Figure 1–2.

response against them. In other words, the immune system must be "tolerant" to self-antigens. If this tolerance breaks down, then disease will occur (autoimmune disease) as either antibodies or lymphocytes destroy normal cells in an attempt to eliminate the offending antigen. Tolerance occurs in both the cell-mediated and antibody-mediated immune systems and can be considered another form of normal immune response. For example, tolerance, as shown by an inability to react to a specific antigen, may be induced by an appropriately administered dose of that antigen. Tolerance is quite specific for the inducing antigen and, like other forms of the immune response, may be boosted only by re-exposure to that same antigen. If not re-exposed to that antigen, then tolerance is gradually lost.

The immune responses may therefore be considered to consist of three general types; they include the antibody and cell-mediated immune responses and tolerance. In considering the necessity for an immune system, it has been pointed out that there is a requirement for self-surveillance as well as for resistance to invasive microorganisms. It is tempting to suggest that the cell-mediated immune responses are a reflection of this surveillance function, whereas the antibody-mediated responses reflect the protective function. Such a distinction is not absolute, however, since antibodies may contribute to graft rejection, and cell-mediated immune responses can participate in resistance to many infectious diseases. Tolerance, on the other hand, represents an essential protective mechanism that serves to prevent an animal from being damaged by an indiscriminate immune response.

MECHANISM OF THE IMMUNE RESPONSES

In some ways the immune system may be compared to a totalitarian state in which foreigners are expelled and citizens who behave themselves are tolerated, but those who "deviate" are eliminated. While this analogy must not be pursued too far, it is readily apparent that such regimes possess a number of characteristic features. These include border defenses and a police force that keeps the population under surveillance and promptly eliminates dissidents. Organizations of this type also tend to develop a pass system, so that foreigners not possessing certain identifying features are rapidly detected and dealt with.

Similarly, when antigen enters the body it first must be trapped in such a way that it can be recognized as being foreign. If so recognized, then this information must be conveyed either to the antibody-forming system or to the cell-mediated immune system. These systems must then respond promptly by the production of specific antibody and/or cells that are capable of eliminating the antigen. The immune systems must also store the "memory" of this event so that on subsequent exposure to the same antigen, their response will be considerably more efficient. In our totalitarian-state analogy, the information would be filed away for future use.

We can therefore consider the basic requirements of the immune systems to include a method of trapping and processing antigen (Fig. 1–4); a mechanism for reacting specifically to the antigen or, in other words, an antigen-sensitive cell; cells to produce antibodies or to participate in the cell-mediated immune responses; cells to retain the memory of the event and to react specifically to the antigen in future encounters; and, finally, cells to eliminate antigen. All of these cell types are recognized within the body. Antigen is trapped, processed and eventually eliminated by cells known as macrophages. Antigen-sensitive cells, both those present at the begin-

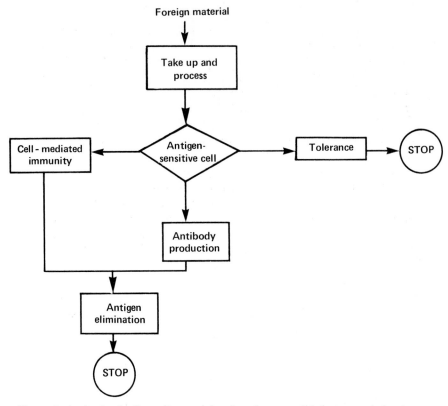

Figure 1–4 A simple flow diagram showing the essential features of the immune responses.

ning of a primary response and those memory cells that initiate a secondary response, as well as the effector cells of the cell-mediated response, are identified as small lymphocytes, while antibody-producing cells are derived from lymphocytes and are known as plasma cells.

In subsequent chapters we will examine each of these basic requirements of the immune responses in turn.

WHERE TO GO FOR ADDITIONAL INFORMATION

Immunology

Basic Immunology Texts Describing the Immune System in Detail

Bach JF. 1981. Immunology, 2nd Ed. John Wiley and Sons, New York. A large comprehensive text that encompasses the whole field of immunology.

Benacerraf B, and Unanue ER. 1979. Textbook of Immunology. Williams & Wilkins Company, Baltimore. A concise review of basic immunology.

Clark WR. 1980. The Experimental Foundations of Modern Immunology. John Wiley and Sons, New York. Arguably, the best available book on basic immunology. It makes extensive use of experimental examples.

Cunningham AJ. 1978. Understanding Immunology. Academic Press, New York. A readable text dealing with basic immunology largely in relation to rodent systems.

Hood LE, Weissman IL, and Wood WB. 1978. Immunology. Benjamin Cummings, Menlo Park, California. An analytical text dealing with the major areas of modern immunology.

Roitt I. 1980. Essential Immunology, 4th Ed. Blackwell Scientific Publications, Oxford. A popular and readable basic and clinical immunology text.

Clinical Immunology Texts

Bellanti JA. 1978. Immunology II. WB Saunders Company, Philadelphia. An excellent account of basic immunology and its clinical applications.

Parker CW. 1980. Clinical Immunology. 2 Vols. WB Saunders Company, Philadelphia. A comprehensive text covering the entire field of human clinical immunology.

Series in Immunology

Advances in Immunology. Academic Press, New York.
Immunological Reviews. Munksgaard, Copenhagen.
Immunology Today. Elsevier North-Holland, Amsterdam.
Progress in Allergy. S. Karger, Basel.

Journals

Many immunology journals contain occasional articles of veterinary interest. Some of the most important of these include: Cellular Immunology, Clinical and Experimental Immunology, European Journal of Immunology, Infection and Immunity, International Archives of Allergy and Applied Immunology, Immunology, Journal of Experimental Medicine, Journal of Immunology, and Parasite Immunology.

Veterinary Immunology

Reviews

The American Veterinary Medical Association organized several symposia between 1969 and 1975 on immunity to infectious diseases in domestic animals. Many of these are now somewhat dated; nevertheless, they remain a useful source of information.

Immunity to selected equine infectious diseases 1969 JAVMA *155* 227–477.
Immunity to selected canine infectious diseases 1970 JAVMA *156* 1661–1817.
Immunity to selected infectious diseases of swine 1972 JAVMA *160* 485–668.
Immunity to selected infectious diseases of cattle 1973 JAVMA *163* 777–924.
Immunity to selected infectious avian diseases 1975 Am J Vet Res *36* 473–604.

Major reviews of veterinary immunology can also be found in:

Veterinary Clinics of North America (1978) *8* 4, WB Saunders Company, Philadelphia.
Advances in Veterinary Science and Comparative Medicine (1979) *23*, Academic Press, New York.
The Ruminant Immune System (1981) Adv. Exp. Med. Biol. *137*, Butler JE ed., Plenum, New York.

Journals

Veterinary journals with frequent articles of immunological interest include Acta Veterinaria Scandinavica, The American Journal of Veterinary Research, The Australian Veterinary Journal, British Veterinary Journal, Canadian Journal of Comparative Medicine, Journal of the American Veterinary Medical Association, Journal of Comparative Pathology, Research in Veterinary Science, Veterinary Bulletin, Veterinary Pathology, The Veterinary Record, and the Cornell Veterinarian.

Two journals that deal specifically with veterinary immunology are:

Veterinary Immunology and Immunopathology, Elsevier North-Holland, Amsterdam, and

Comparative Immunology, Microbiology and Infectious Diseases, Pergamon Press, London.

2

Trapping and Processing
Foreign Material

Animals are faced with the task of permitting the free access of nutrients and oxygen to the body while at the same time excluding potentially damaging foreign material such as bacteria and viruses. In order to serve this function, a number of different protective mechanisms have developed, especially at body surfaces (Chapter 10). In addition, systems have evolved within the body to trap and then eliminate any material that succeeds in evading the outer defenses. These trapping systems act through cells that are able to bind, ingest and destroy foreign material through a process known as phagocytosis (Greek for "eating by cells"). The phagocytic cells of mammals belong to two complementary systems. One system, the myeloid system, consists of cells that act rapidly but are incapable of sustained effort. The second system, the mononuclear phagocytic system, consists of cells that act more slowly but are capable of repeated phagocytosis. These mononuclear phagocytic cells process antigen for the immune response.

MYELOID SYSTEM

The major cell type in the myeloid system is the polymorphonuclear neutrophil granulocyte (neutrophil). Neutrophils are formed in the bone marrow and migrate to the blood stream, where they spend about 12 hours before migrating to the tissues. Their total life-span is only a few days. Neutrophils constitute the major blood leukocyte type in man and carnivores but only about 20 to 30 per cent of ruminant leukocytes.

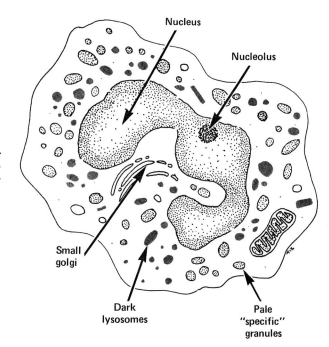

Figure 2–1 The major structural features of a polymorphonuclear neutrophil granulocyte.

STRUCTURE OF NEUTROPHILS

When suspended in blood, neutrophils are round cells about 12μm in diameter. They possess a finely granular cytoplasm at the center of which is a sausage-like or segmented nucleus (Fig. 2–1). Within the cytoplasm are two distinct types of granules. The primary granules, or lysosomes, are electron-dense structures that contain enzymes such as myeloperoxidase and acid hydrolases. The secondary, or "specific," granules are not true lysosomes but nevertheless contain enzymes such as alkaline phosphatase, lysozyme and aminopeptidase. Neutrophils possess a small Golgi apparatus and some mitochondria but no ribosomes or rough endoplasmic reticulum.

FUNCTIONS OF NEUTROPHILS

Phagocytosis. The major function of neutrophils is the destruction of foreign material through the process of phagocytosis. This process is best described by arbitrarily dividing it into stages: chemotaxis, adherence, ingestion and digestion (Fig. 2–2). The first stage in the phagocytic process is the directed movement of neutrophils under the influence of external chemical stimuli. This movement is called chemotaxis. Neutrophils are attracted by many bacterial products, by factors released by damaged cells, and by the products of several immune reactions (Chapters 9 and 17).

Once the neutrophil encounters a particle to be ingested, it must bind it firmly. Normally, this adherence does not happen spontaneously, since both cells and foreign particles suspended in body fluids have a net negative charge (the zeta potential) and hence repel each other. It is therefore necessary to neutralize this charge by coating the particle with a positively charged protein. The best examples of such proteins are antibody molecules and a protein called C3 (the third component of complement)

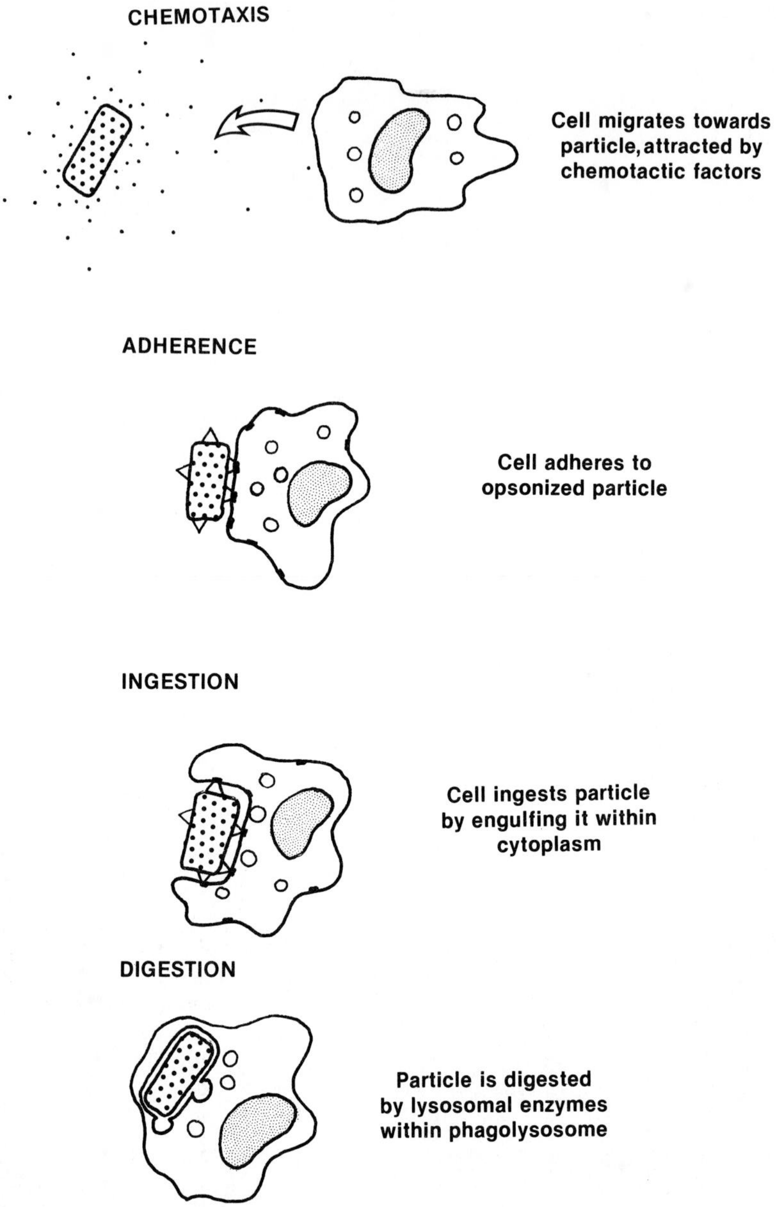

CHEMOTAXIS

Cell migrates towards
particle, attracted by
chemotactic factors

ADHERENCE

Cell adheres to
opsonized particle

INGESTION

Cell ingests particle
by engulfing it within
cytoplasm

DIGESTION

Particle is digested
by lysosomal enzymes
within phagolysosome

Figure 2-2 The process of phagocytosis.

(Chapter 8). A particle coated by antibody or C3 will therefore have a reduced zeta potential, enabling ‎it to make close contact with a negatively charged neutrophil. Neutrophils possess specific receptors for both antibody and C3, which also promote adherence.

Another mechanism that assists in promoting contact between a particle and a phagocytic cell is trapping. Normally, particles are free to float away when they encounter a neutrophil in suspension. In tissues, however, particles may be trapped between a neutrophil and another surface and then be ingested. This process is known as surface phagocytosis.

Once attached firmly to the neutrophil membrane, an adherent particle appears to stimulate local cell-membrane and microtubule activity, which in turn causes the cytoplasm to flow over and around the particle, engulfing it totally (Fig. 2–3). The ease with which this engulfment is accomplished depends, in part, on the nature of the surface of the particle. In general, it is essential that the particle be more hydrophobic than the phagocytic cell. Highly hydrophobic bacteria such as *Mycobacterium bovis* are spontaneously taken into cells. In contrast, *Streptococcus pneumoniae*, which possesses a hydrophilic carbohydrate capsule, is poorly phagocytosed. Fortunately, antibodies and C3 can coat *S. pneumoniae* and render it hydrophobic, so that it may then be readily phagocytosed. Substances that promote attachment and engulfment of particles in this way are known as opsonins (*opson* is Greek for "food preparation").

A particle enclosed within the cytoplasm of a neutrophil finds itself in a space known as a phagosome. Destruction of the particle occurs when hydrolytic enzymes, stored normally within lysosomes, are "emptied" into the phagosome. This occurs as a result of the granules migrating through the cytoplasm and fusing with the phagosome to form a vacuole known as a phagolysosome. The lysosomal enzymes of neutrophils include lysozyme, which can digest some bacterial walls (Chapter 13), proteolytic

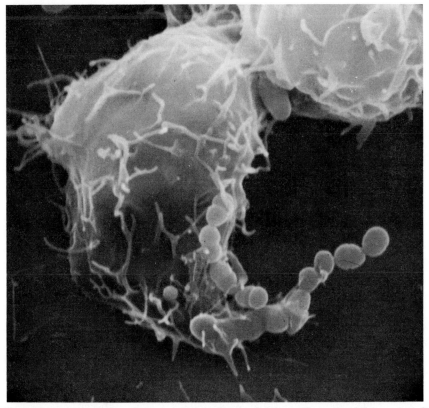

Figure 2–3 A scanning electron micrograph of a bovine milk neutrophil ingesting *Streptococcus agalactiae*. Note how a film of neutrophil cytoplasm appears to flow over the surface of the organism. × 5000.

Table 2–1   SOME OF THE ENZYMES FOUND WITHIN THE LYSOSOMES OF PHAGOCYTIC CELLS*

Enzymes acting on proteins and peptides	Cathepsins Collagenases Elastases Plasminogen activator Kininogen activator Acid phosphatase
Enzymes acting on lipids	Phospholipases Aryl sulfatase
Enzymes acting on carbohydrates	Lysozyme Neuraminidase Glucosidases Galactosidases Hyaluronidase
Enzymes acting on nucleic acids	Acid ribonuclease Acid deoxyribonuclease
Enzymes of the respiratory burst	Myeloperoxidase Superoxide dismutase Catalase

*More than 60 of these enzymes are known.

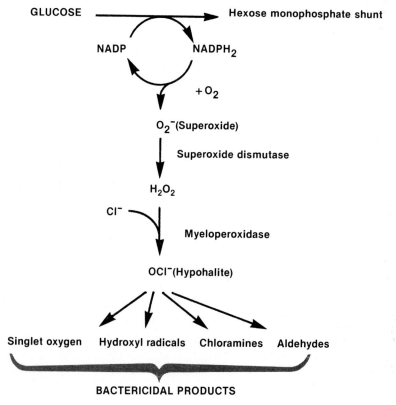

Figure 2–4 The respiratory-burst pathway in neutrophils. Catalase performs the same function as myeloperoxidase within macrophages.

enzymes, myeloperoxidase, ribonuclease and phospholipases (Table 2–1). Taken together, these enzymes are lethal for most microorganisms, but, as might be expected, variations in susceptibility are observed. Gram-positive organisms susceptible to lysozyme are rapidly destroyed. Gram-negative bacteria such as *Escherichia coli* survive somewhat longer, since their outer wall is relatively resistant to digestion. Some organisms such as *Brucella abortus* and *Listeria monocytogenes* are so resistant to the lethal effects of the lysosomal enzymes that they may multiply within phagocytic cells.

The Respiratory Burst.   When a particle is ingested by a neutrophil, a series of biochemical events occur which promote the destruction of the particle.

First, there is enhancement of glycolysis, which results in the production of large amounts of lactic acid within the phagolysosome. This serves to provide an environment that is optimal for the activities of the lysosomal proteolytic enzymes. Second, and more importantly, there is enhancement of the hexose monophosphate shunt, reflected by a marked increase in the cell's oxygen consumption. This "respiratory burst" results in an increased turnover of reduced nicotinamide adenine dinucleotide phosphate ($NADPH_2$) (Fig. 2–4). The recycling of $NADPH_2$ by means of the activities of the enzymes superoxide dismutase and myeloperoxidase results in the generation of highly reactive oxygen metabolites. These include hydrogen peroxide, superoxide anion (O_2^-), singlet oxygen, hydroxyl radicals, chloramines and aldehydes. All of these are very toxic for microorganisms. The importance of the respiratory burst is shown by the observation that animals deficient in either superoxide dismutase or myeloperoxidase suffer from severe recurrent bacterial infections (Chapter 22).

THE FATE OF NEUTROPHILS

Neutrophils possess a limited supply of energy reserves, which cannot be replenished. Therefore, although neutrophils may be very active immediately after release from the bone marrow, they are rapidly exhausted and are usually capable of undertaking only a limited number of phagocytic events. Thus, neutrophils may be considered a first line of defense, moving rapidly toward foreign material and destroying it promptly but being incapable of a sustained effort. Fortunately, a second line of defense is available—the mononuclear phagocytic system. Since neutrophils usually completely destroy any ingested foreign material, they do not process antigen in preparation for presentation to antigen-sensitive cells.

EOSINOPHILS

The second major cell type of the myeloid system is the eosinophil, so-called because its cytoplasmic granules stain intensely with the dye eosin. Eosinophils develop within the bone marrow before migrating into the blood stream, where they circulate with a half-life of only 30 minutes. They subsequently migrate into the tissues, where they have a half-life of about 12 days. The proportion of eosinophils among the blood leukocytes varies with the parasite burden of an animal but ranges from 2 per cent in dogs to 10 per cent in cattle.

Eosinophils are less efficient than neutrophils at phagocytosis, but they do possess lysosomes and mount a respiratory burst when appropriately provoked. They have, in addition, two specialized functions. First, they are uniquely fitted to attack and destroy invading larval helminths. Eosinophil enzymes are particularly effective in destroying larval helminth cuticles (Chapter 15). Second, the enzymes of eosinophils are able to neutralize the inflammatory factors released by mast cells and basophils and therefore regulate the inflammation caused by these cells (type I hypersensitivity) (Chapter 17).

BASOPHILS

Basophils are the least numerous myeloid cells in the blood of domestic animals, constituting about 0.5 per cent of blood leukocytes. Their cytoplasmic granules stain intensely with basophilic dyes such as hematoxylin. Basophils serve a function similar to that of mast cells (see Chapter 17)—namely, to provoke acute inflammation at sites of antigen deposition.

THE MONONUCLEAR PHAGOCYTIC SYSTEM
(Fig. 2–5)

If an animal is injected intravenously with a suspension of carbon particles such as those found in India ink, these particles are taken up from the blood stream by cells throughout the body. Aschoff, the German scientist who discovered this phenomenon, considered that these cells collectively constituted a body system, which he named the reticuloendothelial system. It is now thought, however, that not all the cells that can take up carbon particles in this way actually have the removal of foreign material as their prime function. The cells whose major function is the removal of foreign material

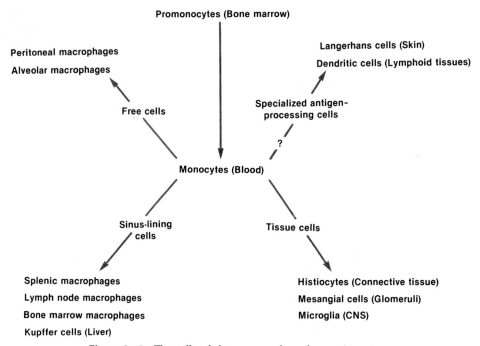

Figure 2–5 The cells of the mononuclear-phagocytic system.

and cell debris are but one component of Aschoff's original reticuloendothelial system, and these cells are now known as the mononuclear-phagocytic system. The mononuclear-phagocytic system consists of a population of cells called macrophages, each containing a single, rounded nucleus.

In contrast to neutrophils, the macrophages of the mononuclear phagocytic system are capable of sustained phagocytic activity, they do process antigen in preparation for the immune response and they make a direct contribution to the repair of tissue damage by removing dead, dying and damaged tissue.

Macrophages are widely distributed throughout the body. Immature macrophages found in the blood stream are called monocytes. They normally constitute about 5 per cent of the total leukocyte population. Mature macrophages may be found in connective tissue, where they are known as histiocytes, or they may be found lining the sinusoids of the liver, where they are called Kupffer cells. The macrophages of the brain are called microglia, and those in the lung are called alveolar macrophages. Major populations of macrophages are found in the spleen, bone marrow, and lymph nodes in close association with sinusoidal endothelium. Nevertheless, irrespective of their name or location, they are all macrophages and they are all part of the mononuclear phagocytic system.

STRUCTURE OF MACROPHAGES

Because of their various habitats, macrophages possess a wide variety of shapes. In general, however, they are round cells, about 14 to 20 μm in diameter when in suspension. They possess abundant cytoplasm, at the center of which is a single, roundish, bean-shaped or indented nucleus (Figs. 2–6 and 2–7; see also Fig. 6–12). The perinuclear cytoplasm contains mitochondria, a Golgi apparatus, large numbers of lysosomes and some rough endoplasmic reticulum, indicating an ability to synthesize protein. The peripheral cytoplasm is usually devoid of organelles, especially in cultured cells, and in living macrophages appears to be in continuous movement, forming and reforming veil-like ruffles. Macrophages can adhere tenaciously to glass surfaces, on which they spread by sending out long, thin cytoplasmic filaments. Some mononuclear phagocytes show variations from this basic macrophage structure. Thus, peripheral blood monocytes tend to have round nuclei, which elongate as the cells mature; alveolar macrophages rarely possess rough endoplasmic reticulum, but their cytoplasm tends to be full of granules; and the microglia of the central nervous system have rod-shaped nuclei and possess very long, thin cytoplasmic processes that are lost when the cell is stimulated into activity by tissue damage.

The structure of macrophages may alter dramatically following cell-mediated immune responses to certain microorganisms. In particular, the macrophages may enlarge and their lysosomes increase greatly in number (see Fig. 6–12). In other situations where foreign material persists for long periods within the body, macrophages may accumulate in large numbers around the persistent material, giving an epithelium-like appearance on histological examination. These cells are therefore referred to as epithelioid cells (Chapter 20). Epithelioid cells are large cells packed closely together and hence are usually polygonal in shape. They possess abundant cytoplasm containing many lysosomes and much endoplasmic reticulum. On occasion these epithelioid cells may fuse together to form multinucleated giant cells in an apparent attempt to totally enclose large particles that cannot be ingested by a single cell.

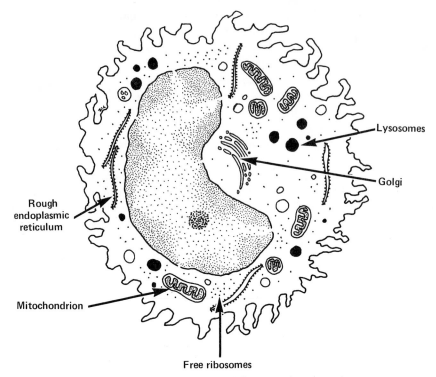

Figure 2−6   The major structural features of a macrophage.

LIFE HISTORY OF MACROPHAGES

All the cells of the mononuclear-phagocytic system arise originally from bone marrow stem cells known as promonocytes. The immediate progeny of these cells are

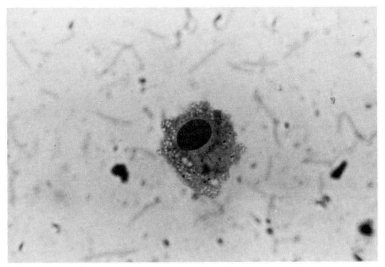

Figure 2−7   Bovine alveolar macrophage containing phagocytosed *Pasteurella hemolytica*. × 900. (From a specimen kindly provided by Dr. B. Wilkie.)

monocytes, which enter the blood stream, where they remain for only a few days (three days in rodents) before entering tissues and developing into macrophages. Under some circumstances and in some species, macrophages may divide to yield daughter macrophages. These tissue macrophages are relatively long-lived cells, replacing themselves at a rate of about 1 per cent per day unless called upon to ingest foreign particles. Their life span in that case depends upon the nature of the ingested material. If, for instance, the ingested particle is easily digested by lysosomal enzymes, the macrophage life span may be unaffected. Some ingested particles, such as the carbon injected in tattoo marks, may be chemically inert. In this case, macrophages may survive for a long time with the inert particle inside, although they may fuse to form giant cells in a further attempt to eliminate the large foreign particles. In some circumstances, such as after intravenous injection of India ink, macrophages may carry the particles to the lung or intestine and from there into the bronchiolar or intestinal lumen whence they are eliminated from the body. In contrast, some particles, although readily phagocytosed, are toxic to macrophages. For example, asbestos particles kill macrophages after phagocytosis and so must be rephagocytosed repeatedly. This continuing destruction of macrophages leads to excessive release of lysosomal enzymes and results in chronic tissue destruction, inflammation and granulation tissue formation. (See also Chapter 20.)

FUNCTIONS OF MACROPHAGES

The major roles of the cells of the mononuclear-phagocytic system are to phagocytose and destroy foreign particles and dead and dying tissues, and to process the foreign material in such a way that it can provoke an immune response. In addition, macrophages can act to regulate the immune response (Chapter 7), to synthesize proteins of the complement system (Chapter 8), and to secrete factors that influence the process of inflammation.

Phagocytosis. Phagocytosis by macrophages is a very similar process to that described previously for neutrophils. Macrophages are chemotactically attracted not only to microbial products and products of the immune reactions, but also to factors released by damaged cells, especially damaged neutrophils. Neutrophils thus not only reach and attack foreign material first, but in dying serve to enhance the accumulation of macrophages at the site of invasion. Antigen is destroyed within macrophages in a manner similar to the process in neutrophils. However, the respiratory burst is much less intense within macrophages. Mature macrophages do not contain myeloperoxidase, but they do contain catalase, which may have an equivalent function.

Antigen-Processing by Macrophages. If all foreign material were totally ingested, digested and destroyed by phagocytic cells, there would be no necessity and no stimulus for the immune responses. It is clear, therefore, that at least some intact antigen must persist in order to stimulate antigen-sensitive cells. When the fate of radioactively labeled antigen is closely followed, it is found that, although most antigen is digested and destroyed, a few molecules remain intact within some macrophages and may be found on the cell surface membrane. The subpopulation of macrophages that do this are characterized by possessing a cell surface antigen called Ia (Chapter 7). Antigen molecules may persist on the macrophage surface for a very long time; it is they that act as the stimulus for the first stage of the immune response—the stimulation of antigen-sensitive lymphocytes.

The processing of antigen in this way serves to regulate the amount of foreign material that reaches the antigen-sensitive cells. If antigen succeeds in evading the macrophages and reaching the antigen-sensitive cells directly, then either tolerance will develop or the resulting immune response will be considerably poorer than normal.

Dendritic Cells. In the cortex of lymph nodes and in the skin, there exists a population of macrophage-like cells which is characterized by an extensive array of long, filamentous cytoplasmic processes. In the lymph nodes, these cells are called dendritic cells; they are called Langerhans' cells in the skin (Fig. 2–8). Dendritic cells and Langerhans' cells can bind antibody to their processes in such a way that it remains free to attach to antigen. As a result, dendritic cells form an extensive antigen-trapping web. Antigen bound to dendritic cells is a very potent stimulant for antigen-sensitive cells, being about ten thousand times more efficient in this respect than unbound antigen. Since the presence of antibody is required for effective antigen trapping by these cells, the dendritic cell system is used only to process antigen for a secondary and subsequent immune response. The enhanced immune responses that occur following a second or subsequent dose of antigen are probably due, at least in part, to the greater efficiency of the dendritic cell system.

Secretory Products of Macrophages. Macrophages secrete a wide variety of biologically important factors into their surroundings. Some of these, such as the complement components C2, C3, C4 and C5 (Chapter 8) and the enzyme lysozyme (Chapter 14), are protective, since they have antimicrobial activity and are secreted continuously. Other factors, such as collagenase, elastase and plasminogen activators, are released during the phagocytic process and may be important in inflammation and

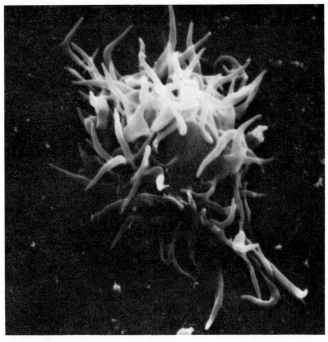

Figure 2–8 A scanning electron micrograph of a cell, possibly a dendritic cell, from a normal guinea pig popliteal lymph node. × 4000. (From Tizard IR, and Holmes WLJ. 1975. Reticuloendothel Soc *17* 333–341. Used with permission.)

wound healing. Finally, macrophages play an important role in regulating the immune responses by secreting regulatory glycoproteins (monokines) such as interferon and interleukin 1 (Chapter 7), hormones such as cyclic AMP, and pharmacologically active agents such as the prostaglandins and leukotrienes (Chapter 17).

FATE OF FOREIGN MATERIAL WITHIN THE BODY

Particulate Antigens Given Intravenously. If colloidal particles, such as the carbon particles of India ink or those of a bacterial suspension, are injected intravenously, they will circulate for a period of time but will be progressively trapped and removed by the macrophages that line the blood sinusoids of the liver, spleen and bone marrow. Most of these cells are found in the liver, which because of its large size will remove the bulk of the injected material. The spleen is a more effective filter than the liver but, being a much smaller organ, it is quantitatively less important. Some of the injected particles will also be trapped by cells as they pass through the pulmonary circulation, so that a significant fraction of the injected material may accumulate in the lung. Bacteria may be rapidly eliminated from the circulation in this way. The rate of clearance is greatly increased if antibodies directed against the bacteria are also present, since opsonization increases trapping efficiency (Fig. 2–9). Some compounds such as bacterial endotoxins, estrogens and simple lipids appear to stimulate macrophage activity and therefore also increase the rate of bacterial clearance.

If antibodies are absent or if the bacteria possess an antiphagocytic polysaccharide capsule, then the rate of clearance is decreased. Drugs, such as steroids, that depress

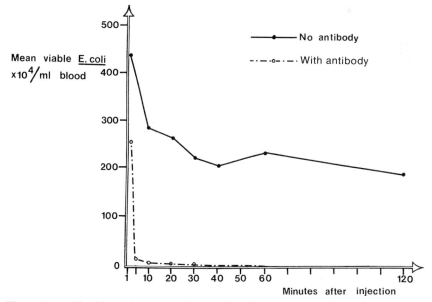

Figure 2–9 The blood clearance of *Escherichia coli* from piglets. One animal had no antibodies; the other had received antibodies to *E. coli*. The importance of antibodies in promoting blood clearance is readily seen. (From Brandenburg AC, and Wilson M. 1974. Res Vet Sci *16* 171–175. Used with permission.)

macrophage activity also depress the clearance rate. If an experimental animal is injected intravenously with a large quantity of a suspension of phagocytosible particles (such as colloidal carbon) then, for a variable period of time subsequently, other particles (such as bacteria) will be very poorly removed from the blood stream. This probably occurs because the first dose of particles effectively absorbs all the nonspecific serum opsonins and so blocks further phagocytosis. In this situation, the mononuclear phagocytic system is said to be blockaded. Blockade of the mononuclear-phagocytic system brought about by massive numbers of bacteria may be a significant factor in reducing the resistance of animals suffering from a severe bacteremia by reducing the rate of clearance of bacteria from the blood stream.

Soluble Antigens Given Intravenously.   Unless very carefully treated, solutions of proteins spontaneously form aggregates as molecules come together. If a solution of a soluble protein antigen is injected intravenously, these aggregates are rapidly removed by the cells of the mononuclear-phagocytic system. The unaggregated remainder, in contrast, is distributed evenly through the animal's blood volume and, if sufficiently small ($\leq$ 100,000 daltons), is also distributed through the extravascular tissue fluids. Once this initial stage of equilibration is achieved, the antigen will be treated like other body proteins and be catabolized, resulting in a slow but progressive decline in antigen concentration. Within a few days, however, the animal begins to mount an immune response to the antigen, and antibodies are produced that combine with the antigen to form immune complexes. These immune complexes are then cleared from the circulation by the mononuclear-phagocytic system. In this way all the antigen is rapidly and completely eliminated (Fig. 2–10).

This triphasic clearance pattern of distribution, catabolism and immune-elimination may be modified under certain circumstances. For example, if the animal has not been previously exposed to the antigen, then the immune response will be a primary one. In this case it takes between five and ten days before antibodies are produced and immune-elimination occurs; if the animal has been previously primed by exposure to the antigen, then a secondary immune response is mounted in two to three days, and the stage of progressive catabolism is therefore relatively short. On the other hand, if antibodies are already circulating in the animal at the time of antigen administration, then immune-elimination occurs immediately and no phase of catabolism is seen. If the material injected is not antigenic or if the immune response does not occur, owing to either tolerance or immunosuppression, then the phase of progressive catabolism continues until all the material is eliminated.

Fate of Antigen Administered by Other Routes.   If insoluble or aggregated antigen is injected into a tissue, some slight damage is bound to occur. As a consequence of this, phagocytic cells—first neutrophils and then macrophages—migrate toward the injection site under the influence of chemotactic factors released from damaged tissue; these cells phagocytose the injected material. This material is then processed, eventually stimulating an immune response. Antibodies and complement (Chapter 8) interact with the antigen, generating more chemotactic factors that attract still more macrophages and in this way hasten the final elimination of the offending material.

If soluble antigen is injected into a tissue, then it will be redistributed by the flow of tissue fluid through the lymphatic system, eventually reaching the blood stream; its final fate is thus similar to intravenously injected material. Any aggregates present are phagocytosed either by tissue macrophages or by the macrophages and dendritic cells of lymph nodes through which the tissue fluid passes.

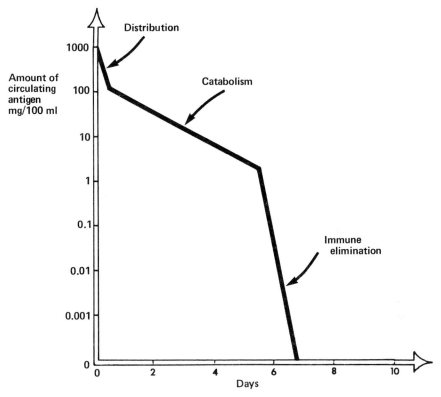

Figure 2–10 The clearance of soluble antigen from the blood stream.

Normally, antigens passing through the intestinal tract are largely catabolized by the digestive enzymes to nonantigenic molecules such as amino acids and monosaccharides. However, some antigenic molecules may remain intact and penetrate the intestinal epithelium. This occurs particularly with the bacterial polysaccharides and those antigens that associate with lipids, since they may be absorbed in chylomicrons. Antigens that succeed in entering the vascular system are promptly filtered out by the Kupffer cells of the liver, whereas those entering the intestinal lymphatics are trapped in the mesenteric lymph nodes. The relatively large size of these nodes in many species testifies to their activity in this respect.

The fate of inhaled antigenic particles depends in large part on their size (see Fig. 10–1). Relatively large particles (greater than 3 μm diameter) are deposited on the mucus layer overlying the respiratory epithelium from the trachea to the terminal bronchioles. These particles are then removed from the respiratory tract by the flow of mucus toward the pharynx or by coughing. Particulate antigens that succeed in reaching the alveoli are mainly ingested by alveolar macrophages that carry them back to the bronchoalveolar junction, where they are also removed from the lung in the mucus layer. Nevertheless, some antigens may be absorbed from the alveoli and diffuse into the interalveolar tissue. Small particles absorbed in this way are cleared to the draining lymph nodes, whereas soluble antigens tend to enter the blood vessels and are therefore distributed throughout the body. When massive quantities of particles are inhaled, as occurs in workers exposed to industrial dusts and to a lesser extent in cigarette smokers, the alveolar macrophage system may be temporarily blockaded and the lung rendered more susceptible to invasion by microorganisms.

ADDITIONAL SOURCES OF INFORMATION

Allison AC. 1978. Macrophage activation and nonspecific immunity. Int Rev Exp Pathol *18* 304–346.

Babior BM. 1978. Oxygen-dependent microbial killing by phagocytes. N Engl J Med *298* 659–668, 721–726.

Bellanti JA, and Dayton DH. 1975. The Phagocytic Cell in Host Resistance. Raven Press, New York.

Birmingham JR, and Jeska EL. 1980. The isolation and long-term cultivation and characterization of bovine peripheral blood monocytes. Immunology *41* 807–818.

Dannenberg AM. 1975. Macrophages in inflammation and infection. N Engl J Med *293* 489–493.

Davies P, and Bonney RJ. 1979. Secretory products of mononuclear phagocytes: A brief review. J Res *26* 37–47.

Hart IR, and Fidler IJ. 1979. The collection, purification and characterization of canine peripheral blood monocytes. J Res *26* 121–133.

Hocking WG, and Golde DW. 1979. The pulmonary-alveolar macrophage. N Engl J Med *301* 580–587, 639–645.

Nathan CF, Murray HW, and Cohn ZA. 1980. The macrophage as an effector cell. N Engl J Med *303* 622–626.

Nelson DS. 1976. Immunology of the macrophage. Academic Press, New York.

Wilkinson PC. 1976. Recognition and response in mononuclear and granular phagocytes: A review. Clin Exp Immunol *25* 355–366.

3

Antigens and Antigenicity

Although neutrophils and the cells of the mononuclear-phagocytic system serve to trap and phagocytose foreign material, not all of this material is capable of subsequently stimulating an immune response. In fact, there appear to be relatively strict limitations on the nature of substances that can do so. The two most important of these limitations are, first, physicochemical restrictions on the types of molecules involved and, second, the nature of the foreign material, which must be such that it can be recognized as not being a normal body constituent.

ESSENTIAL FEATURES OF ANTIGENICITY

Physicochemical Limitations. In order to be antigenic, molecules must be large, rigid and chemically complex. Although small molecules can act as antigens, large molecules are better. For example, serum albumin, with a molecular weight of over 60,000 daltons, is a good antigen, while angiotensin (molecular weight 1031 daltons) is an extremely poor antigen, and a single amino acid such as phenylalanine (molecular weight 165 daltons) is never antigenic by itself. With regard to complexity, macromolecules of complex structure such as the proteins are considerably better antigens than simple large polymers with identical repeating subunits. For this reason, lipids, carbohydrates and nucleic acids, as well as mono-amino acid polymers, are relatively poor antigens. As will be described later, the immune system responds to characteristic stereochemical shapes, and as a result of this response, compounds that have a flexible structure (i.e., those not able to assume a stable configuration) cannot be easily recognized and hence are poorly antigenic. An example of this type of molecule is gelatin, a protein well known for its structural instability, which is a weak antigen unless stabilized by the incorporation of tyrosine or tryptophane molecules. Similarly, flagellin, a protein component of bacterial flagellae, is structurally unstable, and its antigenicity is greatly enhanced by polymerization.

One other physicochemical limitation on antigenicity is degradability. Because the immune response is an antigen-driven process, it follows that if molecules are extremely rapidly catabolized, insufficient quantities may be available to stimulate antigen-sensitive cells. Conversely, the lack of antigenicity of the large inert organic polymers such as the plastics is related not only to their molecular uniformity but also to their metabolic inertness, since they are not degraded and processed by macrophages to a form suitable for initiation of an immune response. A practical consequence of this is seen in the use of glutaraldehyde-fixed porcine heart-valves in human cardiac surgery. The glutaraldehyde "fixes" the valve protein, rendering it metabolically inert and thus non-antigenic.

Foreignness. The second major requirement for antigenicity is foreignness, and antigen-sensitive cells do not respond to material that is not so recognized. The nature of this discrimination is not entirely clear, but it is apparently due to the "turning-off" or "elimination" of cells that may react to self-antigens. It is probable that the lack of response to self-antigens is brought about by exposure of antigen-sensitive cells to these antigens at an early stage in their development (usually early in fetal life). If this exposure does not occur, then self-tolerance does not occur. For example, certain cells such as those in the testes are not in immediate contact with the blood circulation and therefore do not encounter the cells of the immune system. If this isolation is broken down by trauma or by infection, then the testicular cells may encounter antigen-sensitive cells that regard them as foreign and so stimulate an immune response. On a smaller scale, the mitochondria of normal cells not only are removed from direct contact with the circulation, but also have possibly evolved from symbiotic bacteria. As a consequence, if extensive cell destruction occurs in organs such as the liver or heart, antimitochondrial antibodies may be detected in the serum several weeks later.

ANTIGENIC DETERMINANTS AND ANTIGEN SIZE

While complex particles such as bacteria, nucleated cells or erythrocytes can stimulate the immune response, they are obviously composed not of single antigens but of a complex mixture of proteins, glycoproteins, polysaccharides, lipopolysaccharides and lipids. When we observe an immune response against such a particle, we are really observing a number of simultaneous immune responses against each of the antigens on these particles.

On a smaller scale, single protein molecules are not, in themselves, single antigens. Macromolecules have on their surface, areas against which the immune response tends to be directed and with which antibodies tend to bind. These areas are termed antigenic determinants or epitopes. Antigenic determinants on proteins contain about four to six amino acids and are found on exposed or prominent areas on the surface of the molecule (Fig. 3–1). (In general, the number of antigenic determinants on a molecule is directly related to the molecule's size, with about one antigenic determinant for each 5000 daltons.) We can thus narrow our definition of foreignness to the recognition of those antigenic determinants not recognized as self. Identical antigenic determinants may be found on a number of different molecules so that antibody directed against one antigen may be found to react unexpectedly with antigen from an apparently unrelated source. This is known as a "cross-reaction." For example, antibodies to many bacteria are also able to react with animal erythrocytes, since they each possess some surface antigenic determinants in common. Some animals possess antibodies that react with red cells from other animals of the same species. Thus, pigs of blood group O possess antibodies that react with porcine red

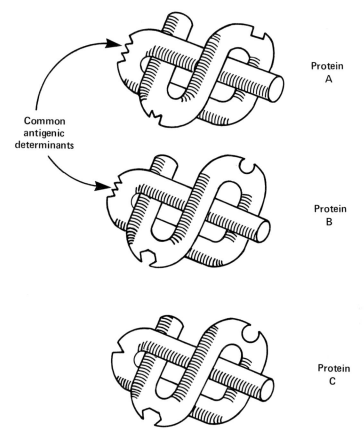

Protein A

Common antigenic determinants

Protein B

Protein C

Figure 3–1 A schematic diagram of three related protein molecules showing how antigenic determinants are found on prominent regions of the molecules. An antiserum to protein A also reacts with protein B because they possess a common antigenic determinant. Similarly, antiserum to protein B reacts with both protein A and protein C, and an antiserum to protein C also reacts with protein B.

cells of blood group A. These "heterophile" antibodies arise not as a response to previous immunization with group A red cells, but in response to antigens found in feed or in the bacterial flora and absorbed from the intestine.

Another example of cross-reactivity occurs between *Brucella abortus* and some strains of *Yersinia enterocolitica*. *Y. enterocolitica*, a relatively unimportant organism, may provoke cattle to make antibodies that react with *B. abortus*. Since brucellosis is detected by testing for the presence of serum antibodies, a yersinia-infected animal may be wrongly thought to carry *B. abortus* and so be killed.

A third example of cross-reactivity occurs between the virus of feline infectious peritonitis (FIP) and pig transmissible gastroenteritis (TGE). It is very difficult to grow the FIP virus in the laboratory. TGE virus, on the other hand, is readily propagated. By detecting antibodies to TGE in cats, it is possible to diagnose FIP without culturing FIP virus.

The degree of cross-reactivity between two antigens is a reflection of the degree of their structural similarity, and this principle may be used to determine relationships between molecules or between species of animals or plants. Thus, in the example

Table 3–1 RELATIVE AMOUNT OF
PRECIPITATE FORMED
WHEN SERUM ALBUMIN FROM EACH
SPECIES IS MIXED WITH
ANTIBODIES TO BOVINE SERUM ALBUMIN

SPECIES	RELATIVE AMOUNT OF PRECIPITATE FORMED
Cattle	+ + + +
Sheep	+ +
Goat	+ +
Pig	+
Chicken	−

given in Table 3–1, it is apparent that, on the basis of antigenic cross-reactivity, goats and sheep are more closely related to cattle than are pigs or chickens.

HAPTENS AND CARRIERS

Although we have already stated that antigens must be large molecules, it has also been pointed out that antigenic determinants are relatively small. It is therefore possible to generate artificial antigenic determinants by chemically linking small organic compounds to macromolecules. If an antigen is modified in this way and used to immunize an animal, antibodies will be formed against any unaltered determinants on the macromolecule, and against the small organic compound itself.

Since small compounds by themselves are not capable of stimulating an immune response, they are not *immunogenic*. Nevertheless, because they can do so when linked to larger molecules and because they can combine with antibodies generated as described above, they must be considered to be *antigenic*. Compounds used in this fashion are known as haptens, and the macromolecules to which they are attached are generally called the carriers. By using haptens of known chemical structure, it is possible to study in great detail the factors influencing the specificity of the reaction between antibody and hapten. For example, the ability of an antiserum to react against one hapten may be compared with its ability to react with structurally related haptens. By means of this simple technique it can be shown that any change in hapten structure that modifies its overall shape reduces its ability to bind antibodies directed against the unmodified molecule. These factors include changes in the hapten's charge, its size or its surface configuration (Table 3–2). Purely chemical changes, which do not alter the shape or the charge distribution of the hapten, do not influence its ability to combine with specific antibody. Since even very minor chemical changes usually result in significant alterations in molecular shape and hence affect the ability of an antibody to combine with a hapten, it has been suggested that an animal must possess the capacity to generate an enormously large variety of antibody molecules in order to account for their apparent ability to combine with all potential haptens. However, because of structural similarities and overlaps, the actual number of different antigenic determinants is probably only about 10 million.

The response of animals to hapten-carrier conjugates has also served to indicate that the antigenic determinants recognized by the antibody-producing system and the

Table 3–2 THE ABILITY OF SPECIFIC ANTISERA TO DISTINGUISH BETWEEN THE STEREOISOMERIC TARTARIC ACIDS*

	HAPTENS		
IMMUNE SERA AGAINST	*l-TARTARIC ACID*	*d-TARTARIC ACID*	*m-TARTARIC ACID*
	COOH | HOCH | HCOH | COOH	COOH | HCOH | HOCH | COOH	COOH | HCOH | HCOH | COOH
l-tartaric acid	+++	±	+
d-tartaric acid	0	+++	+
m-tartaric acid	±	0	+++

*From Landsteiner, K., 1945 (reprinted 1962). The Specificity of Serological Reactions. Dover Publications, New York.

cell-mediated immune system are not identical. As discussed earlier, antibodies may be produced that are specific for a given hapten and that can combine with a hapten irrespective of the carrier molecule to which it is attached. In contrast, if a cell-mediated immune response is mounted against a hapten-carrier conjugate, it is found that this response is directed against the hapten only if it remains bound to the original carrier. Sensitized lymphocytes will not react to the hapten if it is bound to an unrelated carrier molecule. For this reason the cell-mediated immune response is said to be "carrier specific" (Table 3–3).

The concept of haptens and carriers not only provides a basis for much of our knowledge about the specificity of the immune response but is also of clinical importance. Thus, many drugs can combine with proteins and so form hapten-carrier conjugates *in vivo*. Penicillin, for instance, is a small molecule that by itself is nonantigenic. When being degraded in the body, however, a reactive penicilloyl group can be formed, which may bind to serum proteins to form penicilloyl-protein conju-

Table 3–3 SPECIFICITIES OF ANTIBODY AND CELL-MEDIATED IMMUNE RESPONSES FOLLOWING IMMUNIZATION WITH A HAPTEN-CARRIER CONJUGATE*

TEST ANTIGENS	ANTIBODIES	CELL-MEDIATED RESPONSE
Hapten-carrier conjugate	+++	+++
Hapten alone	++	−
Carrier alone	++	+++
Hapten on unrelated carrier	++	−

*Note that the cell-mediated response is specific for the original carrier, i.e., is carrier-specific, whereas the antibody-mediated response is not.

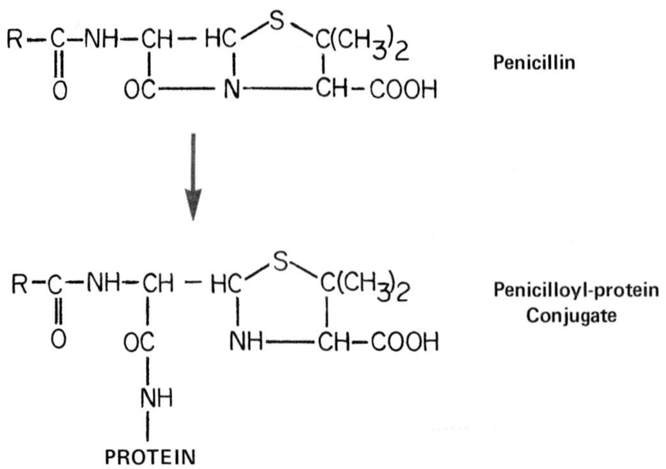

$$R-\underset{\underset{O}{\|}}{C}-NH-CH-\underset{\underset{OC\text{------}N\text{------}}{|}}{HC}\underset{S}{\diagup}\underset{CH-COOH}{\overset{C(CH_3)_2}{|}}$$ Penicillin

$$R-\underset{\underset{O}{\|}}{C}-NH-CH-\underset{\underset{OC}{|}}{HC}\underset{S}{\diagup}\underset{NH\text{------}CH-COOH}{\overset{C(CH_3)_2}{|}}$$ Penicilloyl-protein
Conjugate

$$\underset{\underset{PROTEIN}{|}}{\overset{\overset{|}{NH}}{}}$$

Figure 3–2 Penicillin as a hapten. Penicillin can break down in vivo by a number of pathways to produce several different hapten-protein conjugates. The most important of these is the penicilloyl-protein complex formed by the reaction between penicillenic acid and protein amino groups. At least 95 per cent of the conjugates formed in man are of this type.

gates (Fig. 3–2). The conjugate, not being a normal constituent of the body, is recognized as foreign and therefore induces the formation of antipenicilloyl antibodies, which may participate in hypersensitivity reactions to penicillin (Chapter 17). Another example of a naturally occurring reactive chemical that may bind to body proteins and hence act as a hapten is the toxic component of poison ivy, called urushiol. On contact with skin, urushiol penetrates and binds to dermal proteins and cells. These modified cells are consequently regarded as foreign and attacked in a manner akin to the rejection of a skin graft. The subsequent inflammatory reaction is known as allergic contact dermatitis (Chapter 20), which can be induced by many reactive drugs and chemicals.

SOME SPECIFIC GROUPS OF ANTIGENS

Whereas many different antigens will be discussed in subsequent chapters, some general comments on antigens may be made here. As mentioned earlier, proteins are the best antigens because of their size and structural complexity. Almost all proteins with molecular weights over 1000 daltons are antigenic, although some, like the interferons, are of such uniform structure and so widely distributed among mammals that it is difficult to make good antisera against them. Many of the major antigens of microorganisms, such as the clostridial toxins, bacterial flagellae, virus capsids and protozoan cell membranes, are all proteins. Others include snake venoms, serum and milk proteins and even antibodies themselves when injected into another species.

Polysaccharides are poorer antigens than proteins simply because they tend to consist of structurally mobile polymers containing only a small number of different types of monosaccharide subunits. This is particularly true of the simpler molecules such as starch or glycogen. However, other more complex carbohydrates (particularly those linked to proteins) are of immunological importance. These include the major cell wall antigens of gram-negative organisms and the blood group antigens present on erythrocytes. Many of the so-called "natural" antibodies found in the serum of unimmunized animals are directed against polysaccharide antigenic determinants and probably arise as a result of exposure to antigens derived from the normal intestinal flora or from food.

Lipids, like polysaccharides, are poor antigens because of their relative simplicity. Nevertheless, if linked to proteins or polysaccharides, they may be fully antigenic. Naturally occurring lipid antigens are uncommon. In syphilis, however, antibodies may be produced against cardiolipin, a phospholipid hapten found in heart muscle. The Forsmann antigen, an important cell membrane antigen found in many species of animal, also is a glycolipid (Chapter 18). The cell walls of gram-negative bacteria are composed of complex lipopolysaccharides, but the immune response against these tends to be directed largely against the polysaccharide component.

Because of their relative simplicity and flexibility and also because they are very rapidly degraded, nucleic acids such as DNA or RNA are relatively poor antigens. Nevertheless, it is possible to produce anti–nucleic acid antibodies after artificially stabilizing and linking them to an immunogenic carrier. In certain diseases, such as "systemic lupus erythematosus" in man and dogs (Chapter 21), relatively high levels of antibodies to nucleic acids and nucleoproteins may be found in serum.

ADJUVANTS

Under some circumstances, such as vaccination, it is considered desirable to enhance the normal immune response. Materials that do this are called adjuvants. A large variety of compounds have been employed as adjuvants, although in many cases their mode of action is unclear. The simplest adjuvants are those that function by slowing the release of antigen into the body. As described in Chapter 7, the immune system is antigen-driven. The system responds to the presence of antigen but ceases to respond once antigen is eliminated. It is possible to slow the rate of antigen elimination by first mixing it with an insoluble adjuvant to form a "depot." Examples of depot-forming adjuvants include insoluble aluminium salts such as aluminium hydroxide, aluminium phosphate and aluminium potassium sulfate (alum). When antigen mixed with one of these salts is injected into an animal, a macrophage-rich granuloma is formed in the tissues. The antigen within this granuloma slowly leaks out into the body and so provides a prolonged antigenic stimulus. Antigens that normally persist for only a few days may be retained in the body for several weeks by means of this technique. These adjuvants influence only the primary immune response and have little effect on classical secondary reactions.

An adjuvant with a similar mode of action is beryllium sulfate, which also forms a local granuloma and stimulates antibody formation. This adjuvant has no effect in thymectomized animals and must therefore act to stimulate T cells (Chapter 6); nevertheless, it does not influence cell-mediated immunity. Silica, kaolin and carbon also promote antibody formation when given with antigen, and probably act in a similar fashion.

An alternative method of forming a depot is to incorporate the antigen in a water-in-oil emulsion. The presence of the oil stimulates a local inflammatory response and granulomatous tissue formation around the site of the inoculum while the antigen is slowly leached from the aqueous phase of the emulsion. If killed mycobacteria are incorporated into a water-in-oil emulsion, the mixture is known as Freund's complete adjuvant (FCA), an extremely potent adjuvant. The active fraction of the mycobacteria, which enhances this activity, is known as muramyl dipeptide (n-acetyl-muramyl-L-alanyl-D-isoglutamine). FCA is best given subcutaneously or intradermally, and optimal enhancement is obtained when the antigen dose is relatively low. It acts specifically to stimulate T cell function and thus only enhances responses to thymus-dependent antigens. FCA promotes IgG production over IgM (Chapter 4). It inhibits tolerance induction, favors delayed hypersensitivity reactions, and accelerates graft rejection as well as tumor immunity. FCA is required to induce some experimental autoimmune diseases such as experimental allergic encephalitis and thyroiditis (Chapter 21). It also stimulates macrophage activity, promoting phagocytosis and cytotoxic activity.

Other bacterial products, in addition to muramyl dipeptide, possess adjuvant activity. Endotoxins enhance antibody formation if given at about the same time as the antigen. They have no effect on delayed hypersensitivity but they can break tolerance, and they have a general immunostimulatory activity reflected in a nonspecific resistance to bacterial infections. Endotoxins act as polyclonal B-cell mitogens (Chapter 6), stimulating them to divide while they activate macrophages, making them nonspecifically cytotoxic. Endotoxins may also enhance immune reactivity by promoting interferon release from cells (Chapter 14).

Anaerobic coryneforms, especially *Corynebacterium parvum* (*Propionibacterium acnes*) promote antibody formation in a manner similar to the endotoxins—that is, they promote B cell but not T cell activity and enhance macrophage activity. As a result, they have a general immunostimulating action leading to enhanced antibacterial and antitumor activity. *Bordetella pertussis* also has endotoxin-like activity, but in addition it causes a lymphocytosis in some species as well as rendering rodents highly susceptible to histamine.

Polyribonucleotides consisting of double-stranded nucleic acids such as polyinosinic acid:polycytidilic acid (Poly I:C) act as immunostimulants on mature T cells, probably by functioning as interferon inducers.

Certain surface-active agents such as sodium alginate, lanolin, lysolecithin, vitamin A, saponin and phospholipid liposomes act on cell membranes to enhance immune reactivity. Their mode of action is unknown, but they may reduce antigen destruction by lysosomes.

One related group of compounds that act in an adjuvant-like manner are the immunoenhancing drugs, of which the most widely used is levamisole. A broadspectrum anthelmintic, levamisole appears to function in a manner similar to the thymic hormone thymopoietin (Chapter 5)—that is, it stimulates T-lymphocyte differentiation and their response to antigens. Thus, it enhances cell-mediated cytotoxicity, lymphokine production and suppressor cell function. It also stimulates the phagocytic activities of macrophages and neutrophils. The effects of levamisole are maximal in animals with depressed T-cell function, and it has little or no effect on the immune system of normal animals. Levamisole may therefore be of assistance in the treatment of chronic infections and neoplastic diseases, but it may exacerbate diseases caused by excessive T-cell function.

ADDITIONAL SOURCES OF INFORMATION

Allison CA. 1979. Mode of action of immunological adjuvants. J Res 26 619–630.

Atassi MZ. 1978. Precise determination of the entire antigenic structure of lysozyme. Immunochemistry 15 909–936.

Bomford R. 1980. Comparative selectivity of adjuvants for humoral and cell-mediated immunity. Clin Exp Immunol 39 426–434.

Borek F. 1972. Immunogenicity. Frontiers of Biology Series, Elsevier North-Holland, Amsterdam.

Brunner CJ, and Muscoplat CC. 1980. Immunomodulatory effects of levamisole. JAVMA 176 1159–1162.

Landsteiner K. 1945 (reprinted 1962). The Specificity of Serological Reactions. Dover Publications, New York.

Richards FF, and Konigsberg WH. 1973. How specific are antibodies? Immunochemistry 10 545–553.

Sela M (ed). 1973. The Antigens. Academic Press, New York.

Sela M. 1969. Antigenicity: Some molecular aspects. Science 166 1365–1374.

4

Antibodies

Antibodies are protein molecules produced by plasma cells as a result of the interaction between antigen-sensitive B lymphocytes and specific antigen (Chapter 6). They have the capacity to bind specifically to antigen and hasten its destruction or elimination. Antibodies are found in many body fluids but are present in highest concentrations and are most easily obtained in relatively large quantities for analysis from blood serum.

NATURE OF ANTIBODIES

Antibody molecules, like other proteins, may be classified physicochemically on the basis of their solubility in strong salt solutions, their electrostatic charge and their molecular weight and by their antigenic structure.

Solubility in Salt Solutions. Many years ago when biochemistry was in its infancy, it was found that some of the proteins in serum were precipitated when mixed with an equal volume of a saturated solution of ammonium sulfate, while others remained in solution. Those proteins that precipitate in this way are called globulins; those that remain in solution are called albumins. Antibodies are precipitated from serum by ammonium sulfate and so are classified as globulins. This very simple technique can be readily adapted to provide a means of determining whether antibodies are present in serum, and so may be employed to determine whether a young animal has suckled or not. Unsuckled domestic animals have extremely low levels of antibodies, and therefore addition of a strong salt solution such as sodium, zinc or ammonium sulfate to their serum produces very little precipitate. On the other hand, animals that have successfully suckled have high antibody levels in their serum, and addition of a salt solution results in the development of a dense precipitate. The amount of antibody globulin present in a serum may therefore be estimated from the amount of precipitate formed in the mixture.

Electrostatic Charge. Since protein molecules consist of chains of assorted amino acids, some of which are basic and some acidic, the overall charge on a protein molecule depends on its amino acid composition and is characteristic for that protein. A mixture of proteins may therefore be separated into its constituents by subjecting it to an electrical potential, causing the more positively charged molecules to migrate toward the cathode while negatively charged molecules migrate toward the anode at a rate dependent on their charge. If this technique, known as electrophoresis, is performed so that the protein solution is prevented from diffusing rapidly by the presence of a semisolid matrix such as agar, cellulose acetate or starch gel, then it is possible to fractionate and identify individual proteins in a mixture. When whole serum is treated in this way, it consistently separates into four fractions. The most negatively charged of these consists of a single protein, which also happens not to be precipitated by ammonium sulfate. This is serum albumin. The other three fractions are all globulins and are divided according to their electrophoretic mobility into α, β and γ globulins

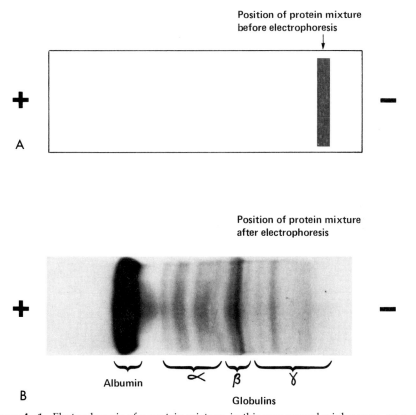

Figure 4–1   Electrophoresis of a protein mixture, in this case normal mink serum, on a strip of cellulose acetate. (Courtesy of Dr. S. H. An.)

(Fig. 4–1). The α globulins are the most negatively charged of these and therefore migrate towards the anode just behind the albumin. They contain serum proteins with various nonimmunological functions; these proteins include the α_1 antitrypsin and α_2 macroglobulin, both of which act as inhibitors of serum proteases. The β globulins are slower, migrating just behind the α globulins. They contain some antibody molecules as well as many of the complement components (Chapter 8). The γ globulins are the least negatively charged serum proteins. They move the shortest distance from the origin, and contain most of the antibodies.

Because antibody molecules are globulins, they are generally known as immunoglobulins (which may be abbreviated to Ig.) The term *immunoglobulin* is used to describe all proteins with antibody activity as well as some proteins that have the characteristic immunoglobulin structure but do not have known antibody activity.

Molecular Weight. In addition to their charge, proteins may also be characterized by their molecular weight. Several techniques are available for measuring this. One commonly used method is to determine the rate at which proteins sediment when ultracentrifuged in solution. Obviously, this sedimentation rate depends on a number of factors, including the viscosity of the suspending fluid and the shape of the protein as well as its molecular weight. Because of the assumptions that must be made, it is common to calculate a "sedimentation constant" for each protein, expressed in Svedberg units and denoted by an S value, rather than attempt to measure accurately the molecular weight in daltons. When immunoglobulins are examined by ultracentrifugation, it is found that most have a sedimentation constant of 7S, but some 11S, 13S and 19S immunoglobulin molecules are also commonly encountered.

As an alternative to ultracentrifugation, it is possible to estimate the size of proteins in a solution by measuring the rate at which they can pass through a glass column filled with beads of cross-linked dextran, in a technique known as gelfiltration. Because very large molecules cannot penetrate the dextran beads, they will pass through the column quickly. In contrast, small molecules penetrate and are retained within the beads and so pass through the column slowly. The rate of passage of a protein molecule through one of these columns is therefore proportional (within limits) to its molecular weight, which may be calculated after reference to a standard curve. When the molecular weights of immunoglobulins are estimated in this way, they are found, like their sedimentation constants, to be heterogeneous. The 7S immunoglobulins have a molecular weight of around 180,000 daltons, the 11S immunoglobulins have a molecular weight of 360,000 daltons, and the 19S immunoglobulins have a molecular weight of 900,000 daltons. Since certain chemical treatments of the 19S molecule can cause it to split into five 7S subunits, it is apparent that this immunoglobulin is a pentamer of the basic 7S unit. Similarly, the 11S immunoglobulin is a dimer, and the 13S immunoglobulin is a trimer of the basic unit.

Antigenic Structure. As proteins, immunoglobulins are excellent antigens when injected into animals of a different species; consequently, antisera can be made that react with immunoglobulin molecules. By using these antisera it is possible to show that immunoglobulins are antigenically heterogeneous and fall into a number of different classes, or isotypes, that appear to be present in all mammals. The four major immunoglobulin classes detected in this way are labeled immunoglobulins M, G, A and E, and each possesses unique antigenic determinants, called μ, γ, α and ϵ respectively. The basic characteristics of each of these major immunoglobulin classes are shown in Table 4–1.

Table 4–1 BASIC CHARACTERISTICS OF THE MAJOR IMMUNOGLOBULIN CLASSES OF THE DOMESTIC ANIMALS

| | *IMMUNOGLOBULIN CLASS* | | | |
PROPERTY	*IgM*	*IgG*	*IgA*	*IgE*
Most usual sedimentation coefficient	19S	7S	11S	8S
Molecular weight	900,000	180,000	360,000	200,000
Electrophoretic mobility	β	γ	β-γ	β-γ
Characteristic heavy chain antigen	μ	γ	α	ϵ
Largely synthesized in:	Spleen and lymph nodes	Spleen and lymph nodes	Intestinal lymphoid tissue	Intestinal and respiratory tracts

STRUCTURE OF IMMUNOGLOBULINS

Immunoglobulin G (IgG) is the immunoglobulin found in highest concentration in serum, and its structure can serve as a model for the other immunoglobulins. IgG has a molecular weight of 180,000 daltons and a sedimentation constant of 7S. On electron microscopy it can be seen to be a Y-shaped molecule, and the "arms" of the Y are capable of binding antigen. If the molecule is treated with chemicals that break disulfide (—S—S—)bonds, it falls apart into four separate polypeptide chains. Two of these chains are "heavy," since they each are of about 50,000 daltons. The other two chains are "light," since they each have a molecular weight of about 25,000 daltons. More information concerning the structure of IgG can be obtained by studying the effect of proteolytic enzymes on the intact molecule. Papain, for example, can split an IgG molecule into three approximately equal-sized fragments, which correspond to the

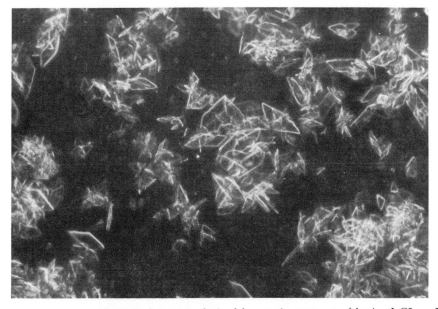

Figure 4–2 Crystallized Fc fragments obtained by papain treatment of bovine IgG2. × 250. (Courtesy of Drs. K. Nielsen and B. Stemshorn.)

Intact IgG molecule

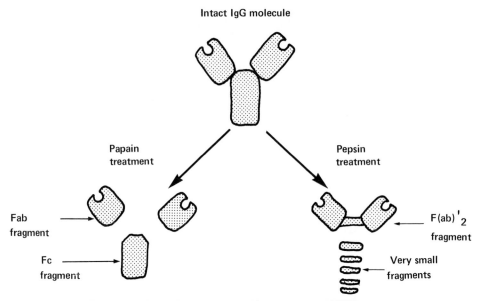

Papain
treatment

Pepsin
treatment

Fab
fragment

F(ab)'₂
fragment

Fc
fragment

Very small
fragments

Figure 4–3 The products of proteolytic enzyme digestion of IgG.

two arms and the tail of the Y-shaped molecule. The two fragments from the "arms"
of the molecule are identical and still possess the capacity to bind antigen; because of
this capacity they are termed the Fab fragments. The third fragment, from the "tail,"
cannot bind antigen but is crystallizable and so is called the Fc fragment (Fig. 4–2). A
second proteolytic enzyme, pepsin, acts on IgG in a slightly different fashion to almost

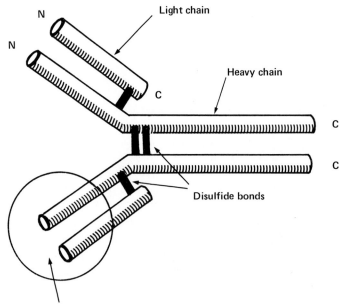

N   Light chain

N

Heavy chain

C

C

C

Disulfide bonds

The antibody combining site is in this region

Figure 4–4 A simple model of an IgG molecule.

completely destroy the Fc region, but it leaves the two Fab fragments joined together to produce a fragment known as F(ab)$'_2$ (Fig. 4–3).

All these observations may be synthesized into a model of IgG structure, seen in Fig. 4–4.

PRIMARY STRUCTURE OF IMMUNOGLOBULINS

The immunoglobulins found in serum are a complex mixture of antibodies directed against a very wide spectrum of antigenic determinants. Because of this heterogeneity, it is impossible to analyze their structure in more than the general terms already described. However, in humans, mice and dogs B cells may become neoplastic, with the result that a clone of cancerous plasma cells may arise from a single precursor cell. Because of their "monoclonal" origin, all these plasma cells synthesize and release a single molecular form of immunoglobulin, which appears in the serum of affected individuals in high concentrations. This plasma cell tumor is known as a myeloma or a plasmacytoma and its immunoglobulin product is a myeloma protein (Chapter 22). Myeloma proteins consist of absolutely homogeneous immunoglobulin molecules so that they may be purified and their chemical and antigenic structure analyzed in detail. In this way each immunoglobulin molecule can be shown to consist of variable regions in the arms of the Y, through which the immunoglobulin binds to antigen; a hinge region where the arms join the tail, which confers flexibility on the molecule; and constant regions in both arms and the tail, in which lie the biological properties of the molecule.

Variable Regions. When the amino acid sequences of a large number of IgG myeloma proteins are compared, it is found that their polypeptide chains, both light and heavy, can be divided into two distinct regions. That portion of the chains situated at the C-terminal end (the end of the peptide chain with a free carboxyl group) has a relatively constant sequence when different myeloma proteins of the same class are compared. In contrast, the N-terminal portion (the end with a free amino group) of each chain is found to be highly variable, so that the amino acid sequence differs greatly between different myeloma proteins. These variable regions are each about 110 amino acid residues long and constitute about half of each light chain and about a quarter of each heavy chain.

When the variable regions are further examined and their degree of variability measured, it is revealed that certain areas within these regions vary considerably more than others and so are considered hypervariable. Between these hypervariable regions are located relatively constant segments. When the three-dimensional structure of this region is examined, it is found that these hypervariable positions lie close to each other on the surface of the molecule (Fig. 4–5). The hypervariable regions on a light and heavy chain act together to form a single antigen-binding site. Consequently, each IgG molecule is functionally bivalent. The specificity of the interactions between antigen and antibody may be explained on the basis that the variations in amino acid sequence in the hypervariable regions give rise to uniquely shaped antigen-binding sites. It is the shape or conformation of an immunoglobulin antigen-binding site that determines the specific antigenic determinants with which it will react.

It has already been discussed in Chapter 3 how the factors that influence the reaction between antibody and antigen can be investigated by means of hapten-carrier conjugates and how, in general, the most important of these factors is the shape of the

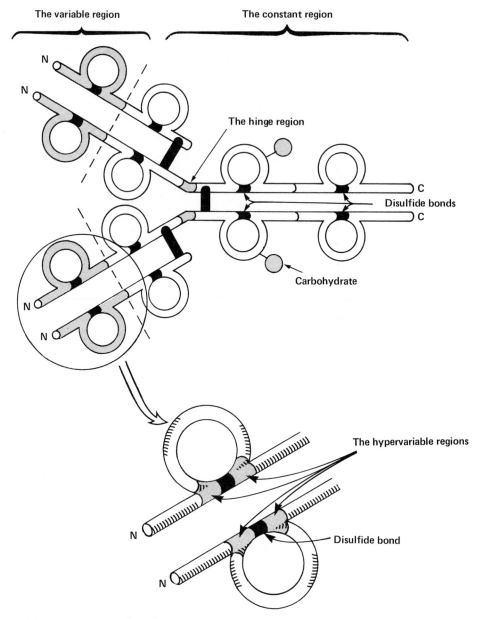

Figure 4–5 A model of an IgG molecule showing the constant, hinge, variable and hypervariable regions.

antigenic determinant. The significance of this factor may be best understood through a study of the forces through which antigen and antibody combine (Table 4–2).

   The binding forces between antigen and its antibody may be grouped together as noncovalent interactions. In classical chemical reactions, molecules are assembled through the establishment of firm, nonreversible covalent bonds. In biological systems, however, these bonds may be insufficiently flexible or adaptable for the body's purposes. In contrast, the formation of noncovalent bonds provides a rapid and

Table 4–2 MAJOR FORCES THROUGH WHICH ANTIGENIC DETERMINANTS AND ANTIBODIES INTERACT

BONDING FORCE	RELATIONSHIP BETWEEN FORCE AND DISTANCE*	STABILIZATION ENERGY** (kcal mole^{-1})
Electrostatic	$1/d^2$	5–10
Hydrogen bonding	$1/d^2$	2–5
Hydrophobic interactions	$1/d^7$	1–5
Van der Waals	$1/d^7$	0.5

*This is the distance between molecules.
**The stabilization energy of a bond is a reflection of the ease with which it is broken. It may be compared with that of covalent bonds, which is in the region of 40–140 kcal mole^{-1}.

reversible way of forming complexes and permits reuse of antibody molecules in a way that covalent bonding does not allow. Noncovalent bonds are generally formed over relatively small intermolecular distances and as a conseqence are only established when two molecules can approach very closely. Thus, the strongest binding between antigen and antibody occurs when the shape of the antigenic determinants and the shape of the antibody-combining site conform very closely. This requirement for a close fit has been likened to the specificity of a key for its lock.

One of the most obvious of the forces that bind antigen to antibody is the electrostatic (ionic) interaction between the negatively charged aspartic or glutamic acids on one molecule and the positively charged lysine, arginine and histidine side-chains on the other. The significance of electrostatic bonding is not completely clear, however, since most biological interactions occur in solutions of relatively high salt concentration, which may serve to neutralize these charges. The major noncovalent force that contributes to antigen-antibody interaction is hydrophobic bonding. Many nonpolar-side-chains of amino acids are hydrophobic, and they tend to come together in such a way that they exclude water and form a stable bond. These hydrophobic interactions are but one example of the mutual attraction of very closely approximated atoms that occurs owing to the presence of Van der Waals forces.

The second group of noncovalent forces that contribute to antigen-antibody bonding is hydrogen bonds. Hydrogen bonds develop when a hydrogen ion attached to one electronegative atom interacts with a second electronegative atom and thus links the two. Hydrogen bonds commonly form during the interactions between many side-chain groups of proteins, and although a single hydrogen bond is relatively weak, a number of them may develop considerable strength.

All the interactions discussed here require that antigen and antibody approach each other extremely closely before firm bonding can occur (Table 4–2) and, in fact, the strength of the bonds so formed will be an indication of this closeness of fit. The strength of binding between an antigenic determinant and an immunoglobulin molecule is termed affinity and may be calculated using the Law of Mass Action, since the interaction between antigen and antibody is reversible. As well as being a measure of the strength of the interaction between antigen and antibody, affinity is also a reflection of the specificity of the antibody. An antibody that binds strongly to a specific antigenic determinant is likely to bind fairly well to other structurally related antigenic determinants and therefore will appear to be relatively nonspecific. In contrast, an antibody that possesses a low affinity for a particular antigenic determinant probably will interact even less strongly with structurally related determinants, and if this cross-reaction cannot be detected, then that weak antibody will appear to be highly specific. During the course of an immune response, the affinity of antibodies for antigen climbs progressively, but as a consequence of this there is an apparent simultaneous decrease in antibody specificity (Chapter 7). Because serum contains a complex mixture of different antibody molecules, it is not correct to use the term *affinity* to describe the strength of reaction of an antiserum with antigen; the term *avidity* is preferable in this context (see Glossary).

By screening myeloma proteins for antibody activity against a very large number of potential antigens, it has been possible to determine their specificity, and it has been found that some myeloma proteins may bind equally well to several apparently unrelated antigenic determinants. This activity may be explained by the fact that the antigen-binding site on an immunoglobulin is considerably larger than a single anti-genic determinant, and each antigen-binding area on an immunoglobulin may be considered to consist of a number of closely associated binding sites for unrelated antigens. When an immune response is mounted against a single antigenic determi-nant, a number of different antibody molecules are produced with a single feature in common—that is, the capacity to bind the inducing determinant. These molecules will also be able to bind other unrelated determinants, but since activity against any one of these unrelated determinants will be present on only a few molecules, it will remain undetected and the antiserum therefore will appear to be specific.

Hinge Region.   On electron microscopy of IgG it can be seen that the Fab regions (the arms of the Y) are mobile and can swing freely around the center of the molecule as if they are hinged. When the amino acid sequence in this part of the molecule is investigated, it is found to contain an unusually large number of proline residues. Because of its unique shape, proline produces a right-angle bend in polypep-tide chains, and since polypeptide chains can rotate freely around peptide bonds, the effect of several linked prolines is to produce a "universal joint" around which the polypeptide chains may swing freely (Fig. 4–6). Proline also tends to "open up" the arrangement of the polypeptide chains, which is why the proteolytic enzymes pepsin

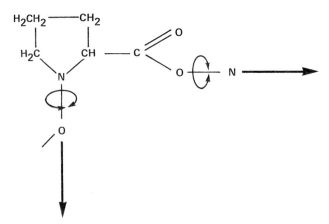

Figure 4–6   The structure of the amino acid proline demonstrating how, when inserted in an amino acid chain, it produces a right-angle bend. Because peptide bonds are free to rotate, three prolines therefore act as a "universal joint."

and papain can attack the molecule in this region. Finally, the interchain disulfide bonds that link the heavy and light chains are also found in the hinge region. This region therefore plays a very significant role in the biological activities of the immunoglobulin molecule.

Constant Regions.   Immunoglobulin constant regions are composed of the C-terminal half of each light chain and the C-terminal three quarters of each heavy chain. The constant region of the light chains (C_L) is about 110 amino acid residues long, whereas the constant region of each heavy chain (C_H) is 330 residues long. When the C_H region of IgG is sequenced, it is found to consist of three similar subunits, or homology regions, called C_H1, C_H2 and C_H3 (IgM and IgE possess a fourth homology region in their Fc, called C_H4). Each constant homology region in both light and heavy chains possesses a single intrachain disulfide bond, which folds the chain into a loop (Fig. 4–7). (Similar loops are also seen in the variable regions where they bring the hypervariable regions together.)

C_L REGION.   Light chains are divided into two types on the basis of their antigenicity and amino acid sequence. These types are called kappa (κ) and lambda (λ). Both light chains on a single immunoglobulin molecule must be identical. The proportion of κ and λ chains varies greatly between species. Dogs, cats, cattle and sheep have 90 per cent λ chains, whereas mice, rabbits and rats have 90 per cent κ chains. Pigs have equal amounts of each type, whereas horses and mink have only λ light chains.

C_H REGIONS.   In addition to binding to specific antigen, immunoglobulins possess a number of other biological activities, most of which are initiated after the immunoglobulin binds to an antigenic determinant. These biological activities include activation of the complement cascade (Chapter 8) and binding of immune complexes to phagocytic cells preparatory to ingestion (opsonization). These and other functions are

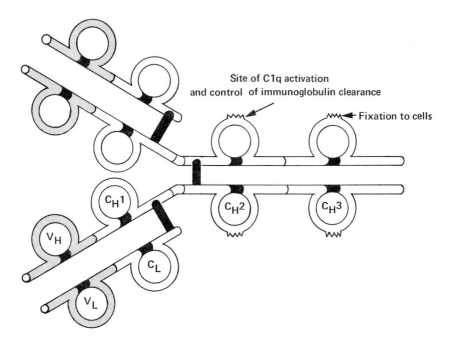

Figure 4–7   The homology regions in an IgG molecule.

mediated through sites on the constant region of immunoglobulin heavy chains. Thus, a small area found on the C_H2 region of IgG is responsible for the initiation of the complement cascade, whereas a similar region on the C_H4 region of IgM performs the same function in that molecule. The fractional catabolic rate of IgG is also controlled by a site on C_H2, whereas adherence to macrophages is mediated through a site on C_H3. Placental transfer of IgG (in humans) and antibody-mediated cell-mediated cytotoxicity (page 92) are also controlled by sites on the heavy chain in the Fc region but probably not by a single homology region.

β2 Microglobulin. A small protein molecule known as β2 microglobulin (11,800 daltons) is found both free in serum and bound to the surface of many cells where it is associated with class I histocompatibility antigens (Chapter 7). β2 microglobulin is remarkable in that its amino acid sequence is very similar to that of an immunoglobulin constant homology region, so much so that it can fix complement and also bind to the Fc receptors of macrophages. For these reasons it is thought that this molecule may be a slightly modified, isolated immunoglobulin constant homology region.

IMMUNOGLOBULIN CLASSES

Immunoglobulin G. IgG is the immunoglobulin class found in highest concentration in blood serum (Table 4–3) and for this reason plays the major role in antibody-mediated defense mechanisms. It is a 7S immunoglobulin with a molecular weight of 180,000 daltons and γ antigenic determinants on its heavy chains. Because of its relatively small size, it can escape from blood vessels more easily than can the other immunoglobulin molecules, and therefore it readily participates in the defense of tissue spaces and body surfaces. IgG can opsonize, agglutinate and precipitate antigen (Chapter 9), but it can activate the complement cascade only if sufficient molecules have accumulated in a correct configuration on the antigen surface (Chapter 8). Some subclasses of IgG may bind to mast cells and therefore participate in type I hypersensitivity (Chapter 17).

Immunoglobulin M. IgM is the immunoglobulin found in second highest concentration in the serum of most animals. It is a 19S molecule with a molecular weight of 900,000 daltons, made up of five 7S subunits. Each of these subunits is structurally similar to the basic Y-shaped immunoglobulin molecule, except that they possess four,

Table 4–3 SERUM IMMUNOGLOBULIN LEVELS IN DOMESTIC ANIMALS AND MAN

SPECIES	*IMMUNOGLOBULIN LEVELS (mg/100 ml)*					
	IgG	*IgM*	*IgA*	*IgG(T)*	*IgG(B)*	*IgE*
Horse	1000–1500	100–200	60–350	100–1500	10–100	—
Bovine*	1700–2700	250–400	10–50	—	—	—
Sheep	1700–2000	150–250	10–50	—	—	—
Pig	1700–2900	100–500	50–500	—	—	—
Dog	1000–2000	70–270	20–150	—	—	2.3–42
Chicken	300–700	120–250	30–60	—	—	—
Human	800–1600	50–200	150–400	—	—	0.002–0.05

*Cattle show very significant seasonal differences in serum immunoglobulin levels.

rather than three, C_H homology units and they carry μ antigenic determinants. The IgM monomers are linked by disulfide bonds in a circular fashion to form a star, and a small cysteine-rich polypeptide called the J chain (15,000 daltons) links two of the units (Fig. 4–8). IgM molecules are secreted intact by plasma cells, and the J chain must therefore be considered to be an integral part of this molecule.

IgM is the major immunoglobulin produced in a primary immune response. It is also produced in a secondary response, but this tends to be masked by the massive production of IgG in this response. Although produced in a relatively small quantity, IgM is considerably more efficient (on a molar basis) than IgG at complement activation, opsonization, neutralization of viruses and agglutination. Because of their very large size, IgM molecules are confined essentially to the blood vascular system

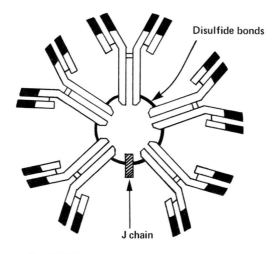

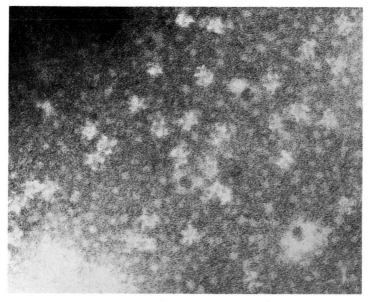

Figure 4–8 The structure of IgM and an electronmicrograph of this immunoglobulin from bovine serum. Approximate magnification × 240,000. (Courtesy of Drs. K. Nielsen and B. Stemshorn.)

and are therefore probably of little importance in conferring protection in tissue fluids or body secretions. IgM monomers (7S IgM) also function as antigen receptors on B cells (Chapter 6).

Immunoglobulin A. IgA is a carbohydrate-rich immunoglobulin of conventional structure. It tends to form polymers so that 11S dimers, 13S trimers and higher polymers are found in addition to the basic 7S molecule (see Fig. 10–2). The most common of these components is a dimer consisting of two 7S units joined by a J chain. While IgA is the second most concentrated immunoglobulin in human serum, it is usually only a minor component in animal serum (Table 4–3). However, IgA is the major immunoglobulin found in the external secretions of the body. As such, it is of critical importance in protecting the intestinal, respiratory and urogenital tracts, the udder and the eyes against microbial invasion. IgA does not activate the complement cascade nor can it act as an opsonin. It can, however, agglutinate particulate antigen and neutralize viruses. It is thought that its major mode of action is to prevent the adherence of antigens to the body surfaces. Because of its importance, IgA is dealt with in greater detail in Chapter 10.

Immunoglobulin E. IgE is a typical Y-shaped, four-chain immunoglobulin with an additional homology region in the heavy chain near the hinge region. As a result, it has a molecular weight of 196,000 daltons and a sedimentation constant of 8S. This immunoglobulin is found in extremely low concentrations in the serum of many species (for example, 20 to 500 ng/ml in humans) but is nevertheless of major importance in that it mediates type I hypersensitivity reactions (allergies and anaphylaxis) (Chapter 17), and it is also associated with the immune response to many helminth infestations (Chapter 15). IgE possesses a unique Fc region that enables it to bind to certain tissue cells, most notably mast cells and basophils, and together with antigen it mediates the release of vasoactive agents from these cells. IgE is also unique among immunoglobulins in that it is destroyed by heating to 56° C for 30 minutes.

Immunoglobulin D. IgD is a 7S immunoglobulin found mainly on the surface of some B lymphocytes, where it functions as an antigen receptor. IgD has been demonstrated in man, laboratory animals and chickens. It has not yet been shown to be present in the major domestic mammals.

IMMUNOGLOBULINS AS ANTIGENS

Immunoglobulins are proteins and are therefore antigenic when taken from one animal and inoculated into an unrelated species. When the resulting anti-immunoglobulin antibodies are analyzed, several major categories of antigenic determinants may be recognized.

First, as described earlier, some of these antibodies are directed against major determinants on the immunoglobulin heavy chains—i.e., against γ, μ, α or ϵ determinants—and these antibodies can thus delineate immunoglobulin classes. However, closer examination of these antibodies shows that these major classes may be divided into subclasses (Table 4–4). For example, bovine IgG is a mixture of two antigenically distinct subclasses, called IgG1 and IgG2. Not only are these two subclasses antigenically different, but IgG1 has a faster electrophoretic mobility than IgG2 and so can be readily distinguished from it by immunoelectrophoresis (Chapter 9). The importance of these immunoglobulin subclasses lies in the fact that they are involved in different biological activities; for example, bovine IgG2 clumps particulate antigen well,

Table 4–4   IMMUNOGLOBULIN CLASSES AND SUBCLASSES OF
DOMESTIC ANIMALS AND MAN

SPECIES	IMMUNOGLOBULIN CLASSES					
	IgG	IgA	IgM	IgE	IgD	
Horse*	Ga, Gb, Gc, G(B), G(T)a, G(T)b	A	M	E	?	
Cattle	G1, G2	A	M	E	?	
Sheep	G1, G1a, G2	A1, A2	M	E	?	
Pig**	G1, G2, G3, G4	A1, A2	M	E	?	
Dog	G1, G2a, G2b, G2c	A	M	E	?	
Cat	G1, G2	A	M	E	?	
Chicken	G1, (G2, G3)?	A	M	?	D	
Man	G1, G2, G3, G4	A1, A2	M	E	D	

*A γ 10S molecule and two immunoglobulins of fast γ mobility have been reported.
**A γ 18S molecule and a 4S "half" Ig molecule have also been reported.

whereas IgG1 does not. This can be of significance in the immunological diagnosis of
infectious diseases such as brucellosis (Chapter 9). The collective term for antigenic
determinants found on the immunoglobulins of all animals of a species is *isotypes*. The
term thus includes classes, subclasses and light-chain types.

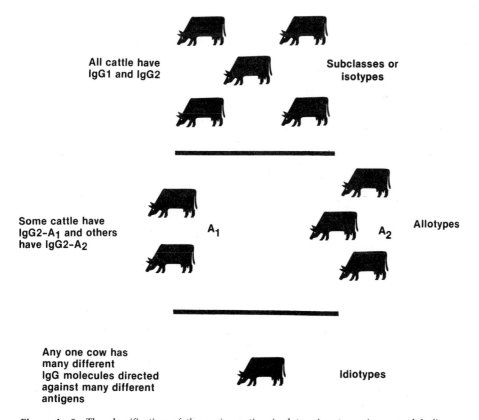

Figure 4–9   The classification of the major antigenic determinants on immunoglobulins.

The second group of antigenic determinants recognized by anti-immunoglobulin sera are those found on the constant regions of the light and heavy chains in the immunoglobulins of some, but not all, animals of a species. These determinants arise as a result of minor changes in amino acid sequences, are inherited by individuals in mendelian fashion, and are known as allotypes (Fig. 4–9). Allotypes are stable genetic markers that can be of use in identifying animals in cases of disputed paternity.

The third group of antigenic determinants are those found within the hypervariable regions. These are known as idiotypes. In most cases the antigen-binding site itself forms the major idiotypic antigenic determinant. Since any one animal possesses a mixture of immunoglobulins directed against a wide variety of antigenic determinants, it must possess an equally wide spectrum of idiotypes. Antisera directed against specific idiotypes are of great use in investigating the nature of antigen recognition by antigen-sensitive cells.

IMMUNOGLOBULINS OF DOMESTIC ANIMALS

All domestic animals possess IgG, IgM and IgA, and it is probable that they also possess IgE and IgD (Table 4–4). The basic characteristics of each of these classes do not differ among species, and their properties and functions are as described previously. Nevertheless, they do differ in the number and types of subclasses present in each species as well as in the possession of allotypes.

HORSE.   In the horse there exist five IgG subclasses—IgGa, IgGb, IgGc, IgG(B) (sometimes called IgB), and IgG(T) (sometimes called IgT). IgG(T) is interesting in that it is rich in carbohydrate and, because it is found in high concentrations in body secretions, was orginally thought to be the equine homologue of IgA. Its designation T was derived from the observation that it was greatly elevated in horses employed for tetanus antitoxin production. However, analysis of its antigenic structure and amino acid sequence shows that it is closely related to IgG and so is best considered an IgG subclass. IgG(T) does not fix guinea pig complement and reacts in a precipitation reaction by a rather characteristic flocculation (see Fig. 9–7). Other unclassified immunoglobulins detected in the horse include a 10S γ_1 molecule and two immunoglobulins of fast γ mobility.

CATTLE.   In cattle, as discussed earlier, IgG is divided into two subclasses, IgG1 and IgG2, on the basis of antigenicity and electrophoretic mobility. The IgG1 constitutes about 50 percent of the serum IgG and is remarkable for being the predominant immunoglobulin in cow's milk rather than IgA. IgG2 levels are highly heritable and thus concentrations vary greatly between cattle. Allotypes have been reported to occur in cattle. One allotype, known as B1, is found on light chains of some cattle but is relatively uncommon. Several other allotypes have been reported; they include G_2A^1 and G_2A^2, found on IgG2 heavy chains and inherited as autosomal dominants, and G_1A^1, found on IgG1 heavy chains. IgE has also been identified in cattle.

SHEEP.   The immunoglobulins of sheep are similar to those of cattle. Sheep possess IgG1, IgG2 and an IgG3. Some sheep have been reported to possess an IgG1a, but this is probably an allotype. Sheep also possess a heat-labile IgE with a molecular weight of 210,000 daltons.

PIGS.   Pigs possess three IgG subclasses, named IgG1, IgG2 and IgG3. In addition, adult pigs may possess a $\gamma 1$, 18S macroglobulin antigenically similar to IgG2, and newborn piglets possess a 5S IgG, which may not have light chains. Four

IgG allotypes have been reported in sows, and spontaneously occurring antibodies to these have been found in the serum of young piglets. It is thought that the piglets may become sensitized to the sow's immunoglobulins following neonatal absorption of these from colostrum. IgE has been reported to occur in the pig.

DOGS AND CATS.   Dogs possess four IgG subclasses named IgG1, IgG2a, IgG2b and IgG2c, whereas cats possess two (IgG1 and IgG2). An IgM allotype has been reported to occur in the dog and IgE also has been identified in this species.

CHICKENS.   Although the IgG in this species has some unique properties (so much so that it has been named IgY by some workers) it is the functional counterpart of IgG in mammals and will therefore be called that here. Chicken IgG has a sedimentation constant of 8S and a molecular weight of 200,000 daltons. Some workers have reported the existence of three subclasses, termed IgG1, IgG2 and IgG3, although this has not been completely substantiated. Chickens also possess IgA, which is present in secretions and, like its mammalian equivalent, tends to form polymers. Chicken IgM is a 19S molecule formed predominantly during the primary immune response, and it contains a J chain. A 7S IgM can be detected in the amniotic fluid of eggs and in day-old chicks. It is thought to be derived from oviduct secretions in the hen. An avian homologue of IgD has also been identified.

Chickens have three immunoglobulin allotype loci. The G-1 locus codes for IgG heavy chain allotypes. The M-1 locus codes for IgM heavy chain allotypes, and the L-1 locus codes for light chain allotypes. There may be as many as fourteen different allotypes coded at the G-1 locus.

THE GENERATION OF ANTIBODY DIVERSITY

One immediate result of the studies on antisera to hapten-carrier conjugates described in Chapter 3 was the realization that antibodies could distinguish among antigenic determinants differing only in minor structural configurations (see Table 3–2). It was subsequently realized that an enormous number of different antigens existed and that the number of different antibodies required to combine with these antigens must also be extremely large.

One difficulty raised by this finding was the assumption that an impossibly large amount of genetic material would be required to code for every potential antibody molecule. When the structure of immunoglobulins was clarified, however, it became clear that the specificity of an antibody for its complementary antigenic determinant lay only in the structure of the variable regions of the light and heavy chains. It also became clear that coding for immunoglobulin molecules was accomplished by at least two major groups of genes: variable region genes, which code for the variable regions, and constant region genes, which code for the remainder of the molecule. In order to explain the specificity of antibodies, we must account for the variation within the variable regions, especially the hypervariable areas. In order to explain the differential synthesis of different immunoglobulin isotypes, we must account for variations in constant region genes. Much of the information that follows is derived from studies in mice. Nevertheless, it is anticipated that similar mechanisms are operative in all mammals.

Variable (V) Region Diversity.   At least three different genes are required to construct a single immunoglobulin light chain. One gene, the V_L gene, codes for the bulk of the variable region; another gene, the C_L gene, codes for the constant region;

and a third gene, the J_L gene, codes for the portion of the light chain joining the two regions.

In the germ-line genome of a mouse there is a "library" of about 100 to 1000 different V_L genes and about 5 different J_L genes. As a B lymphocyte differentiates in an animal, one of these V_L genes and one of the J_L genes are selected from the library at random and are joined with the single C_L gene. This combination then codes for the entire light chain (Fig. 4–10). It is clear that between 500 and 5000 different V_LJ_L combinations are available. In addition, the joining of V_L to J_L is imprecise; indeed, there are six different ways for these genes to join. This increases the number of possible different V_LJ_L combinations, and hence the number of different variable regions, to between 3000 and 30,000. By the time a B cell has matured, it is committed to making only the light chain coded for it by its selected genes.

Similar considerations apply to the genetics of heavy chain variable regions. In addition to V_H and J_H genes, a small additional gene segment, called D, is inserted between V_H and J_H. There are about 300 to 500 different V_H genes, several D genes and several J_H genes. The joins between V_H and D and between D and J_H are also imprecise, and many different connections may be made. It is clear, therefore, that an extremely large number of V_HDJ_H combinations may be generated and bound to a C_H gene to make complete heavy chain genes.

Since the antigen-binding site of an immunoglobulin consists of the variable regions of both light and heavy chains acting together, the total possible number of gene combinations and hence of immunoglobulins with different antigen-binding sites synthesized by an animal is also extremely large. One estimate places it in the region of 10^8 different combinations. In order to place this figure in perspective, it should be pointed out that a mouse possesses around 10^{12} lymphocytes and a cow considerably more.

(The site of V_LJ_L and V_HDJ_H joining coincides with the position of only one of the hypervariable regions. Unfortunately, it is not clear how the other hypervariable regions are generated. It may be through somatic mutation—i.e., random mutations in V genes—occurring while a B cell is maturing. If this is the case, then the available antibody diversity would obviously increase still further.)

Constant Region Diversity The immunoglobulin class that predominates in a primary immune response is IgM. When a second dose of the same antigen is

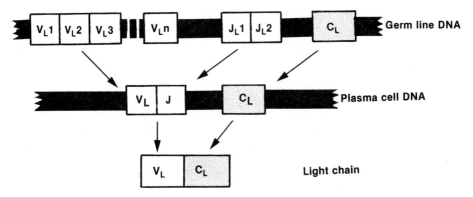

Figure 4–10 The genetic basis of immunoglobulin light-chain diversity. In the germ-line DNA there exists a large number of variable and J-region genes. In an individual plasma cell only one of each is required and translated to generate a light chain.

administered, the major antibody class switches usually to IgG, but IgA or IgE may also be synthesized. This switch is accomplished without changing the specificity of antibody, by attaching a new constant region onto a pre-existing variable region. It is probable that the genome of an antibody-producing cell contains the genes for all constant regions arranged in linear fashion: —$C\mu$—$C\gamma$—$C\epsilon$—$C\alpha$—. When IgM is produced, the cell utilizes only the $C\mu$ gene. On switching to IgG production, the $C\mu$ gene is deleted and $C\gamma$ used instead. On switching to IgA production, the $C\mu$, $C\gamma$ and $C\epsilon$ genes are deleted and the variable region genes attach directly to the $C\alpha$ gene. It is interesting to speculate whether this switch might be triggered by specific enzymes within a particular tissue or organ. Thus, it is possible that antibody production could be regulated at body surfaces by an enzyme that deletes the intervening $C\mu$ and $C\gamma$ genes and thus permit B cells in those tissues to synthesize only IgA or IgE.

ADDITIONAL SOURCES OF INFORMATION

Davies DR, Padlan EA, and Segal DM. 1975. Three-dimensional structure of immunoglobulins. Ann Rev Biochem 44 639–667.

Feinstein A. 1979. Immunoglobulins and histocompatibility antigens. Nature (London) 282 230.

Frieden E. 1975. Non-covalent interactions. J Chem Educ 52 754–761.

Gottlieb PD. 1980. Immunoglobulin genes. Mol Immunol 17 1423–1435.

Halliwell REW, Schwartzman RM, Montgomery PC, and Rockey JH. 1975. Physicochemical properties of canine IgE. Transplantation Proc 7 537–543.

Heddle RJ, and Rowley D. 1975. Dog immunoglobulins, immunochemical characterization of dog serum, parotid saliva, colostrum, milk and small bowel fluid. Immunology 29 185–195.

Higgins DA. 1975. Physical and chemical properties of fowl immunoglobulins. Vet Bull 45 139–154.

Osler AG. 1978. On the precedence of 19S antibodies in the early immune response. Immunochemistry 15 714–720.

Porter P. 1979. Structural and functional characteristics of immunoglobulins of the common domestic species. Adv Vet Sci Comp Med 23 1–21.

Robertson M. 1980. Chopping and changing in immunoglobulin genes. Nature 287 390–392.

Seidman JG, Leder A, Nau M, et al. 1978. Antibody diversity. Science 202 11–17.

Schultz RD, Scott FW, Duncan JR, and Gillespie JH. 1974. Feline immunoglobulins. Infect Immun 9 391–393.

Spiegelberg HL. 1974. Biological activities of immunoglobulins of different classes and subclasses. Adv Immunol 19 259–294.

Proposed rules for the designation of immunoglobulins of animal origin. 1978. Bull WHO 59 815–817.

5

Cells and Tissues of the Immune System

Although antigen is trapped and processed by the macrophages of the mononuclear-phagocytic system, the mounting of an immune response is a function of lymphocytes. These lymphocytes are the relatively featureless small round cells that constitute the predominant cell type in organs such as the spleen, lymph nodes and thymus (see Fig. 6–1). Because their morphology has provided no clues as to their function, very little was known about the role of lymphocytes until relatively recently. They have now been shown, however, to be extraordinarily complex, and their major function appears to be the production of antibodies or specific effector cells in response to macrophage-bound antigen. These responses occur within lymphoid organs (Fig. 5–1), which therefore must provide an environment for efficient interaction between lymphocytes, macrophages and antigen. In addition, control systems must be provided in order to regulate the immune responses, and this regulation can occur at two levels. On the first level, the production of lymphocytes must be controlled so that their numbers are appropriate for the tasks involved. In addition, some form of "editing" of these cells must occur so that those produced are reactive only to foreign antigenic determinants and not to "self" antigens. On the second level, the magnitude of the response of each lymphocyte also must be regulated so that it is sufficient but not excessive for the body's requirements.

The tissues of the lymphoid system may therefore be classified on the basis of their roles in generating lymphocytes, in regulating the production of lymphocytes and in providing a suitable environment for the interaction between processed antigen and antigen-sensitive cells (Fig. 5–2).

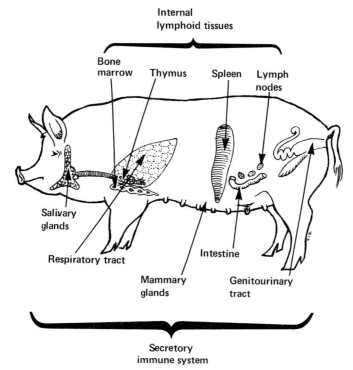

Figure 5−1 The lymphoid tissues of animals.

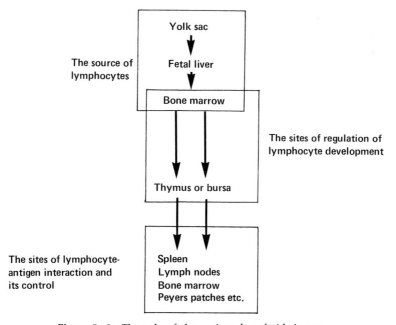

Figure 5−2 The role of the various lymphoid tissues.

SOURCES OF LYMPHOID CELLS

In the very young fetus, lymphoid stem cells are produced first by the yolk sac membrane and later by the fetal liver (Chapter 11). In the older fetus and adult animals, the bone marrow serves as the major source of lymphoid cells. The central role of the bone marrow is emphasized by the observation that, of all the tissues in the adult animal, it alone is able to prevent the death of animals that have been lethally irradiated. Therefore, it is presumably capable of providing all the cells necessary to restore the functions of the other lymphoid organs.

The bone marrow in adult animals serves two functions. Not only is it a hematopoietic organ serving as the source of all blood cells, including lymphocytes, but like the spleen, liver and lymph nodes it also contains many mononuclear-phagocytes and thus serves to remove particulate antigens from circulating blood. Because of this dual function, the bone marrow has two compartments, a hematopoietic compartment and a vascular compartment. These two compartments alternate, like slices of cake, in wedge-shaped areas within long bones. The hematopoietic areas contain precursors of all the blood cells as well as macrophages and lymphocytes and are enclosed by a layer of adventitial cells. In older animals these adventitial cells may become so loaded with fat that the hematopoietic tissue is masked, and the marrow may have a fatty yellow appearance. The vascular compartment consists of blood sinuses lined by endothelial cells and crossed by reticular cells and macrophages.

PRIMARY LYMPHOID ORGANS

The organs whose function is to regulate the production and differentiation of lymphocytes are known as primary lymphoid organs. They include the thymus, found in both mammals and birds, and the bursa of Fabricius, found only in birds. These organs arise early in fetal life from outgrowths at the ectoendodermal junctions. The thymus arises from the third and fourth pharyngeal pouches, whereas the bursa develops from the cloaco-dermal junction. Because of this, each organ consists of a mass of epithelial cells. Lymphoid stem cells from the yolk sac, the fetal liver and eventually the bone marrow migrate into these organs via the bloodstream, and it is in them that recognizable lymphocytes are first observed in the fetus (Chapter 11) (Table 5–1).

Table 5–1 COMPARISON OF PRIMARY AND SECONDARY
LYMPHOID ORGANS

	PRIMARY LYMPHOID ORGAN	SECONDARY LYMPHOID ORGAN
Origin	Ectoendodermal junction	Mesoderm
Time of development	Early in embryonic life	Later in fetal life
Persistence	Involutes after puberty	Persists through adult life
Effect of removal	Loss of lymphocytes	No effect or only minor
	Loss of immune responses	consequences
Response to antigen	Unresponsive	Fully reactive
Examples	Thymus; bursa	Spleen; lymph nodes

THYMUS

The thymus is an organ found in the anterior mediastinal space. In horses, cattle, sheep, pigs and chickens, however, it also extends up the neck as far as the thyroid gland. The size of the thymus can vary considerably, its relative size being greatest in the newborn animal and its absolute size being greatest at puberty. After puberty, atrophy of the thymic parenchyma occurs and the cortex is replaced by adipose tissue, but remnants of the thoracic thymus may persist in many animals until old age. In addition to this age-related involution, the thymus also atrophies rapidly in response to stress, so that the thymus of animals dying after prolonged sickness may be abnormally small.

Structure of the Thymus (Fig. 5–3). The thymus consists of a series of lobules of loosely packed epithelial cells, and each lobule is covered by a connective tissue capsule. The outer part of each lobule, the cortex, is densely infiltrated with lymphocytes, but in the inner part, the medulla, the epithelial cells are clearly visible. Within the medulla are round bodies known as thymic (Hassall's) corpuscles, whose function is not known. They contain keratin and perhaps represent an abortive attempt at keratinization by the epithelial cells. Occasionally, the remains of a small blood vessel may be observed at their center, and in cattle they may contain high concentrations of IgA (Chapter 10). The blood supply to the thymus is derived from arteries that enter through connective tissue septa and run as arterioles along the cortico-medullary junction. The capillaries that arise from these arterioles enter the cortex and loop back to the medulla. These capillaries are covered by a barrier composed of an endothelium, an abnormally thick basement membrane and a continuous outer layer of epithelial cells. It appears that this barrier may effectively prevent circulating antigens from entering the thymic cortex. No lymphatics enter the thymus.

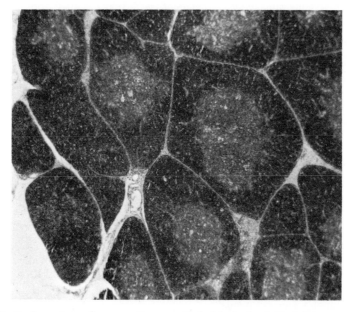

Figure 5–3 A section of puppy thymus. Each lobule is divided into a cortex rich in lymphocytes, hence staining darkly, and a paler medulla consisting largely of epithelial cells. × 45. (From a specimen kindly provided by Dr. S. Yamashiro.)

Function of the Thymus. The function of the thymus was unknown until relatively recently, since its removal in adult animals has no immediately obvious effect. If, however, it is removed from newborn rodents, then a number of important consequences result.

NEONATAL THYMECTOMY. Thymectomy performed on newborn mice within a day of birth results in these animals becoming much more susceptible to infection and occasionally becoming runted. Closer examination of these neonatally thymectomized animals reveals that there is a drop in the number of circulating lymphocytes and a marked depression in the ability of the animals to mount some types of immune response (Table 5–2). In particular, their capacity to reject grafts is severely compromised, reflecting a total loss of the cell-mediated immune response. Antibody-mediated immunity is depressed also, but to a lesser extent.

ADULT THYMECTOMY. Removal of the thymus from adult animals produces no immediately obvious results. If, however, animals are kept for several months after this operation, there is a progressive decline in the number of their circulating lymphocytes and in the capacity of lymphocytes to mount cell-mediated immune responses. We may interpret these results to suggest that, although the adult thymus is still functional, there exists a reservoir of thymus-derived cells that must be exhausted before the effects of thymectomy become apparent.

The results of thymectomy indicate that the neonatal thymus acts as a source of many of the circulating blood lymphocytes. These are called thymus-derived lymphocytes or T cells. These thymus-derived lymphocytes actually originate in the bone marrow but are "processed" in the thymus after being attracted by hormones secreted by thymic epithelial cells. Once within the thymus, these lymphocytes divide at a rapid rate. (This division is unaffected by the presence of antigen.) Of the new cells produced within the thymus, most appear to die there, while others (about 5 per cent of the total in rodents and about 25 per cent in calves) emigrate and so colonize the secondary lymphoid organs with T cells.

The thymus also functions as an endocrine gland. Several different hormones are secreted by thymic epithelial cells, the most important of which are thymosin, the thymopoietins and FTS (facteur thymique serique). Thymosin is a mixture of small polypeptides that act on bone marrow precursor cells to make them mature into cells possessing at least some T-cell characteristics. There are two thymopoietins. These are polypeptides that provoke T-cell precursors to differentiate and enhance T-cell function

Table 5–2 EFFECTS OF NEONATAL THYMECTOMY AND
BURSECTOMY ON THE IMMUNE RESPONSES AND ON LYMPHOID TISSUES

FUNCTION	THYMECTOMY	BURSECTOMY
Numbers of circulating lymphocytes	↓ ↓ ↓	—
Presence of lymphocytes in thymus-dependent areas	↓ ↓ ↓	—
Graft rejection	↓ ↓ ↓	—
Presence of lymphocytes in thymus-independent areas and germinal centers	↓	↓ ↓ ↓
Plasma cells	↓	↓ ↓ ↓
Serum immunoglobulins	↓	↓ ↓ ↓
Antibody formation	↓	↓ ↓ ↓

by depressing cyclic AMP levels. FTS is a peptide secreted by thymic epithelial cells, which can partially restore T-cell function in thymectomized animals. (Its sequence in the pig is Gln–Ala–Lys–Ser–Glu–Gly–Ser–Asn.) The precise interrelationships between these factors are unclear, but it is possible that each acts to regulate the activities of the T cell during different stages of its maturation.

BURSA OF FABRICIUS

The bursa of Fabricius (Fig. 5–4) is a lymphoepithelial organ found in birds but not in mammals. It arises from the ectoendodermal junction as a round, sac-like structure just dorsal to the cloaca. Like the thymus, the bursa reaches its maximal size in the chick about one to two weeks after hatching and then undergoes gradual involution.

Structure of the Bursa.   Like the thymus, the bursa consists of lymphoid cells embedded in epithelial tissue. This epithelial tissue lines a hollow sac connected to the cloaca by a duct. Inside this sac, large folds of epithelium extend into the lumen, and scattered through these folds are follicles of lymphoid cells. Each lymphoid follicle is divided into a cortex and medulla. The cortex contains lymphocytes, plasma cells and macrophages. At the cortico-medullary junction there is a basement membrane and capillary network on the inside of which are epithelial cells. These medullary epithelial cells show frequent mitotic figures, and toward the center of the medulla appear to be replaced by lymphoblasts and lymphocytes, so that the center of the follicle may appear to consist solely of lymphocytes.

Function of the Bursa.   The bursa may be removed either surgically or by infecting newborn chicks with a virus that causes bursal destruction (infectious bursal disease). Since the bursa involutes when chicks become sexually mature, premature bursal atrophy may also be provoked by administration of testosterone. When treated in these ways, birds show only a slight drop in the numbers of circulating lymphocytes, but they produce only very small quantities of antibody, and there is a loss of antibody-producing plasma cells. Since bursectomized birds can still reject foreign skin grafts, there appears to be little effect on the cell-mediated immune response. These birds are more susceptible than normal to leptospirosis and salmonellosis but not to bacteria against which cell-mediated immunity is important, such as *Mycobacterium avium*. (Interestingly enough, birds with a large bursa tend to be relatively more resistant to many diseases.)

These results have been interpreted to suggest that the bursa is a primary lymphoid organ whose function is to serve as a maturation and differentiation site for the cells of the antibody-forming system. These cells are therefore called B cells. However, more recent studies have suggested other interpretations. For example, it can be shown that spleen cells from neonatally bursectomized birds, if transplanted into a normal bird, cause the recipient to lose its ability to make antibodies. It has been demonstrated that this results from the development of a population of suppressor cells in the bursectomized bird. It is probable that the loss of antibody production in bursectomized birds is due, therefore, to the actions of these suppressor cells.

In addition, the bursa also functions as a secondary lymphoid organ—that is, it can trap antigen and undertake some antibody synthesis. Indeed, it also contains a small focus of T cells just dorsal to the bursal duct opening.

It is probable, therefore, that the bursa has a number of different functions and can no longer be considered to be a pure primary lymphoid organ.

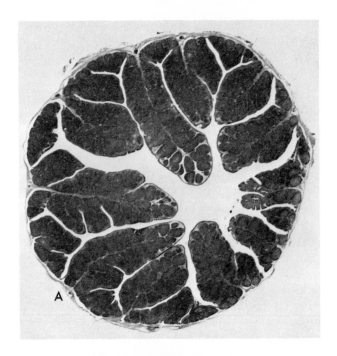

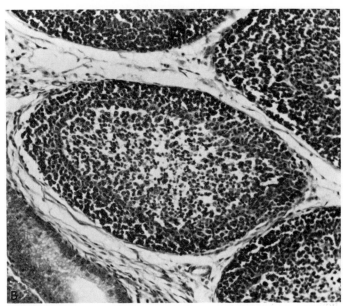

Figure 5−4 Photomicrographs showing the structure of the bursa of Fabricius. *A,* Low-power photomicrograph showing the bursa of Fabricius of a 14-day-old chick. × 5. *B,* A single follicle. × 360. (From a specimen kindly provided by Dr. S. Yamashiro.)

Bursal Equivalent of Mammals. Mammals do not possess a bursa, and consequently investigators have searched for an organ with equivalent function. In order to conform to the criteria of a primary lymphoid organ (see Table 5–1), the bursal equivalent might be expected to arise from an ectoendodermal junction and to atrophy at puberty, and the removal of such an organ from a newborn animal might be expected to prevent antibody production. No such organ has been identified. It now seems probable that bursal functions in the mammal are the joint responsibility of the intestinal lymphoid tissue, such as the Peyer's patches, and the bone marrow.

SECONDARY LYMPHOID ORGANS

In contrast to the thymus and bursa, the other lymphoid organs of the body arise from mesoderm late in fetal life and persist through adult life (see Table 5–1). They are responsive to antigenic stimulation and thus are poorly developed in germ-free animals. This is in marked contrast to the primary lymphoid organs, which do not normally respond to antigen and are thus of normal size in germ-free animals. Removal of secondary lymphoid organs does not significantly reduce an animal's immune capability. Examples of these secondary lymphoid organs include the spleen, the lymph nodes and the lymphoid nodules of the gastrointestinal, respiratory and urogenital tracts. These organs are rich in macrophages and dendritic cells that trap and process antigens and in T and B lymphocytes, which mediate the immune responses. The overall anatomical structure of these organs is therefore designed to facilitate antigen trapping and to provide maximal opportunities for processed antigen to be presented to antigen-sensitive cells.

LYMPH NODES

Structure of Lymph Nodes. Lymph nodes are round or bean-shaped structures strategically placed on lymphatic channels in such a way that they can trap antigen being carried from the periphery of the body to the blood stream. Thus, lymph nodes consist of a reticular network filled with lymphocytes, macrophages and dendritic cells through which lymphatic sinuses penetrate (Fig. 5–5). A subcapsular sinus is found immediately under the connective tissue capsule of the node; other sinuses pass through the body of the node but are particularly prominent in the medulla. Lymphatic vessels enter the node at various points around its circumference, and efferent lymphatics leave from a depression or hilus on one side. The blood vessels to and from a lymph node also enter and leave via the hilus.

The interior of a lymph node is divided into a peripheral cortex, a central medulla and an ill-defined area between these two regions termed the paracortical zone. The cells in the cortex are predominantly B lymphocytes and are arranged in nodules. Prior to exposure to antigen these nodules are termed primary follicles. In lymph nodes that have been stimulated by antigen, the cells within primary follicles expand to form characteristic structures known as germinal centers. A follicle containing a germinal center is known as a secondary follicle. Some T cells are found in the cortex, distributed in an area immediately surrounding each germinal center.

The cells in the paracortical zone are mainly T lymphocytes and are arranged in poorly defined nodules called tertiary follicles. In neonatally thymectomized or congenitally athymic animals, this area is deprived of cells and so can be considered a thymus-dependent area (Fig. 5–6).

The cells of the medulla include B lymphocytes, macrophages, reticulum cells and plasma cells. These are arranged in cellular cords between the lymphatic sinuses.

In the pig, the lymph nodes are structurally inverted so that the afferent lymphatics enter the node through the hilus and the lymph passes from the cortex at the center

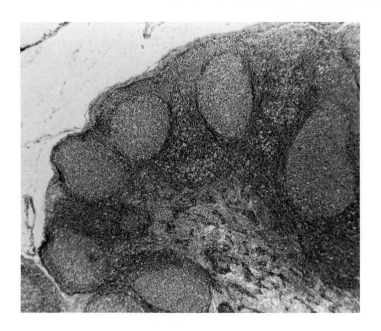

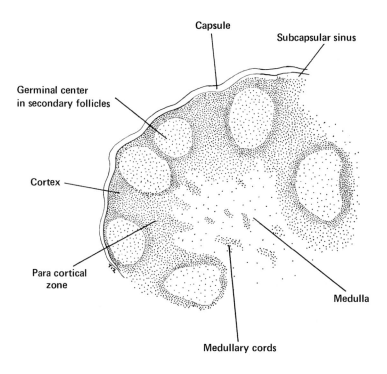

Figure 5–5 A section of dog lymph node. × 100. (From a specimen kindly provided by Dr. S. Yamashiro.)

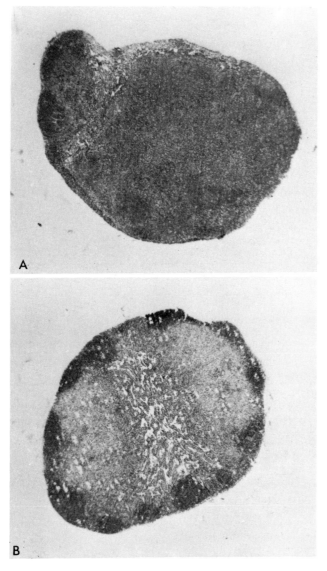

Figure 5–6 Sections of lymph nodes. *A,* from a normal mouse. *B,* From a nude mouse. Nude mice are congenitally athymic and are therefore devoid of T cells. This may be seen in this photomicrograph as a lack of cellular density in the paracortical zone. × 60.

of the node to the medulla at the periphery before leaving through the efferent vessels (Fig. 5–7).

Lymphocyte Circulation. Lymph flows through the calf thoracic duct at 500 ml per hour, and it contains about 1×10^8 lymphocytes per milliliter. If the thoracic duct is cannulated and the lymph removed, a calf will become severely lymphopenic within a few hours. When the lymphoid tissues of such an animal are examined, it can be shown that cells have disappeared from lymph node paracortical zones. Because of the rapid depletion of lymphocytes by this technique, it is clear that thoracic duct cells must normally recirculate back to the lymphoid tissues (Fig. 5–8). In fact, the

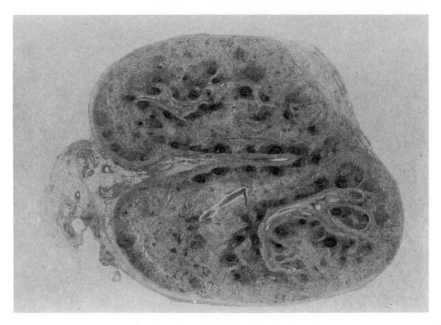

Figure 5–7 A section of a lymph node of a pig showing its structural inversion. The germinal centers in this lymph node are therefore in the cortical region in the center of the node. The medulla is at the periphery. × 15. (From a specimen kindly provided by Dr. S. Yamashiro.)

lymphocytes that enter the vena cava from the thoracic duct spend only between two and twelve hours in blood before returning to the lymphoid tissues. They leave the blood stream by way of the venules of the lymph node paracortical zone. These venules (usually called, somewhat unnecessarily, post-capillary venules) possess an

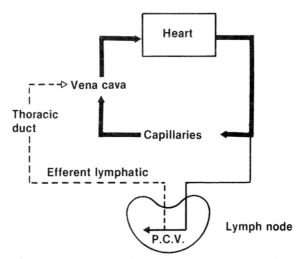

Figure 5–8 A schematic diagram depicting the circulation of lymphocytes. Lymphocytes found in the peripheral blood may be newly formed cells passing from the bone marrow to the primary lymphoid organs, cells passing from the primary to the secondary lymphoid organs, or recirculating cells. It is this latter group that constitutes the major portion of the circulating blood lymphocytes. (P.C.V.—post-capillary venule.)

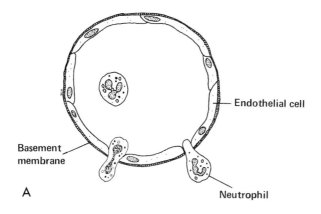

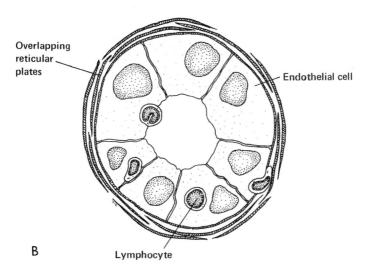

Figure 5—9 A diagram comparing the migration of neutrophils from a conventional capillary, as occurs in acute inflammation (*A*), with the migration of lymphocytes from a "postcapillary" venule within the paracortical zone of a lymph node (*B*). Neutrophils, when migrating from conventional capillaries, pass between endothelial cells and then directly through the basement membrane. In contrast, lymphocytes appear to migrate through the cytoplasm of the tall endothelial cells lining "postcapillary" venules and then infiltrate between overlapping reticular plates before gaining access to the node.

extremely tall endothelium. Circulating lymphocytes adhere to these endothelial cells and then pass into the node, either by penetrating through their cytoplasm or, more likely, between the endothelial cells (Fig. 5–9). T cells re-enter the lymphatic circulation via the efferent lymph; there is thus a continuing recirculation of these cells between lymph and blood. It is tempting to suggest that this is most appropriate for lymphocytes whose function is to survey the body for aberrant cells. As a result of this circulation, the majority of lymphocytes found in peripheral blood are T cells (see Table 6–3).

A small proportion of the circulating T cells do not return to lymph nodes but leave the circulation from venules within the lymphoid tissues located on body surfaces, such as the lung or intestine. These cells are specifically involved in the development of immune responses at body surfaces.

Response of Lymph Nodes to Antigen.   Antigen deposited in tissues is carried by the flow of tissue fluid to local lymph nodes. Its fate within these nodes depends upon whether the animal has had previous exposure to the antigen. Lymph nodes possess two separate antigen-trapping systems. One system uses the macrophages present in the medulla, and since these cells can take up antigen in the absence of antibodies, this system can function relatively effectively on first exposure to antigen. The other system involves dendritic cells, which are found in the lymph node cortex and in particular within secondary follicles. Dendritic cells possess a large array of cytoplasmic processes (see Fig. 2–8) and can thus form a web through which antigen must pass as it filters through the cortex. The efficiency of this web as an antigen-trapping device does depend, however, upon the presence of antibody, which is required for antigen to adhere to the dendritic cell processes.

If an animal possesses no antibodies to an injected antigen, then most of the antigen entering the node will be phagocytosed by macrophages situated in the medulla. The antigen-carrying macrophages then migrate to the cortical follicles, where antigen-sensitive cells are present, and it is the antibody-producing progeny of these cells that subsequently move to the medulla. Some of these antibody-producing cells are also released into the efferent lymph and in this way colonize other lymph nodes downstream. Some time after antibody production is first observed in the medulla, germinal centers appear in the cortex, arising as a result of proliferation of cells within primary follicles. The dividing cells are usually relatively large and pale-staining but compress the surrounding lymphocytes into a dense mantle around the germinal center (Fig. 5–10). Dendritic cells may form a cap on the peripheral side of the germinal center. Antigens that do not stimulate antibody production do not usually cause germinal center formation.

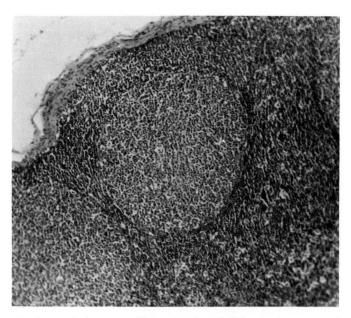

Figure 5–10 A germinal center within secondary follicles in the cortex of a dog lymph node. × 240. (From a specimen kindly provided by Dr. S. Yamashiro.)

On second exposure to antigen, adherence to follicular dendritic cells is the predominant means of antigen trapping. In a secondary response the germinal centers tend to become less obvious as the activated cells migrate from the cortex to the medullary cords and out in the efferent lymph. Once this stage is completed, the germinal centers then show hyperplasia and, to a limited extent, antibody production. All this movement of cells within the lymph node ensures that antibody-producing cells are kept well away from antigen-sensitive cells. As will be discussed later (Chapter 7) this prevents an immediate inhibition of the immune response through the negative feedback exerted by the antibody.

When responding to antigens that stimulate a cell-mediated rather than an antibody-mediated immune response, such as skin grafts, the T cell–rich paracortical areas respond by the production of large pyroninophilic cells (i.e., they stain with pyronin, which is a stain for RNA; thus, a cell with pyroninophilic cytoplasm is rich in ribosomes and is probably a protein-producing cell). These large pyroninophilic cells give rise, in turn, to more small lymphocytes, which participate in the cell-mediated immune responses.

SPLEEN

Just as lymph nodes serve to "filter" antigen from lymph, so the spleen "filters" blood. The filtering process removes both antigenic particles and effete blood cells. In addition, the spleen stores erythrocytes and platelets and undertakes erythropoiesis in the fetus. It is therefore divided into two compartments: one for storage of erythrocytes, for antigen trapping and for erythropoiesis, which is called the red pulp; and one in which the immune response occurs, known as the white pulp (Fig. 5–11).

Structure of Splenic White Pulp. The white pulp of the spleen consists of lymphoid tissue and is intimately associated with its vasculature. Vessels entering the spleen travel through muscular trabeculae before entering its functional areas. Immediately on leaving the trabeculae each arteriole is surrounded by a sheath of lymphoid tissue known, naturally enough, as the periarteriolar lymphoid sheath. The arteriole eventually leaves this sheath and branches into penicillary arterioles, which possess a characteristically thickened wall forming a structure known as an ellipsoid. These arterioles then open, either directly or indirectly, into venous sinuses that drain into the splenic venules. The periarteriolar lymphoid sheath consists largely of T cells and is depleted following neonatal thymectomy. However, scattered through the sheath are primary follicles consisting largely of B cells. On antigenic stimulation these follicles develop germinal centers and so become secondary follicles. Each follicle is surrounded by a layer of T cells in what is known as the mantle layer or zone. The white pulp as a whole is separated from the red pulp by a marginal sinus, a reticulum sheath and a marginal zone of cells.

Response of the Spleen to Antigen. Intravenously administered antigen will be trapped, at least in part, in the spleen, where it is taken up by macrophages found both in the marginal zone and lining the sinusoids of the red pulp. These cells carry antigen to the primary follicles of the white pulp from which, after a few days, antibody-producing cells migrate. These antibody-producing cells colonize the marginal zone and the red pulp, and it is in these regions that antibody production is first detected. Germinal center formation also occurs within the primary follicles within a few days, although this is not directly associated with antibody production. In an animal already

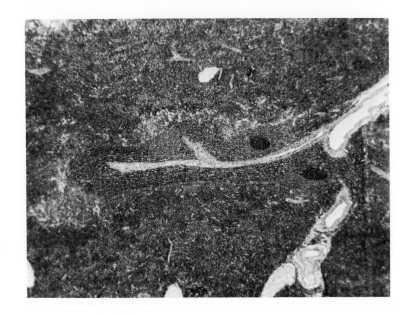

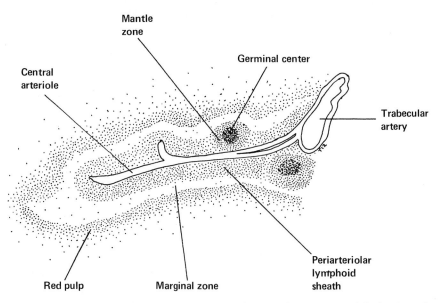

Figure 5–11 A histological section and diagram showing the structure of the bovine spleen. × 50. (From a specimen kindly provided by Dr. J. R. Duncan.)

possessing circulating antibody, trapping by dendritic cells within the secondary follicles becomes significant. As in a primary immune response, the antibody-producing cells migrate from these follicles to the red pulp and the marginal zone where antibody production largely occurs, although some antibodies may also be produced within the hyperplastic secondary follicles.

Lymphocyte Trapping. When antigen enters the spleen or lymph nodes, it initiates lymphocyte trapping. That is, lymphocytes that normally pass freely through these organs get trapped so that they cannot leave. The nature of the trapping process is not clear, but the process probably occurs as a result of the interaction between antigen and macrophages, leading to the release of a "monokine" (Chapter 6) that influences the movement of lymphocytes in some way. Presumably, trapping serves to concentrate antigen-sensitive cells in close proximity to sites of antigen accumulation and so increases the efficiency of the immune responses. Many adjuvants may also "spring" this trap, and it is possible that herein lies one explanation of adjuvanticity. After about 24 hours the lymph node begins to release the trapped cells and shows increased cellular output for about seven days. Toward the end of this time, many of these released cells become antibody producers and memory cells.

OTHER SECONDARY LYMPHOID TISSUES AND THE SITES OF ANTIBODY PRODUCTION

As the foregoing discussion indicated, antibodies are produced in the secondary lymphoid tissues. These tissues include not only the spleen and lymph nodes but also the bone marrow, tonsils (see Fig. 10–4) and lymphoid tissues scattered throughout the body, particularly in the digestive (Fig. 5–12), respiratory and urogenital tracts.

Although its scattered nature makes it difficult to measure, the bone marrow constitutes the largest mass of secondary lymphoid tissue in the body. Therefore, if antigen is given intravenously, it will be trapped and will stimulate antibody production not only in the spleen, but also in the bone marrow. Although the spleen produces the greatest amount of antibody in relation to its size, the bone marrow produces the greatest total amount of antibody, accounting for up to 70 per cent of the antibody produced in response to some antigens (Fig. 5–13). The lymphoid tissues of the lung

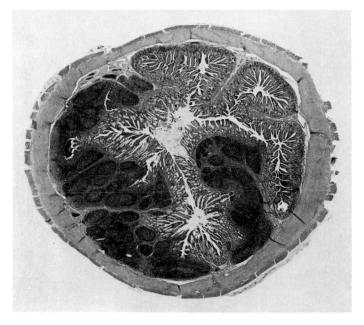

Figure 5–12 A section of dog intestine showing a Peyer's patch in the wall of the ileum. × 5. (From a specimen kindly provided by Dr. S. Yamashiro.)

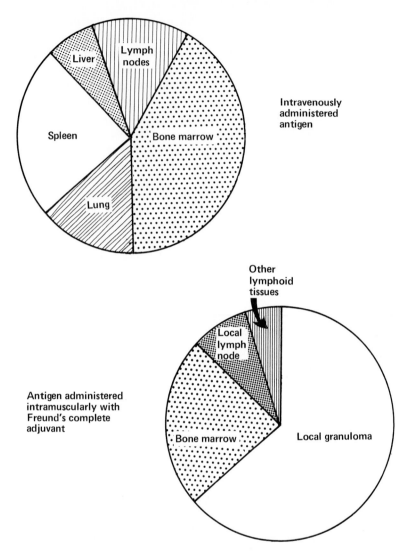

Figure 5–13 The relative contribution of different organs or tissues to antibody production following the administration of antigen.

may also contribute significantly to the immune response against intravenously administered antigen.

Antigen administered orally, if it can penetrate the intestinal wall without being degraded, may stimulate the intestinal lymphoid tissues. As a result, sensitized lymphocytes leave the intestine, circulate in the bloodstream and then colonize surfaces throughout the body. Antigenic stimulation of one part of the intestine may thus provoke antibody formation throughout the digestive tract as well as in the lung, the udder and the urogenital tract (Chapter 10). Antigen introduced directly into the nonlactating mammary gland stimulates local antibody synthesis in lymphoid nodules within the gland and in the draining lymph nodes. Antibody is therefore found in relatively high levels in milk during the subsequent lactation. Antigen administered by inhalation stimulates local antibody production in the lymphoid tissues of the respiratory tract and, if adsorbed into the blood stream, will provoke a systemic immune response.

Many adjuvants, such as those containing alum or water-in-oil emulsions, act by forming an insoluble antigen-containing depot. It is usual for this foreign material to stimulate granulation tissue formation. Antibody-forming cells may develop within this granulation tissue and may contribute a significant proportion of the antibody formed in these cases (Fig. 5–13).

ADDITIONAL SOURCES OF INFORMATION

Butcher EC, Scollay RG, and Weissman IL. 1980. Organ specificity of lymphocyte migration: Mediation by highly selective lymphocyte interaction with organ-specific determinants on high endothelial venules. Eur J Immunol *10* 556–561.

Cahill RNP, Poskill DC, Frost H, and Trinka Z. 1977. Two distinct pools of recirculating T lymphocytes: Migratory characteristics of nodal and intestinal T lymphocytes. J Exp Med *145* 420–428.

Goldstein AL, Thurman GB, Low TKL, Rossio JL, and Trivers GE. 1978. Hormonal influences on the reticuloendothelial system: Current status of the role of thymosin in the regulation and modulation of immunity. J Res *23* 253–266.

Firth GA. 1977. The normal lymphatic system of the domestic fowl. Vet Bull *47* 167–179.

Ham AW. 1974. Histology. JB Lippincott Company, Philadelphia.

Odend'hal S, and Breazile, JE. 1980. An area of T cell localization in the cloacal bursa of white leghorn chickens. Am J Vet Res *41* 255–258.

Owen RL, and Nemanic P. 1978. Antigen processing structures of the mammalian intestinal tract: An SEM study of lymphoepithelial organs. Scanning Electron Microscopy *II* 367–378. SEM Inc., O'Hare, Illinois.

Sharbaugh RJ, Ainsworth SK, and Fitts CT. 1976. *In vitro* response of bovine thoracic duct lymphocytes to phytohemagglutinin following adult thymectomy. Clin Exp Immunol *25* 342–346.

Torres-Medina A. 1981. Morphologic characteristics of the epithelial surface of aggregated lymphoid follicles (Peyer's patches) in the small intestine of newborn gnotobiotic calves and pigs. Am J Vet Res *42* 232–236.

Weiss L. 1972. Cells and tissues of the immune system: Structure, functions, interactions. Foundations of Immunology Series. Prentice-Hall, Inc., Englewood Cliffs, New Jersey.

6

The Cellular Basis of the Immune Response

It is clear from our observation of immune responses that certain cells must be able to recognize antigen and then respond to specific antigenic determinants. It is also clear that the response of these antigen-sensitive cells must result in either the production of antibodies or in the production of cells that can participate in the cell-mediated immune responses (specific effector cells). In addition, cells must be generated that can respond even more effectively to a second exposure to the same antigen—in other words, memory cells.

The hypothesis that accounts for the ability of an animal to mount a specific immune response against any one of a very wide variety of antigens is known as the clonal selection theory. This theory was put forward by Nobel Prize winner Sir Macfarlane Burnet in 1959 and has now been amply confirmed. The basic postulates of this theory are as follows:

1. Lymphoid stem cells differentiate randomly to produce clones of lymphocytes, each of which is committed to respond to a single antigenic determinant.
2. Antigen binding to lymphocyte receptors triggers them to proliferate and differentiate into effector cells and memory cells.
3. The specificity of antibodies produced by a lymphocyte is identical to that of its antigen receptors.
4. Tolerance results when a clone of antigen-binding lymphocytes is destroyed or suppressed.

It is now recognized that antigen-sensitive cells do exist. They occur in two populations: the B cells, which eventually give rise to antibody production; and the T cells, which give rise to cell-mediated immunity. Antigen binding to these cells induces them to proliferate and is the initiating event in the immune responses.

DIFFERENTIATION BETWEEN T AND B CELLS

B cells and T cells look identical, and it is not possible to distinguish between them on the basis of morphology (Fig. 6–1). It is therefore necessary to identify some functional features characteristic of each cell population in order to differentiate them (Table 6–1).

One method of differentiating lymphocytes is to identify characteristic cell-surface antigens. This may be done by preparing specific antisera against lymphocyte sub-populations. Thus, thymus cells may be inoculated into an animal of a different species, which then responds by making specific anti–T cell antibodies. These antibodies can be chemically linked to a fluorescent dye. If lymphocytes are immersed in this fluorescent antiserum, then the antibodies will bind only to T cells. If the treated cell suspension is then washed and examined using an ultraviolet microscope specially adapted for this purpose, the T cells, having bound fluorescent antibody, will be seen to glow in the dark.

This fluorescent antibody technique (which is described in greater detail in Chapter 9) may also be used to identify B cells. We know that B cells possess cell-surface immunoglobulin molecules. By using a fluorescent anti-immunoglobulin serum as described in the previous paragraph, it is possible to identify B cells within a cell mixture.

When properly applied, the fluorescent antibody technique is capable of identifying not only T cells and B cells, but also of identifying subpopulations within these groups. T cells, for example, possess a large number of specific cell-surface antigens (Ia, Thy-1, Lyt-1, 2 and 3, etc.) that are found in characteristic patterns among the T-cell subclasses. B cells may be subdivided on the basis of the immunoglobulin class (IgM, IgG, IgA, etc.) on their cell surfaces.

A second group of techniques used to distinguish T cells from B cells involves the demonstration of characteristic cell-surface receptors (Table 6–2). Thus, T cells, but not B cells, of most species possess receptors enabling them to bind foreign erythrocytes. For example, if mouse T cells and sheep erythrocytes are centrifuged gently together and resuspended, then the erythrocytes stick to the T cells to form "rosettes." In contrast, B cells possess receptors for immunoglobulin-Fc regions. B cells therefore form rosettes with antibody-coated erythrocytes (Fig. 6–2). It may also be shown by using complement-coated erythrocytes that B cells but not T cells possess receptors for certain complement components (Chapter 8).

A third technique by which T and B cells may be distinguished involves comparing their responses to certain proteins called lectins. Lectins—which come from many different sources, especially plants—have an affinity for cell-surface sugars. Since these sugars may differ between T and B cells, some lectins bind only to T cells, others bind only to B cells and some bind to both. Lectins that bind to lymphocytes commonly provoke them to divide. Thus, the lectin phytohemagglutinin, which is extracted from the kidney bean (*Phaseolus vulgaris*), stimulates T cells (and B cells to a much lesser extent) to divide, as does concanavalin A, a lectin extracted from the Jack bean (*Canavalia ensiformis*). Pokeweed mitogen, a lectin from the pokeweed plant (*Phytolacca americana*), stimulates both B and T cells.

Other non-lectin products also function as mitogens; for example, the bacterial endotoxins stimulate B cells to divide, whereas BCG vaccine stimulates only T cells to divide.

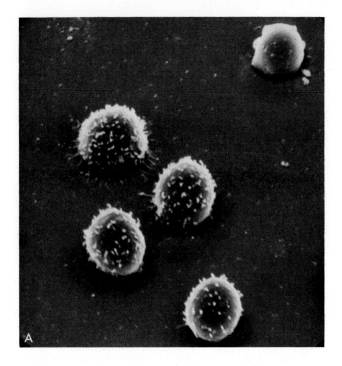

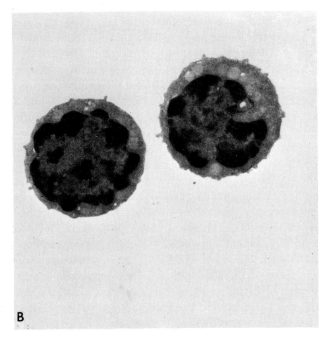

Figure 6–1 *A,* Scanning electron micrograph of lymphocytes from a mouse lymph node. × 1500. *B,* Transmission electron micrograph of lymphocytes from a mouse peritoneal cavity. × 3000.

Table 6–1 THE IDENTIFYING FEATURES OF T AND B LYMPHOCYTES

PROPERTY	B CELLS	T CELLS
Distribution	Lymph node cortex Splenic follicles	Lymph node paracortex Spleen periarteriolar sheath Peripheral blood

Cell surface receptors for
  Antigen
  Immunoglobulin Fc
  C3b
	
	+++
	+++
	+
		
		++
		+
		−

Foreign erythrocytes	−	+++
Cell-surface antigens	Immunoglobulin	Thy 1, Lyt
Divide in response to:	Pokeweed mitogen Bacterial lipopolysaccharide	Phytohemagglutinin Concanavalin A BCG vaccine Pokeweed mitogen
Antigen receptor	Immunoglobulin	V_H region linked to class II antigen
Antigens preferentially recognized	Foreign macromolecules	Histocompatibility antigens
Tolerance induction	Difficult	Relatively easy
Progeny cells	Plasma cell Memory cells	Effector lymphocytes Memory cells
Major secreted products	Immunoglobulins	Lymphokines

These techniques enable investigators to characterize mixed lymphocyte populations. Thus, about 70 per cent of mouse or human peripheral blood lymphocytes can be shown to be T cells and about 20 per cent B cells. The remaining lymphocytes are neither typical T nor typical B cells. In the absence of characteristic markers, they are called "null" cells. Unfortunately, the techniques described above for distinguishing T

Table 6–2 CELL SURFACE RECEPTORS ON CELLS OF THE IMMUNE SYSTEM

		RECEPTORS FOR:				
CELL TYPE	ANTIGEN	IMMUNO-GLOBULIN Fc	COM-PLEMENT COM-PONENTS	HISTAMINE	INSULIN	ERYTHRO-CYTES
Macrophages	−	+++	++	+	+	−
Neutrophils and eosinophils	−	+	+	+	−	−
B cells	+++	+++	+	−	+	−
T cells	+++	(+)*	−	+	+	+
NK cells	+	(+)	−	−	−	(+)

*(+) — only present under certain circumstances or in very small amounts.

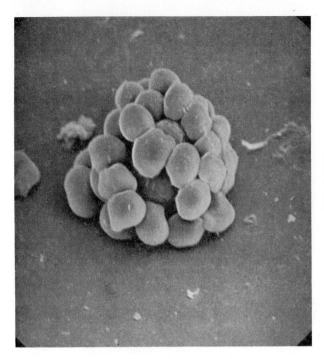

Figure 6–2 Scanning electron micrograph of a "rosette" formed by allowing antibody-coated sheep erythrocytes to come into contact with a mouse lymphocyte. × 2250.

from B cells were first worked out in mice and subsequently modified for use in humans. The reliability of these techniques in distinguishing T from B cells in the major domestic animals remains unclear (Table 6–3). Most results suggest that the relative proportions of T, B and null cells in the blood of domestic animals are approximately 30:20:50. The high proportion of null cells is probably a reflection of the inadequacies of the techniques presently available. It is anticipated that this proportion will drop as techniques are improved.

Table 6–3 PERIPHERAL BLOOD LYMPHOCYTES OF THE DOMESTIC ANIMALS*

SPECIES	PERCENTAGE OF IMMUNOGLOBULIN NEGATIVE CELLS FORMING ROSETTES WITH ERYTHROCYTES (PROBABLY T CELLS)	PERCENTAGE OF IMMUNOGLOBULIN POSITIVE CELLS (PROBABLY B CELLS)
Bovine	32–63	11–38
Equine	38–66	20
Ovine	28–80	15–35
Porcine	30–46	7–19
Canine	26–56	23–32
Feline	30–33	30–40
Chicken	45	30

*The great range of published figures reflects the inadequacy of the currently available techniques. The percentage figures do not add up to 100 per cent because of the occurrence of null (non–T, non–B) cells.

THE CELLULAR BASIS OF ANTIBODY PRODUCTION*

THE B CELL ANTIGEN RECEPTOR

B cells can respond to antigen because they have specific antigen receptors on their surface. These receptors are immunoglobulin molecules attached to the cell membrane and positioned so that their antigen-binding (Fab) sites are exposed, whereas the Fc region is buried within the cell membrane. There are about 10^4 to 10^5 of these receptor immunoglobulin molecules on the surface of each B cell. Normally, unprimed B cell receptors are of the monomeric (7S) IgM class, although some B cells (at least in mice and humans) possess IgD surface receptors. As an immune response progresses, the class, but not the specificity of B cell antigen receptors, may change. Because all the receptor immunoglobulins on a single B cell are identical and of a single specificity, an individual B cell can bind and respond only to the antigenic determinants against which its receptor immunoglobulins are directed.

B cells of differing specificities are, apparently, generated at random from bone marrow. It has been shown that an adult mouse spleen, for example, contains about 2 $\times$ 10^8 B cells capable of responding to at least 10^7 different antigens. For some of these antigens there may be only one or two responsive cells; for others there may be several thousand.

THE RESPONSE OF B CELLS TO ANTIGEN

The binding of antigen to a B cell–receptor immunoglobulin is not sufficient in itself to trigger an immune response. The proliferation of B cells is rigorously controlled and will normally occur only if certain critical conditions are met. These conditions are, first, that the antigen is processed by certain macrophages and presented to the B cell while fixed to the macrophage surface and, second, that certain nearby T cells, called helper T cells, must also be responding to the same antigen (Fig. 6–3).

Macrophage Help. Although all macrophages phagocytose antigen, only some have the ability to process the antigen in such a way that it can stimulate B cells. These antigen-processing macrophages are characterized by possessing a cell-membrane antigen called Ia in mice. (Ia is a class II histocompatibility antigen; see Chapter 7.) Ia positive macrophages permit residual antigen to remain on the cell membrane, where it is up to 10^4 times more effective than unbound antigen in promoting an immune response. Both B cells and helper T cells will respond to antigen only if it is bound to an Ia positive macrophage (Fig. 6–4). These macrophages also promote the B-cell response by releasing a soluble "helper" substance known as interleukin 1, which activates the helper T cells.

T-Cell Help. When helper T cells encounter macrophage-bound antigen, they also secrete "helper" substances. These are complex mixtures of proteins; some, such as interleukin 2, act in a non–antigen-specific fashion, enhancing the responses of B

---

*Most of our knowledge of the cellular interactions that occur in the immune response has been derived from experiments conducted in mice, and the following sections should be read bearing this in mind.

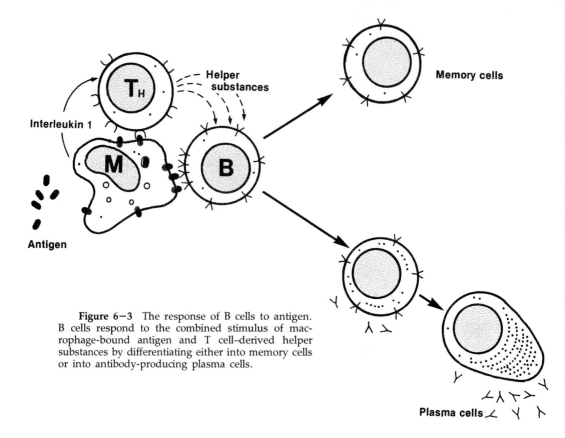

Figure 6–3 The response of B cells to antigen. B cells respond to the combined stimulus of macrophage-bound antigen and T cell–derived helper substances by differentiating either into memory cells or into antibody-producing plasma cells.

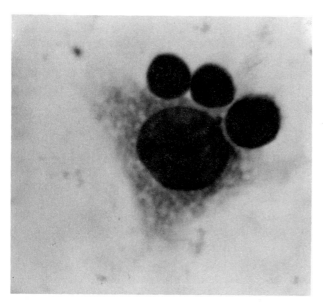

Figure 6–4 Macrophage-lymphocyte interaction. The lymphocytes are from an animal sensitized to the hapten dinitrophenol (DNP) linked to the carrier bovine serum albumin. The macrophage was coated with DNP linked to the unrelated carrier ovalbumin by means of cytophilic antibodies to ovalbumin. The three lymphocytes are therefore binding to an antigen-coated macrophage. (See Fig. 6–3.) × 1300.

cells in general to antigen. Other T cell–derived helper substances are antigen specific, promoting the response of B cells to only a single antigen. Antigen-specific helper factors consist of a single immunoglobulin heavy chain variable region (V_H) linked to an Ia molecule. The precise mode of action of these V_H-Ia factors is unclear, although it is assumed that the V_H region can bind antigen. It is possible that the Ia protein not linked to V_H might function as a non–antigen-specific helper factor. (It is clear that genes that regulate the production of Ia could also effectively regulate immune responsiveness; see Chapter 7.)

The B-Cell Response. As noted, B cells will respond to antigen if it is on the surface of an Ia-positive macrophage in the presence of macrophage-derived and helper T cell–derived helper substances. Once stimulated by these, the B-cell surface commences to flow and the membrane-bound antigen becomes concentrated into a small region (or cap) on the cell surface (Fig. 6–5). The antigen may then be taken into the B cell or released into the surrounding medium.

Following capping, the responding B cell enlarges and commences to divide repeatedly. After a few days, the progeny of the original responding cell gradually differentiates into two morphologically and functionally discrete cell populations. The cells in one of these populations acquire the capacity to manufacture large quantities of antibody and are called plasma cells. The cells in the other population remain morphologically unchanged and function as memory cells (Fig. 6–6).

PLASMA CELLS. Because plasma cells arise by differentiation from B cells, it is possible to identify a series of stages that are morphologically intermediate between lymphocytes and plasma cells. Plasma cells are ovoid, 8 to 20 μm in diameter (Figs. 6–7 and 6–8). They are widely distributed throughout the body but are concentrated in

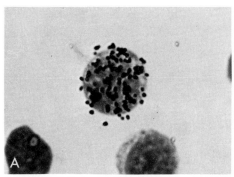
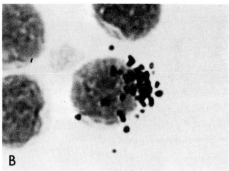
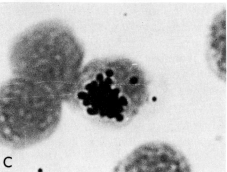

Figure 6–5 The capping phenomenon: Autoradiographs of lymph-node cells from an immunized mouse incubated with bound, tritiated, polymerized flagellin. *A*, Uniform distribution of antigen after incubation at 0°C for 30 minutes. *B* and *C*, Aggregation of antigen at a polar region after incubation at 37°C for 15 minutes. *A*, *B* and *C*, × 2400. (From Diener E, and Paetkan VH. 1972. Proc Nat Acad Sci, *69* 2364. Used with permission. Courtesy of Dr. Diener.)

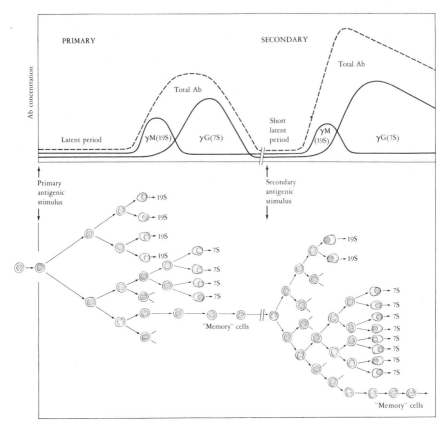

Figure 6–6 The response of antigen-sensitive B cells to antigen. (From Bellanti JA. 1979. Immunology. WB Saunders Company, Philadelphia. Courtesy of Dr. Bellanti.)

the red pulp of the spleen, the medulla of lymph nodes, and in bone marrow. They possess a round, eccentrically situated nucleus whose chromatin is distributed unevenly, so that the nucleus may resemble a clockface or cartwheel. They possess extensive cytoplasm that is strongly basophilic and pyroninophilic, as befits a cell rich in ribosomes that produce antibodies. Because these antibodies must be rapidly secreted, these cells also possess a large, pale-staining Golgi apparatus. Plasma cells are capable of synthesizing as many as 300 molecules of antibody per second, and on occasion this antibody may accumulate within cells to form vesicles known as Russell bodies. Normally, however, antibodies are secreted through reverse pinocytosis soon after they are formed. The specificity of the immunoglobulin produced by these plasma cells is identical to that of the original antigen receptor on the parent B cell. Once fully differentiated, plasma cells die after three to six days, and this population therefore disappears. This disappearance is reflected in serum antibody levels as the immunoglobulins produced by these cells decline gradually through catabolism.

It is now a relatively simple matter to identify individual cells producing antibody against sheep erythrocytes. The test (known as a Jerne plaque assay, after its originator) can be performed by mixing a suspension of antibody-producing cells (usually spleen cells from an inoculated animal) with sheep erythrocytes and stabilizing the mixture in an agarose gel (agarose is a purified form of agar). When the mixture is incubated at 37°C,

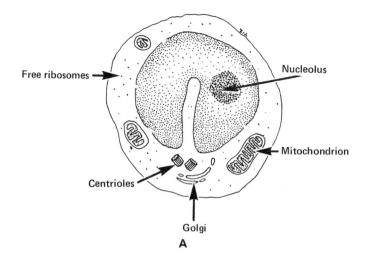

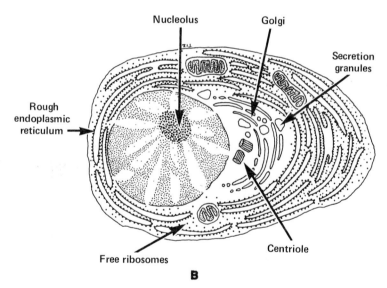

Figure 6–7 The major structural features of a lymphocyte (*A*) and a plasma cell (*B*).

antibodies released from the producing cells diffuse into the agarose and combine with nearby red cells. If hemolytic complement (Chapter 8) is incorporated in the agarose, and if the antibody being produced is IgM (Chapter 4), then antibody-coated red cells will be lysed. As a result, there appears a clear zone or plaque owing to the local lysis of red cells around each antibody-producing cell (Fig. 6–9). The test may be modified to detect cells producing antibodies of other immunoglobulin classes by incorporating specific antiglobulins in the agarose. Thus anti-IgA will reveal IgA-producing cells, and so on. It may also be employed to detect antibodies to soluble antigens, if these antigens are first chemically linked to the erythrocytes.

MEMORY CELLS. The other population of cells derived from a stimulated antigen-sensitive B cell comprises small lymphocytes and so remains morphologically

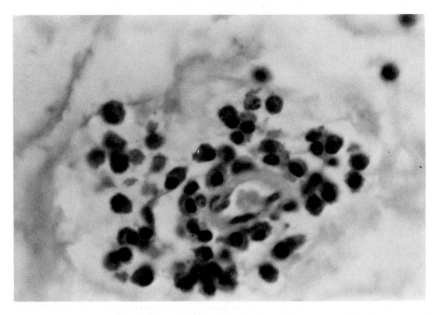

Figure 6—8 Plasma cells in the medulla of a dog lymph node. × 450. (From a specimen kindly provided by Dr. S. Yamashiro.)

indistinguishable from the parent cell. These cells possess immunoglobulin receptors of an identical specificity to those of the parent, although the surface-immunoglobulin class switches from IgM to IgG, IgA or IgE. These cells live for many months or years after the first exposure to antigen. As a result, if a second dose of antigen is given to an animal, it will encounter and stimulate many more antigen-sensitive cells than did the first dose. Consequently, a secondary immune response is quantitatively greater than a primary response, and the immunoglobulin produced is primarily of the IgG rather than the IgM class. The lag period is shorter in a secondary as opposed to a primary response, because more antibody is produced and because the lymphoid organs can process antigen much more effectively (Chapter 5).

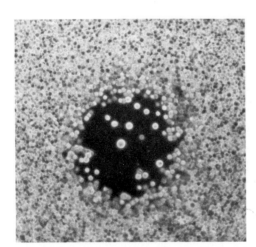

Figure 6—9 A zone of hemolysis surrounding a mouse spleen cell producing antibodies against sheep erythrocytes. The Jerne plaque technique.

THE CELLULAR BASIS OF CELL-MEDIATED IMMUNITY

In the previous section we discussed how B cells, upon encountering specific antigen, respond by multiplication and differentiation. The result of this response is the development of two different cell populations, one of which comprises long-lived memory cells whereas the other comprises very short-lived antibody-producing plasma cells. This section describes how T cells respond in a parallel fashion and also react to antigen by differentiation and division. As a consequence, two cell populations are produced—one of long-lived memory cells, the other of effector T cells. Instead of synthesizing and releasing antibody in the same way as B cells, the T cells either release a number of biologically active factors, the most important of which are proteins known as lymphokines, or, alternatively, attack and destroy foreign (allogeneic) target cells.

T-CELL HETEROGENEITY

T cells are much more heterogeneous than B cells, particularly with respect to their life span and the functions they serve. Some T cells act as effectors in the cell-mediated immune response by producing biologically active lymphokines, and others are capable of destroying foreign cells in grafts or tumor cells. Some T cells act to enhance the response of other T or B cells to antigen and are therefore known as helper cells. Others function as suppressor cells and inhibit the responses of other T and B cells. Even within these subgroups there are subdivisions. For example, some helper cells are non–antigen specific, whereas others help the response to a specific antigen only. It is sometimes possible to characterize these subgroups by their cell-surface antigens, their receptors and their life span. For example, suppressor T cells possess Fc receptors for IgG, whereas helper T cells have Fc receptors for IgM. If an animal is thymectomized in adult life, then the T-cell population of the secondary lymphoid organs can be shown to fall into two general categories. One group of cells, found largely in the spleen, is short lived and disappears within a few days. These cells, known as T1 cells, can function as both helpers and suppressors. They are not capable of direct cytotoxic activity. In contrast to the T1 cells, the remaining T cells, known as T2 cells, are much longer lived and thus persist for many months after adult thymectomy. T2 cells are found largely in the lymph nodes and, recirculating in the blood stream, they are capable of direct cytotoxic activity.

It is not entirely clear whether T1 cells are the precursors of T2 cells or, alternatively, whether both populations are generated simultaneously by the thymus.

Notwithstanding this complexity, all T cells possess the common property of having been processed in the thymic environment during their maturation process.

THE T-CELL ANTIGEN RECEPTOR

T cells can recognize and respond to antigen in a manner similar to B cells. The precise structure of the T-cell antigen receptor, however, remains unclear. It probably consists of two closely linked molecules. One of these molecules has a specific antigen-binding site and probably consists of an isolated V_H immunoglobulin region.

The second portion of the receptor consists of an Ia antigen. This is a single 30,000-dalton polypeptide chain. Its structure is coded for by genes at the class II locus of the major histocompatibility complex (Chapter 7). The function of the Ia portion of the receptor is unknown, but it probably serves to regulate the response of the T cell to antigen. The difficulties encountered in characterizing the T-cell antigen receptor are compounded by the small number (100 to 1000) of them on the T-cell surface.

THE RESPONSE OF T CELLS TO ANTIGEN

On binding to the T-cell antigen receptor, antigen stimulates the T cell to divide and differentiate. Like the B-cell response, the T-cell response is regulated by the presence of interleukins released from macrophages and from T helper cells.

The antigenic determinants to which T cells respond appear to differ from those recognized by B cells. Thus, the immune responses to foreign grafts or to cells modified by virus infection or chemical treatment are all primarily cell-mediated. T cells, in fact, appear to react optimally to antigen presented in close association with histocompatibility antigens (Fig. 6–10). It is possible that this reaction accounts for the necessity for macrophage processing, since macrophage surface-bound antigen will be presented in this way. The importance of histocompatibility antigens in initiating the T-cell response is emphasized by the observation that up to 10 per cent of mouse T cells will respond to a single foreign histocompatibility antigen, although only one in 10^4 to 10^5 cells will respond to a more conventional antigen. In addition, T cells, when exposed to a hapten-carrier conjugate, tend to respond in a way that is carrier-specific,

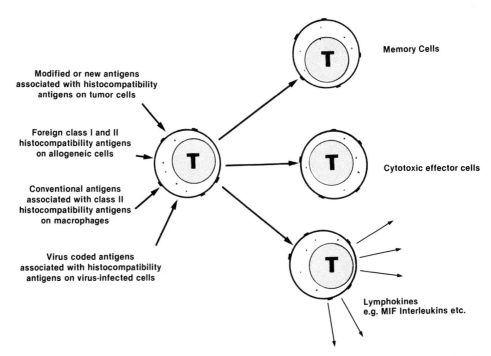

Figure 6–10 The response of T cells to antigen. T cells respond to antigens associated with histocompatibility antigens by differentiating into memory cells, cytotoxic effector cells or lymphokine-producing cells.

in contrast to B cells, which are able to respond to haptenic determinants alone (see Table 3–3). This may indicate that the T-cell antigen receptor recognizes a different antigenic determinant than does the corresponding B-cell antigen receptor.

Antigen-sensitive T cells respond to antigen by dividing and eventually generating both memory cell and effector cell populations (Fig. 6–10). The effector cells are somewhat larger than unstimulated lymphocytes, and their cytoplasm is pyroninophilic, suggesting a capacity for protein synthesis. These cells are capable of performing a number of different activities; for example, they can synthesize and secrete various non–antigen-specific, biologically active proteins, known as lymphokines; they can generate antigen-specific non-immunoglobulin factors that possess potent biological activity, known as transfer factors; and they can participate in direct cytotoxic reactions on contact with allogeneic target cells.

Lymphokines. Lymphokines are proteins with molecular weights of between 25,000 and 75,000 daltons. They are released mainly from activated T cells, but B cells may produce them in response to nonspecific stimulants such as bacterial lipopolysaccharides or PPD tuberculin. Lymphokines possess a wide range of biological activities (Table 6–4), and at least 90 different lymphokine-mediated activities

Table 6–4 SOME OF THE NON–ANTIGEN-SPECIFIC LYMPHOKINES PRODUCED BY T CELLS FOLLOWING *IN VITRO* ANTIGENIC STIMULATION

TYPE OF FACTOR	FACTOR	CHARACTERISTIC
Factors affecting macrophages	Migration inhibition factor (MIF)	Prevents migration of macrophages
	Macrophage aggregating factor (MAF)	Causes macrophages to aggregate
	Macrophage disappearing factor (MDF)	Makes peritoneal macrophages adhere to serosa
	Macrophage chemotactic factor (MCF)	Attracts macrophages
	Specific macrophage-arming factor (SMAF)	Stimulates macrophage cytotoxic activity
	Macrophage stimulating factor (MSF)	Stimulates macrophage migration
Chemotactic factors for:	Neutrophils Eosinophils Basophils	
Cytotoxic and growth inhibitory factors:	Lymphotoxins (LT)	Kills target cells
	Inhibitor of DNA synthesis (IDS)	Inhibits target-cell division
	Proliferation inhibiting factor (PIF)	Inhibits target-cell proliferation
	Suppressor factors	Suppress immune reactivity
Growth stimulating factors:	Mitogenic factor (MF)	Stimulates lymphocyte division
	Lymphocyte activating factor (LAF)	Stimulates the lymphocyte response to antigen
	Interleukin 2 (IL2)	Required for T helper activity
	Helper factors	Mediate T helper activity
	Interferon (IFN)	Promotes immune reactivity

have been recognized. Unfortunately, it is not yet clear whether these activities are a true reflection of their heterogeneity or of the many different methods used to assay them. In general, lymphokines are neither antigen-binding nor antigen-specific. Lymphokines act on a number of cell populations to induce functional changes that serve, in general, to influence cellular activities.

LYMPHOKINES AND MACROPHAGES. The lymphokine that was discovered first and that has been most thoroughly studied acts *in vitro* to prevent macrophages from migrating out of capillary tubes. It is therefore known as macrophage migration inhibition factor, or MIF. The activity of MIF can be shown by packing a glass capillary tube with a suspension of macrophages and lymphocytes. (This is easily obtained by washing out the peritoneal cavity of a laboratory animal with tissue culture fluid). If this capillary tube is then placed horizontally on a flat surface and immersed in tissue culture fluid, then the macrophages will migrate out to form a fan of cells on the surface (Fig. 6–11). This migration occurs if cells from an unsensitized donor are allowed to migrate in the presence of antigen. Similarly, cells from a sensitized donor migrate normally in the absence of antigen. However, cells from a sensitized animal do not migrate when incubated in the presence of antigen. The inhibition of migration is due to the release of MIF from T cells exposed to antigen. The MIF formed by these cells acts by making macrophages clump and is possibly identical to macrophage disappearing factor (MDF) (Table 6–4). MIF is a mixture of glycoproteins that range

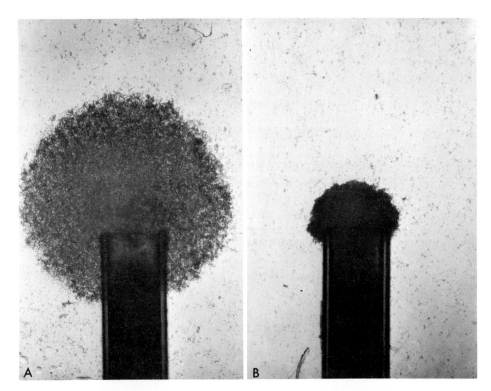

Figure 6–11 The macrophage migration inhibition test using bovine MIF. Normally, guinea pig peritoneal macrophages are free to migrate from a glass capillary tube (*A*). MIF may be produced by exposing peripheral blood lymphocytes from a sensitized calf to appropriate antigen. In the presence of this factor, macrophage migration is inhibited (*B*). (Courtesy of Dr. B. N. Wilkie.)

in size from 35,000 to 55,000 daltons. They can be isolated and the purified material used to prevent the migration of normal macrophages in the absence of antigen. MIF may be detected *in vivo* in the lymph draining the sites of delayed hypersensitivity skin reactions (which are a form of localized cell-mediated immune response). Although "classical" MIF is generally considered to be non–antigen specific, MIF-like factors specific for the inducing antigen have been reported to exist. (See also Chapter 20.)

On reacting with allogeneic (foreign) target cells, sensitized T cells release a soluble factor that confers on macrophages the capacity to kill these specific target cells. This soluble factor is known as specific macrophage arming factor (SMAF), and it may be classified as a lymphokine. Once macrophages armed by SMAF meet antigen, they may become further activated so that not only are they capable of killing allogeneic cells in a nonspecific fashion, but their bactericidal capacity is also greatly enhanced. This form of macrophage activation is of significance in the development of resistance to certain intracellular pathogenic microorganisms. For example, some bacteria, notably *Mycobacterium tuberculosis, Brucella abortus, Listeria mono-cytogenes* and the salmonellae, as well as the protozoan parasite *Toxoplasma gondii*, are normally capable of proliferation within macrophages, since they block phago-some-lysosome fusion. It has been suggested that this blocking is accomplished by the release of cyclic AMP from the organism into the phagosome. Because of their intracellular location, antibodies cannot confer resistance to disease caused by these organisms. However, during the course of these infections, a cell-mediated immune response is stimulated, in which T cells interact with antigen and release SMAF-like lymphokines. These factors cause the animal's macrophages to increase in both size and metabolic activity. The lysosomes in these cells enlarge and contain increased amounts of hydrolytic enzymes (Figs. 6–12 and 6–13), and the phagosome-lysosome block is removed so that destruction of the intracellular organisms occurs. Activated macrophages also acquire membrane Ia antigen and thus become capable of processing antigen for activation of T lymphocytes (page 79).

Other lymphokines that modify macrophage behavior include macrophage chem-otactic factor (CF), which attracts these cells to sites of antigen–T cell interaction, and a factor that stimulates macrophage migration (MSF). Therefore, it is not surprising that intradermal inoculation of some lymphokine preparations into an animal leads to the development of an inflammatory reaction characterized by mononuclear cell infil-tration and resembling delayed hypersensitivity (Chapter 20).

IMMUNOREGULATORY LYMPHOKINES. Lymphocyte-derived helper and suppressor factors can be considered to be lymphokines. They are discussed in detail in Chapter 7.

LYMPHOKINES THAT ACT ON OTHER CELLS. One form of cell-mediated skin reaction that may be induced by the intradermal inoculation of certain antigens is known as cutaneous-basophil hypersensitivity, because the reaction site is extensively infiltrated with basophils (Chapter 20). It has been shown that this reaction is due in some cases to the release of a basophil-chemotactic lymphokine from sensitized T cells. Similarly, in certain systemic helminth infestations such as Trichinosis, it has been suggested that the massive eosinophilia so characteristic of this condition may be mediated, at least in part, by an eosinophil-mobilizing lymphokine.

TRANSFER FACTOR

In order to demonstrate that an immune reaction is cell mediated, it is usually necessary to demonstrate that it can be transferred from a sensitized animal to a nor-

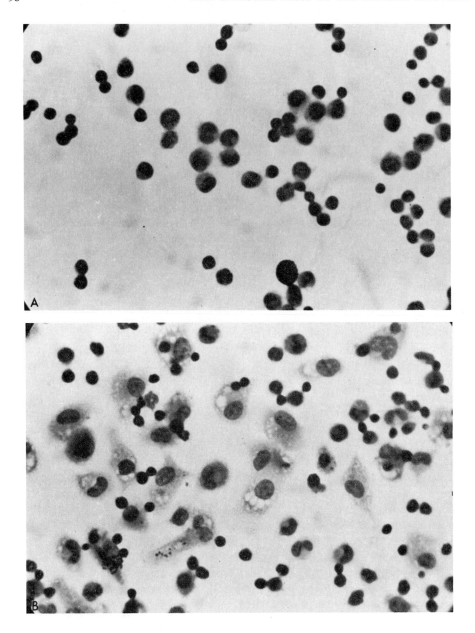

Figure 6—12 Giemsa-stained monolayers of mouse peritoneal macrophages. *A*, From a normal mouse. *B*, From a mouse infected 10 days previously with a sublethal dose of *Listeria monocytogenes*. These macrophages have been "activated" in a form of cell-mediated immune response. × 450.

mal animal by means of washed lymphocytes. In humans, cattle, sheep and dogs, and to a lesser extent in rodents, successful and specific transfer may be achieved by means of lymphocyte extracts. The activity in these extracts, known as transfer factor, will pass through a dialysis membrane and must therefore have a molecular weight of less than 10,000 daltons. A single injection of transfer factor may confer specific cell-mediated reactivity on a normal recipient, lasting for over a year in some cases. Trans-

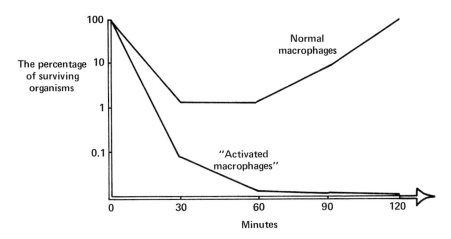

Figure 6–13 The destruction of *Listeria monocytogenes* when mixed with cultures of normal macrophages and "activated" macrophages from Listeria-infected mice.

fer factor is a complex riboprotein that contains part of a class II histocompatibility antigen (Chapter 7) and that can bind antigen. Because of its small size it is difficult to conceive of it as an informational macromolecule. It has been suggested that it may contain very small quantities of antigen and that the rest of the molecule may act as a powerful adjuvant, but this has not been substantiated and its precise mechanism of action remains unknown. Transfer factor has been used therapeutically in humans to confer immunity toward antigens to which patients are unreactive. An example of this is the treatment of chronic mucocutaneous candidiasis. This is a disfiguring fungal infection occurring in individuals who are unable to respond immunologically to the invading organism. Administration of transfer factor from immune individuals permits recipients to mount a successful immune response.

CELL-MEDIATED CYTOTOXICITY (Table 6–5)

Some T cells develop the ability to attach to allogeneic or altered tissue cells and destroy them. This can be a very rapid process. Within seconds following contact between a T cell and its target, all the organelles and the nucleus of the target cell disrupt simultaneously. The T cell can then disengage itself and move on to find

Table 6–5 MECHANISMS OF TARGET-CELL DESTRUCTION

EFFECTOR CELL	*MECHANISM INVOLVED*
T cell	Cell-target contact
T cell	Soluble lymphotoxins
Activated macrophage	Cell-target contact, specific or non-specific
Neutrophils Macrophages B cells K cells	Through Fc receptor and antibody (ADCC); possibly also involving complement
NK cells	Cell-target contact

another victim. The mechanisms involved in this dramatic process are unclear. It is speculated that the T cell attaches to the target and destroys it by producing cytotoxic lymphokines or lymphotoxins. The lymphocyte may insert its lymphotoxins into the target membranes in such a way that they form transmembrane channels or holes. As a result, all cell membranes then rupture simultaneously.

Under some circumstances the lymphocyte need not come into direct contact with the target, instead releasing its lymphotoxins into the surrounding fluid. When these come into contact with the target cell, they cause its lysis. This process is, of course, much less efficient than cytotoxicity mediated by direct contact, and it suffers from the additional problem of nonspecificity. Any cell, including the cytotoxic lymphocyte, that is in the neighborhood when free lymphotoxin is released may also be destroyed. Under other circumstances, macrophages may acquire the capacity to destroy target cells under the influence of lymphocyte mediators such as SMAF. However, this form of cytotoxic reaction is considerably less efficient than direct T cell–mediated cytotoxicity, taking hours rather than minutes.

Two other mechanisms of cell-mediated toxicity, although not mediated by T cells, may be mentioned here for comparison. Cells that possess receptors for the Fc region of immunoglobulins may bind to allogeneic target cells or bacteria by means of specific antibody and when bound to targets in this way may be cytotoxic. Cells capable of this include monocytes, eosinophils, neutrophils and a population of non-T, non-B small lymphocytes, which may be called killer (K) or null cells and which are probably identical to NK cells (see page 254). The mechanism of this antibody-dependent cell-mediated cytotoxicity (ADCC) is unknown. However, neutrophils and eosinophils probably act through a respiratory burst mechanism (Chapter 2), which causes destruction of target-cell membranes. This reaction is also considerably slower and less efficient than direct T cell–mediated cytotoxicity.

Finally, normal animals possess a population of natural killer (NK) cells, which have the ability to destroy virus-infected or tumor cells in the absence of previous sensitization. NK cells are not T cells, but they may be related to them. Their mode of action is unknown, but their activity is greatly enhanced by the lymphokine interferon (Chapter 7).

ADDITIONAL SOURCES OF INFORMATION

Greaves MR, Owen JJT, and Raff MC. 1975. T and B lymphocytes. Origins, Properties and Roles in Immune Responses. Elsevier North-Holland Publishers, New York.

Hafeman DG, and Lucas ZJ. 1979. Polymorphonuclear leukocyte–mediated, antibody-dependent cellular cytotoxicity against tumor cells: Dependence on oxygen and the respiratory burst. J Immunol *123* 55–62.

Klesius PH, Fudenberg HH, and Smith CL. 1980. Comparative studies on dialyzable leukocyte extracts containing transfer factor: A review. Comp Immun Microbiol Infect Dis *3* 247–260.

Klinman NR. 1976. The acquisition of B cell competence and diversity. Am J Pathol *85* 694–703.

Matter A. 1979. Microcinematographic and electron microscopic analysis of target cell lysis induced by cytotoxic T lymphocytes. Immunology *36* 179–190.

McCluskey RT, and Cohen S. 1974. Mechanisms of Cell-Mediated Immunity. Basic and Clinical Immunology Series. John Wiley & Sons, New York.

Robertson M. 1979. Recognition, restriction and immunity. Nature *280* 192–193.

Rowlands DT, and Daniele RP. 1975. Surface receptors in the immune response. N Engl J Med *293* 26–32.

Unanue ER. 1980. Cooperation between mononuclear phagocytes and lymphocytes in immunity. N Engl J Med *303* 977–985.

7

Regulation of the Immune Responses

The interactions of T cells and B cells with each other or with other cell populations, such as macrophages, form a complex pattern, and our understanding of the ramifications of these interactions is currently in a state of dynamic change. Students studying this area for the first time may find its complexity discouraging. It should, however be, borne in mind that all bodily processes are subjected to careful and rigorous controls. It is most probable that the immune system is by no means unique in its complexity and that the patterns of interaction that we are now discovering are only a reflection of the superb sophistication of biological systems in general.

THE CONTROL OF CELLULAR ACTIVITY

Most cellular activities are regulated through manipulation of the ratio of two cyclic nucleotides—adenosine 3',5' cyclic monophosphate (cyclic AMP) and guanosine 3',5' cyclic monophosphate (cyclic GMP). If the relative level of cyclic AMP is raised or the level of cyclic GMP lowered, then cellular functions tend to be inhibited. In contrast, if cyclic GMP is raised or cyclic AMP lowered, then cellular activities are enhanced. Many, if not all, of the mechanisms that regulate immune responses do so by either directly or indirectly modulating the cyclic AMP/cyclic GMP ratio within cells (Table 7–1).

Table 7–1 ROLE OF CYCLIC AMP IN SOME IMMUNOLOGICAL PHENOMENA*

CELL	STIMULUS THAT ELEVATES CYCLIC AMP	EFFECT OF ELEVATED CYCLIC AMP
Lymphocyte	Antibodies Immune complexes Suppressor cells Prostaglandins	Inhibition of antigen-stimulated differentiation and division
Macrophage	Some ingested bacteria and protozoa?	Inhibition of lysosome-phagosome fusion
Mast cells	E prostaglandins Histamine	Inhibition of antigen-induced histamine release

*Cyclic AMP generally acts to inhibit cellular activities, although the overall effect is modulated by the cyclic AMP/cyclic GMP ratio.

THE REGULATION OF THE IMMUNE RESPONSES

The immune responses, both cell- and antibody-mediated, while essential for the protection of the body, have the potential to cause severe damage if permitted to act in an unregulated fashion. Failure to control the specificity of an immune response may result in the production of autoantibodies and autoimmune disease. Failure to mount an adequate level of response may cause immunodeficiency and increased susceptibility to infection. In contrast, an excessive immune response may cause a disease such as amyloidosis. Failure to control the burst of lymphocyte proliferation that occurs in the immune responses may lead to the development of lymphoid tumors. Failure to control the mother's immune response to the fetus may lead to abortion. It is obvious, therefore, that the immune responses must be carefully regulated to ensure that the only responses permitted to occur are appropriate in terms of both quality and quantity. As might be anticipated, a number of different control mechanisms exist in order to accomplish this task (Fig. 7-4).

REGULATION OF IMMUNE RESPONSES BY ANTIGEN

In general, the immune responses are antigen driven. Once antigen is eliminated, then the stimulus for cell proliferation (but not immunoglobulin synthesis) is removed and that particular immune response ceases. If antigen persists, then the stimulus persists, and as a consequence the immune response tends to be prolonged rather than terminating abruptly. This type of prolonged response is observed after immunization with poorly metabolized antigens, such as the bacterial polysaccharides, or with antigen incorporated in oily or insoluble adjuvants. The amount of antigen available to stimulate B cells also exerts a selective influence on antibodies produced during the immune response. Thus, in the early stages of an immune response, antigen is relatively plentiful. As the immune response progresses and the quantity of available antigen declines, the remaining antigen is likely to bind and stimulate those cells whose surface immunoglobulins have the highest affinity for it. As a result, selective stimulation of high-affinity cells occurs, and consequently there is a tendency for the antibodies produced during the course of an immune response to increase gradually in affinity for the inducing antigenic determinant. As discussed earlier (page 46), this process also results in an apparent decrease in antibody specificity.

Antigen-sensitive cells will respond to antigen by producing antibodies or specific effector cells only if that antigen is presented to them in an appropriate dose and manner. If the amount of antigen encountered by an antigen-sensitive cell is either excessive or inadequate or if the antigen is presented to the cells in an inappropriate fashion, then, instead of responding to antigen by division and differentiation, cells may become unreactive or even be eliminated and a state of tolerance will result.

Tolerance is a state in which an animal becomes specifically unresponsive to a particular antigen. The most obvious example of this is the failure of animals to make antibodies against normal body components. Burnet and Fenner suggested in 1948 that this self-tolerance was associated with the state of maturation of antigen-sensitive cells at the time they first encounter the antigen. They suggested that antigen-sensitive cells became specifically unresponsive if exposed to an antigen during fetal life but that after birth these cells responded to new antigens by mounting conventional immune responses. As evidence for this suggestion they pointed to the existence of chimeric calves. In about 90 per cent of dizygotic twin calves, the placental circulations fuse and the blood of these calves mixes freely. Any circulating hematopoietic stem cells are also free to intermingle in each calf. Consequently, when these calves are born they carry a mixture of erythrocytes, some from one animal and some from its twin. Yet in spite of being genetically and antigenically dissimilar, the calves are fully tolerant to each other's blood cells.

A variation on this "natural" experiment can be performed in the laboratory if cells from one inbred strain of mice are inoculated into the fetuses of a second inbred strain. When the inoculated mice are born they are found to be completely tolerant to cells of the donor strain, so they can, for instance, accept skin grafts indefinitely from that strain. This experiment confirms Burnet and Fenner's suggestion that antigen given *in utero* provokes tolerance rather than immunity. The "switch" from tolerance induction to normal immune responses occurs soon after birth in laboratory rodents. In domestic mammals, the young are born at a much more mature stage of immunological development and this "switch" occurs at a much earlier stage of fetal life (Chapter 11). The existence of this phenomenon explains how self-tolerance occurs, since most self-antigens are present in the fetus and thus can induce tolerance long before an animal is exposed to extrinsic antigens.

Tolerance may also be induced in adult animals. As pointed out earlier, the conditions under which a T cell or a B cell will respond to an antigen are highly restrictive—that is, the antigen must be presented to these cells in an appropriate dose and manner.

If antigen doses ranging from very small to very large are given to an animal, it is found that very low and very high doses are tolerogenic whereas medium doses provoke immune responses. Very low doses of antigen induce tolerance only in T cells, whereas high doses render both B cells and T cells unresponsive. Because of the requirement for T helper cells in the immune response, tolerance of either type will block antibody production.

Most solutions of proteins contain a mixture of aggregated and monomeric molecules. The aggregated molecules are readily phagocytosed by macrophages and are thus highly immunogenic. If a protein solution is ultracentrifuged so that these aggregates are removed, it becomes highly tolerogenic. It is believed that this may be because of antigen reaching antigen-sensitive cells directly without having undergone macrophage processing.

Another type of tolerance is provoked by high doses of polysaccharide antigens. These antigens can bind tightly to B cell antigen receptors and block the further response of these cells to antigens.

Although it is possible to identify a number of different mechanisms by which tolerance may be induced, the precise mechanisms involved at the cellular level remain unclear. In tolerance induced in fetal animals, the specific T cells do not appear to be completely eliminated, since some self-reactive cells can be detected in adults if very sensitive techniques are used. In tolerance induced by inappropriate dosage of antigen or macrophage avoidance, it is possible that suppressor cells are preferentially stimulated. In tolerance provoked by high doses of polysaccharide, the mechanisms appear to involve a form of receptor blocking.

In general, all these forms of tolerance gradually wane as antigen is eliminated. If antigen persists, as in self-tolerance, then the tolerant condition may be maintained indefinitely. Once antigen is eliminated, B cells regain their reactivity rapidly whereas T cells take considerably longer to recover.

REGULATION OF IMMUNE RESPONSES BY ANTIBODY

Antibody or immune complexes generally exert a negative feedback on immune responses. For example, specific IgG antibody can depress the further production of IgM or IgG to the same antigen, and high levels of IgM antibody depress the further synthesis of IgM. This feedback process ensures that immunoglobulin levels in normal animals remain relatively constant regardless of the degree of antigenic stimulation to which they are subjected. It was once considered that this negative feedback was mediated by antibody, which combined with antigen to mask its antigenic determinants and so removed the stimulus for cell proliferation. It is likely, however, that this is but a minor mechanism, since negative feedback requires the presence of intact Fc regions on the inhibitory immunoglobulin molecules. B cells possess Fc receptors, and it is possible that the binding of antibodies or immune complexes to these receptors causes these cells to "turn off," perhaps by increasing intracellular levels of cyclic AMP (Fig. 7–1). Suppressor T cells also possess Fc receptors, and it is possible that antibody or immune complexes may act through these to stimulate suppressor cell activities.

When serum immunoglobulin levels are abnormally elevated, as in plasma cell tumors (myelomas, Chapter 22), these feedback mechanisms depress normal immunoglobulin synthesis; as a result, animals with myelomas are very susceptible to secondary infection. A similar phenomenon occurs in young animals that have acquired immunoglobulins passively from their mother. The presence of maternal antibody, while conferring immunity, prevents the successful vaccination of these newborn animals, since it effectively inhibits immunoglobulin production (Chapter 11). It is also of interest to note that antibody-producing cells migrate away from the lymph-node cortex and the lymph follicles of the spleen, where the antigen-sensitive cells react with antigen (Chapter 5). Presumably, if this movement did not take place, then the presence of high concentrations of immunoglobulin in close proximity to antigen-sensitive cells might prematurely "switch off" an immune response.

The class as well as the quantity of immunoglobulin produced during an immune response is also regulated. Most unstimulated B cells have IgD or IgM surface

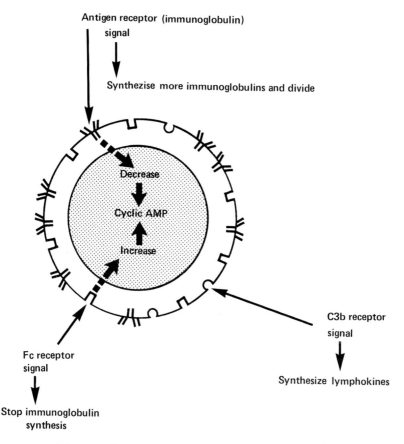

Figure 7–1 Schematic diagram showing how the immune response might be controlled through surface receptors on B cells. It should be pointed out that the signal from the antigen receptor must be complemented by signals from helper factors for maximal efficiency.

immunoglobulin. During an immune response these cells switch to the production of IgG, IgA or IgE, and this switch is regulated by T cells. In the absence of T cells the switch is inefficient, and only IgM production persists at a relatively low level. Antigens such as bacterial lipopolysaccharides, polymerized flagellin and pneumococal polysaccharide, which do not stimulate T cells readily and which can induce B cells to respond in the absence of T cells, generate a persistent IgM response with no switch to IgG production. As might be anticipated, neonatal thymectomy does not depress the immune responses to these antigens, which may therefore be considered "thymus independent." Neonatal bursectomy may also result in a failure of the IgM-to-IgG switch, suggesting that the bursa is responsible for this process in birds.

Immunological Networks. It has been suggested, and there is some evidence to show, that the idiotypes produced during an immune response may function as antigens and provoke antibodies against themselves. The new idiotypes on anti-idiotype antibodies provoked in this way may then, in their turn, function as antigens and also provoke antibody formation, and so forth. This concept has been developed into a suggestion that a network of interacting idiotype–anti-idiotype reactions are provoked in any immune response and that these may serve to regulate immune reactivity.

REGULATION OF IMMUNE RESPONSES BY HISTOCOMPATIBILITY GENES

When cells or tissues are transplanted between genetically non-identical animals, they provoke an immune response. The antigens against which this response is directed are glycoproteins that are found on the surface of all nucleated cells and are called histocompatibility antigens. Cells possess a large number of antigens on their surface. Some of these are much more immunogenic than others and are called major histocompatibility antigens. Grafts that differ from the host in these major antigens are rejected much more promptly than are grafts differing in the minor antigens. These major histocompatibility antigens are detected most easily on blood leukocytes and consequently, are denoted by the initials of the species followed by L (for "leuko-cyte"), and A (denoting the first and most important histocompatibility antigens). Thus, HLA denotes the major histocompatibility antigens in humans; DLA denotes those in dogs; BoLA, those in bovines; SLA, those in swine, and so forth. In mice and chickens the major histocompatibility antigens are known as H2 and B respec-tively, since they were first recognized as blood-group antigens (Table 7–2).

TERMINOLOGY

The following definitions are offered as an aid to those who may have forgotten any genetics they once knew.

Genes are units of DNA that code for the amino acid sequence of a polypeptide chain. Genes can exist in two or more alternative forms known as *alleles*. Alleles are located on chromosomes at sites called *loci*. In any individual a single locus can contain only one gene. Because chromosomes are paired, one being inherited from each parent, loci are also inherited in pairs.

A *gene complex* is a cluster of multiple genes, related structurally or functionally and occupying a restricted area of a chromosome. The term *haplotype* is used to describe the complete set of alleles at all loci within a gene complex on a single chromosome.

Table 7–2   THE HISTOCOMPATIBILITY ANTIGENS OF DOMESTIC ANIMALS*

| SPECIES | NAME | NUMBER OF LOCI IDENTIFIED | | |
		CLASS I	CLASS II	CLASS III
Dogs	DLA	5(A, B, C, D, E)†	1(Ir)	–
Swine	SLA	2(A,C)	1(D or Ia)	1
Cattle	BoLA	1(A)	1	–
Sheep	OLA	2(A, B)	–	–
Goats	GLA	2(A_1A_2)	1	–
Chickens	B	2(B–F, B–G)	1	1
Horses	ELA	1		
Mice	H2	2(K, D)	1(I)	1(S)
Humans	HLA	4(A, B, C, D)	1(Dr)	2(CH, RG)

*Currently accepted names for these loci are in parentheses.

†In many cases, the number of identified loci is highly debatable. The figures given here will almost certainly be modified in the future.

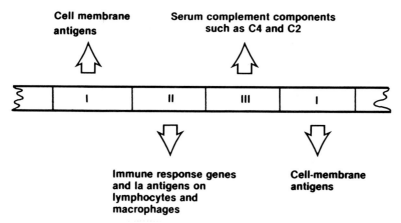

Figure 7–2 The basic structure of the major histocompatibility complex of the mouse. This species has two class I loci flanking single class II and class III loci.

The major histocompatibility antigens possessed by an individual animal are inherited through the activities of a gene complex (Fig. 7–2). Within the major histocompatibility complex are found three important classes of loci. Class I loci contain genes that code for molecules that are the target antigens in transplantation reactions. Class II loci contain genes that regulate lymphocyte proliferation and interactions as well as the strength of the immune responses. Class III loci contain genes that control the production of some complement components and their receptors.

The antigens coded for by genes in class I loci are membrane-bound glycoproteins with a molecular weight of 45,000 daltons. Each antigen is associated with a single molecule of β_2-microglobulin, which, you may remember, is very closely related to a single C_H homology region (Fig. 7–3). The overall structure of the antigen bears a superficial resemblance to half an immunoglobulin molecule without variable regions.

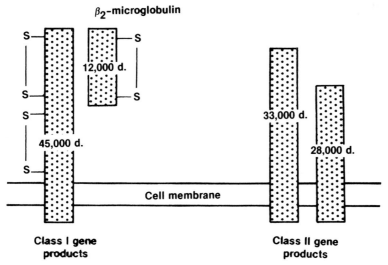

Figure 7–3 The structure of class I and class II histocompatibility gene products. The class I products may occur in pairs and thus bear a superficial resemblance to an immunoglobulin molecule.

Class I antigens are found on all cells except those in the very early embryo and some that are very highly differentiated, such as erythrocytes and sperm. Some cells, especially lymphocytes and macrophages, have much more class I antigen than others. When a tissue or organ is grafted onto a genetically unrelated recipient, the class I molecules provoke a strong immune response that contributes to the graft rejection. Indeed, T cell–mediated cytotoxicity in graft rejection is largely directed against the class I antigens. Since the intensity of this reaction is determined by these antigens, it may be suggested that they regulate T cell–mediated cytotoxicity.

Within each class I locus there is a tremendous amount of genetic polymorphism—that is, the antigens coded for by these loci are highly variable. In pigs, for example, there are 20 to 25 alleles at each class I locus. Since there may be three or more class I loci and no more than two alleles inherited at each locus in any individual animal, the potential number of different antigen combinations is very large. Class I antigens are identified by means of specific antisera and are therefore called serologically defined (SD) antigens (Chapter 16).

Class II genes control lymphocyte proliferation and interaction and thus regulate the immune responses. They do this by coding for certain lymphocyte and macrophage surface glycoprotein antigens, which are necessary for lymphocyte-lymphocyte and macrophage-lymphocyte interactions. Some of these antigens function as histocompatibility antigens on lymphocytes. They are detectable by means of the mixed lymphocyte culture technique and are therefore called lymphocyte-defined (LD) antigens (Chapter 16). LD antigens are very potent at stimulating graft rejection as well as the graft-versus-host response.

Another group of class II antigens controls the immune responses by being an integral part of the T cell–antigen receptor and the T cell–derived helper and suppressor substances. In mice these are known as Ia antigens and the genes coding for them are immune response (Ir) genes. Only macrophages that bear Ia molecules are capable of cooperating with T cells and presenting antigen to B cells. The Ir locus may be divided into several subloci, whose products control several different aspects of T-cell function. For example, in mice the products of sublocus I-J are essential constituents of T cell–derived suppressor factors. Class II antigens consist of two membrane-bound polypeptide chains of 33,000 and 28,000 daltons. They do not contain β_2-microglobulin (Fig. 7–3).

Class III loci contain genes coding for the levels of complement components C1, C2 and C4 as well as the development of the C3 receptor on lymphocytes (Chapter 8). They do this by coding for the precursor molecules of these proteins. These precursor molecules are very large but are split to generate the functional complement components.

Class I, II, and III loci are always grouped together to form a major histocompatibility complex. The precise arrangement of these loci, the number of alleles at each locus and the number of loci vary between species (Table 7–2).

Histocompatibility Antigens and Disease.   Since the overall function of the major histocompatibility complex is to regulate immune function, it is logical to assume that these genes will also influence susceptibility to diseases in which immune responses play a significant role. Thus, in chickens possession of the histocompatibility antigen B^{21} is linked to resistance to Marek's disease, whereas possession of B^2 is associated with resistance to lymphoid leukosis. Chickens homozygous for B^1 generally have high adult mortality, are highly susceptible to Marek's disease and respond poorly to such antigens as *Salmonella pullorum* or human serum albumin. In the OS strain of chickens, homozygous B^1 birds are much more susceptible to autoimmune thyroiditis (Chapter 21) than are B^4 birds.

Similar associations have been observed in humans. It is clear, therefore, that selection for specific histocompatibility antigens has great potential for use in the genetic selection of disease-resistant strains of domestic animals.

REGULATION OF IMMUNE RESPONSES BY REGULATORY CELLS (Fig. 7–4)

It has already been described how helper T cells are needed if B cells are to respond optimally to antigen. In addition, there also exist subpopulations of T cells whose function is to inhibit the immune response. These are known as suppressor T cells. They act to suppress B- and T-cell responses to antigen by releasing soluble suppressor factors, at least fifteen of which have been described. Some of these factors act directly on antigen-sensitive B and T cells; others act to inhibit helper T cells. Some of these factors are antigen-specific and others are not. The antigen-specific

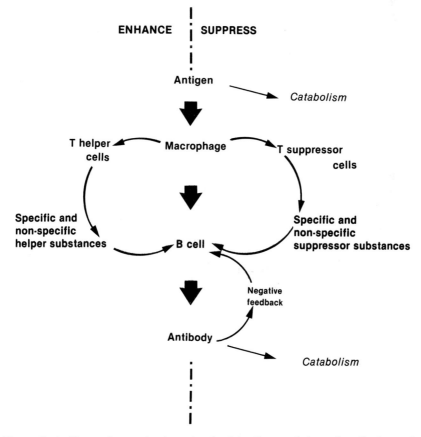

Figure 7–4 The major mechanisms involved in the regulation of antibody production. These include antigen catabolism. Regulation of activity by helper and suppressor cells and negative feedback by antibody.

suppressor factors, like the antigen-specific helper factors, consist of a V_H region linked to a class II histocompatibility antigen (I–J).

Suppressor cells function throughout an animal's life. Thus, the inability of newborn animals to mount an immune response is due in part to suppressor cell activity, as is the decline in immune competence in old animals. Part of the unreactivity of pregnant animals towards the fetus is ascribed to suppressor cells, as is the normal decline in the primary immune response. Tolerance may in some cases be due to suppressor cell activity. Thus, tolerance to self-antigens is largely suppressor-cell mediated. Loss of suppressor cell populations can therefore result in the development of autoimmune responses. The immunodepression seen in some virus diseases, in cancer and following trauma or burns has been shown, at least in part, to be due to suppressor cell activity. Some individuals, such as those who suffer from type I hypersensitivity conditions, appear to have depressed suppressor cell function. The administration of desensitizing "shots" by promoting suppressor cell function can lead to clinical improvement. There is, indeed, no doubt that suppressor T cells function as major regulators of immune reactivity.

REGULATION OF IMMUNE RESPONSES BY OTHER FACTORS

In recent years it has been possible to show that many normal body constituents may have the ability to regulate immune reactivity. In some cases subsequent investigation has shown that this regulation is due to an ability to influence suppressor cell populations. For example, α fetoprotein, a protein synthesized in large quantities by the fetal liver, is potently immunosuppressive and may therefore contribute to the immunological acceptance of the fetus by the mother. α Fetoprotein has been shown to be a potent stimulator of suppressor cell activity.

Another immunosuppressive factor is known as C-reactive protein (CRP). This is a protein, found normally in low concentrations in serum, whose level increases rapidly within hours of infection, inflammation or tissue damage. In addition to being immunosuppressive, CRP can promote phagocytosis, inhibit platelet function and activate complement. Its function is unknown, but it has been suggested that CRP prevents the occurrence of autoimmunity to intracellular antigens released from damaged tissue.

Prostaglandins are ubiquitous hydroxyaliphatic fatty acids, some of which, especially prostaglandin E, may be immunosuppressive since they effectively raise intracellular cyclic AMP levels. Since prostaglandins are produced by macrophages, these cells may, under some circumstances, serve to inhibit the immune response and thus act as suppressor cells.

Histamine, another ubiquitous pharmacologically active agent, can bind to T cells through specific H2 receptors (Table 6–2). In doing so, the cyclic AMP level within these cells rises and their activity is depressed. Conversely, if the histamine binds to lymphocyte H1 receptors, it enhances their activity. It may therefore serve to regulate T-cell activity in general.

Interferon. Interferon is a term applied to small proteins with nonspecific antiviral activity. Recently, it has become clear that these proteins have a number of other functions. Some, known as α and β interferons, are released by virus-infected cells and protect normal cells from virus invasion (Chapter 14). Others, known as γ interferons, are lymphokines that serve to regulate immune reactivity in addition to

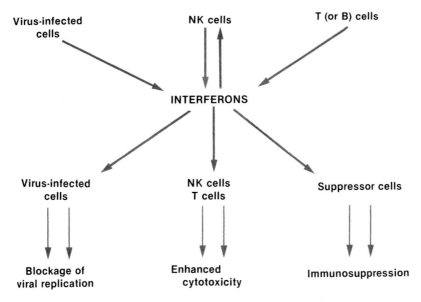

Figure 7-5 The sources and functions of the interferons.

possessing antiviral activity (see Table 14–2). γ Interferons act more slowly than α or β interferon but are less species-specific and are effective against a wider range of viruses. γ Interferons are derived from T cells and from NK cells. They act to suppress the immune response by depressing lymphokine synthesis and by stimulating suppressor cell activity, but they also act on both NK cells and T cells to enhance cell-mediated cytotoxicity (Chapter 16). Thus, paradoxically, interferons may be immunosuppressive while at the same time they increase host resistance to tumors and to viruses (Fig. 7–5).

IMMUNE REGULATION

It should be clear to the reader that there exists a great and complex system of interacting factors that control immune reactivity. A moment's consideration should reveal that this is an inevitable and consistent feature not only of the immune system but also of all body systems.

In order for any complex multicellular organism to survive and function, it is essential that an efficient yet flexible control system must exist. In this respect the immune system is not unique. It happens to be the first of the body's systems to have been analyzed in detail, but it may be predicted that other body systems will be found to be equally complex.

ADDITIONAL SOURCES OF INFORMATION

Auerbach R, and Clark S. 1975. Immunological tolerance: transmission from mother to offspring. Science *189* 811–812.
Bloom BR. 1980. Interferons and the immune system. Nature *284* 593–595.
Calderon J, Kiely JM, Lefko JL, and Unanue ER. 1975. The modulation of lymphocyte function by molecules secreted by macrophages. J Exp Med *142* 151–164.

David CS. 1979. Role of Ia antigens in immune response. Transplantation Proc *11* 677–682.

Edelman GM (ed). 1974. Cellular Selection and Regulation in the Immune Response. Society of General Physiologists Series, Vol 29. Raven Press, New York.

Festenstine H, and Demant P. 1978. Basic immunogenetics: biology and clinical relevance. Current Topics in Immunology, Vol. 9. Edward Arnold, London.

Playfair JHL. 1974. The role of antibody in T-cell responses. Clin Exp Immunol *17* 1–18.

Raff M. 1977. Immunological networks. Nature *265* 205–207.

Rosenthal AS. 1980. Regulation of the immune response—role of the macrophage. N Engl J Med *303* 1153–1156.

Taniguchi M, Takai I, and Tada T. 1980. Functional and molecular organization of an antigen-specific suppressor factor from a T-cell hybridoma. Nature *283* 227-228.

8

Physiological and Pathological Consequences of the Immune Responses

Up to this point, the immune responses have been considered part of an isolated system concerned solely with the elimination of antigen from the body. However, body systems rarely, if ever, act in total isolation, and the immune system is no exception, since it acts in conjunction with many other systems to produce a wide variety of different effects. Although most of these consequences may be considered to be physiological when operating normally, it is not uncommon for them, when operating in apparent excess of the normal body requirements, to produce lesions that are considered to be pathological. It should, however, be pointed out that in declaring a reaction to be pathological, we must consider not only the immediate discomfort of an animal, but also the influence of this reaction on the animal's long-term survival and therefore on the survival of the species as a whole. For example, antigen-antibody interactions commonly lead to the development of acute inflammatory reactions. If these reactions involve critical locations such as the walls of blood vessels or the upper respiratory tract, they may be extremely uncomfortable or even life-threatening. Nevertheless, they do serve to hasten the elimination of antigen, and this may greatly outweigh the risks incurred by not eliminating antigen.

ANTIGEN-ANTIBODY INTERACTION AS AN INITIATING EVENT IN PHYSIOLOGICAL PROCESSES

The properties of antibody molecules complexed with antigen are very different from those of free antibody (Fig. 8–1). For example, antigen-bound antibody acquires the capacity to bind to phagocytic cells and thus functions as an opsonin. Similarly, new antigenic determinants appear on antigen-bound antibody. These determinants are regarded by the immune system as foreign and therefore provoke the formation of autoantibodies known as rheumatoid factors (Chapter 21). The development of these new antigenic determinants and new biological activities are a function of the immunoglobulin Fc region. Normally, the Fc region is masked by the Fab regions. When the antibody binds antigen through the Fab regions, the shape of the molecule changes and the Fc region is exposed. The active sites on the Fc region thus become available and free to exert their biological functions.

A second mechanism involved in the development of the biological activity of immunoglobulins probably relates to the number of available active sites. A single active site may be unable to initiate reactions by itself. Only when several antibody molecules bind closely together on an antigen may the combined stimulus be sufficient to initiate subsequent reactions.

THE COMPLEMENT SYSTEM

There are a number of physiological processes that, if activated in the absence of effective controls, could lead to disastrous consequences. Examples of these include the clotting system, the fibrinolytic system and the kinin system. Uncontrolled activa-

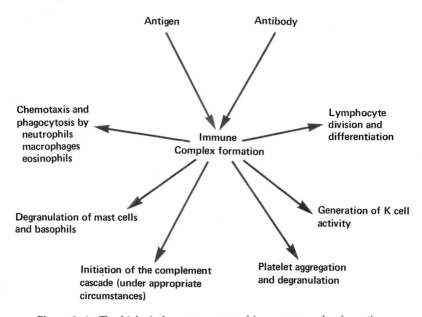

Figure 8–1 The biological consequences of immune-complex formation.

tion of these systems could lead to uncontrollable hemorrhage, extensive intravascular thrombosis or severe disturbances in vascular permeability, respectively. Therefore, in order to ensure that uncontrolled activation does not occur, all these systems are regulated by mechanisms that involve a series of interlinked enzyme reactions. The general principle of these interlinked reactions is that the products of one reaction catalyze a second reaction whose products then catalyze a third reaction and so on (Fig. 8–2). Since many of these intermediate products either are present in limiting quantities, have a very short half-life or are easily inhibited, it is possible to ensure that the reaction does not proceed to completion in an uncontrolled fashion. Chain reactions of this type are known as "cascade" reactions and usually require some form of "trigger" to initiate the reaction chain. For example, in the case of the blood clotting cascade, it is activation of Hageman factor by altered surfaces that serves as the initiating event that sets the cascade in motion. In addition to the systems mentioned previously, there exists a system whose activation may result in the disruption of cell membranes and, as a consequence of this disruption, cause the destruction either of cells or of organisms. This system is termed "complement." The complement system must be carefully regulated, since uncontrolled generation of the products of the system may lead to massive cellular destruction.

The complement system may be considered to consist of three distinct pathways. Two of these pathways represent alternative procedures for the activation of the third component of the cascade. The third, or terminal, pathway is not a true cascade reaction but a series of aggregations by which a membrane-damaging complex is generated from the activated third component. Complement components are either labeled numerically with the prefix C—i.e., C1, C2, C3, etc., or designated by letters of the alphabet—i.e., B, D, P etc. There are at least 15 of these components; they are all serum proteins and together they make up about 10 per cent of the globulin fraction of serum. The molecular weights of the complement components vary between 80,000 daltons for C9 to 400,000 daltons for C1q. Their serum concentrations in humans vary between 3 mg/100 ml of C2 to 130 mg/100 ml of C3. Complement components are

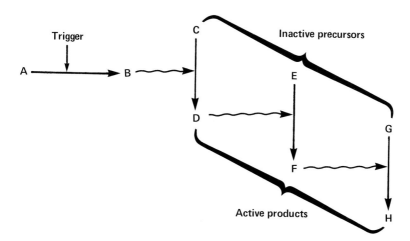

Figure 8–2 The principle of cascade reactions. A trigger initiates the conversion to an inactive proenzyme A to an active enzyme B. This enzyme B acts to convert proenzyme C to enzyme D. Enzyme D in turn converts proenzyme E to enzyme F, and so forth.

synthesized at various sites throughout the body; for example, all of the C1 subcomponents are synthesized in intestinal epithelium; C2, C5, C3, H, P, D, B and C4 in
macrophages; and C3, C6 and C9 in the liver. The levels of C1, C4 and C2 in serum
are controlled by genes in the major histocompatibility complex (Chapter 7).

"Classical" Pathway for Activation of C3 (Fig. 8–3). The "classical" pathway
of complement activation, so called because it has been known for many more years
than the "alternate" pathway, is initiated by antigen-antibody interaction on surfaces
such as cell membranes. The process may be initiated by combination of antigen with
either a single molecule of IgM or two closely spaced IgG molecules. The active sites
on the Fc region of the immunoglobulin molecules exposed by combination with
antigen in this way can bind and activate the first component of complement (C1). C1
is a trimolecular complex containing three subcomponents—Clq, Clr and Cls—which
are held together as a single unit by calcium. The binding of Clq to antibody initiates
a series of changes in each component in turn so that, eventually, Cls develops
proteolytic activity. The natural substrates of Cls are the complement components C4

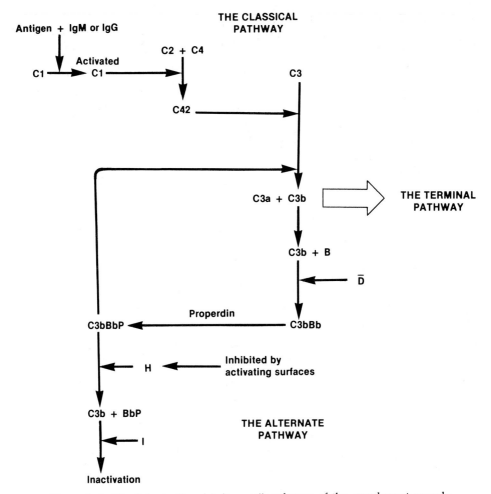

Figure 8–3 The "classical" and "alternate" pathways of the complement cascade.

and C2, and C1s acts on both of these to generate a new enzyme, C42. C42 binds to cell surfaces, and since it is proteolytic, it acts on the next component, C3, to split it into two fragments, known as C3a and C3b. One molecule of C42 (also known as C3 convertase) may act on several hundred molecules of C3 in this way, resulting in a relatively large quantity of C3b being deposited on the antigen surface.

"Alternate" Pathway for Activation of C3. The alternate pathway (whose factors are denoted by letters of the alphabet B, D, P, etc.) provides a mechanism by which C3 convertase activity may be generated in the absence of antibody but in the presence of certain foreign surfaces such as bacterial and fungal cell walls or helminth cuticles.

In normal plasma C3 slowly, continuously and spontaneously breaks down to C3a and C3b (Fig. 8–3). The C3b thus formed binds to surfaces where it complexes with factor B. This C3b,B complex is then split by an enzyme D to form C3b,Bb. C3b,Bb can act as a C3 convertase, but it is extremely unstable and must be stabilized by addition of factor P, also known as properdin. However, in normal serum there exist two inhibitors, factor H, which splits the C3b,Bb,P complex into C3b and Bb,P, and factor I which can then inactivate the C3b. Thus, the products of the alternate pathway are normally destroyed as soon as they are formed.

Factor H is strongly inhibited, however, by the presence of surfaces that do not contain sialic acid. These include bacterial and fungal cell walls, helminth cuticles, some tumor cell membranes and aggregated immunoglobulins. Consequently, if any of these surfaces are present, factor H will not be active; thus, C3b,Bb,P will not be destroyed but will remain able to act on native C3 to generate C3a and C3b (Fig. 8–4). Because of the cyclic nature of the reaction, very large quantities of C3b can be

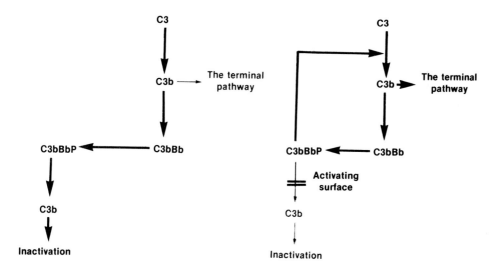

In normal serum

In the presence of
an activating surface

Figure 8–4 The activation of the alternate pathway in the presence of activating surfaces results in the generation of large quantities of C3 convertase, which would otherwise be destroyed.

generated in this way. Thus, the alternate pathway provides a route by which potential invaders—bacteria, fungi or helminths—can activate complement despite the absence of antibody.

Terminal Complement Pathway (Fig. 8–5). The final stage of the complement pathway differs from the processes involved in the production of C3 convertase in that it is not a cascade reaction in the strict sense. Apart from the enzymatic activation of C5, the terminal pathway involves the self-aggregation of complement components out of solution and into a large macromolecular complex bound to the cell surface. Thus, C3b acts on C5 to split it into C5a and C5b. C5b, C6 and C7 then aggregate to form a stable complex, C567. C8 can bind to this complex to form a structure with some membrane-damaging properties (it possibly activates cell membrane phospholipases). However, several molecules of C9 combine with C5678 to form a very potent cytolytic complex. This final complex is a large "doughnut"-shaped structure that can insert itself into a cell membrane. It is either through the central "hole" or around the complex that the cell contents escape, resulting in its destruction.

Inhibitors of the Complement System. As might be expected, there exist a number of naturally occurring inhibitors of the complement pathways. One of the most important of these is the inactivator of C1. Normally, when C1 acts on C2 it splits off a small polypeptide with kinin-like activity, the amount of kinin produced being controlled by the C1 inactivator. In individuals who suffer from a congenital deficiency of this inactivator, excessive amounts of this C2 kinin are produced. The C2 kinin increases vascular permeability, and affected individuals therefore suffer from attacks

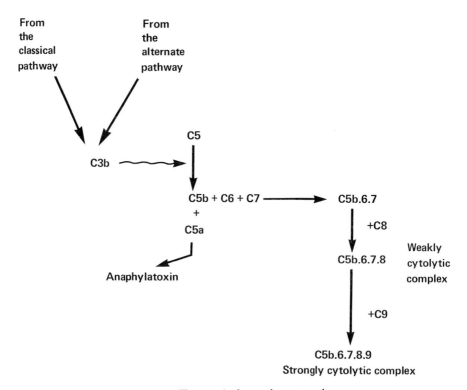

Figure 8–5   The terminal complement pathway.

of widespread noninflammatory edema. In humans, this condition is known as hereditary angioedema. If this edema involves the larynx, it may cause the victim to suffocate. In addition to the C1 inhibitor there also exists a C4 inhibitor and a C6 inhibitor as well as factors H and I.

BIOLOGICAL CONSEQUENCES OF COMPLEMENT ACTIVATION (Fig. 8–6).

If activation of the complement pathways takes place on a cell surface, then lesions will develop in the target cell membrane and cell death will result. There is little restriction on the nature of the target, and complement can damage or kill nucleated cells, erythrocytes, gram-positive bacteria, gram-negative bacteria in the presence of the enzyme lysozyme (Chapter 13) and viruses, particularly those with lipid envelopes. While these lytic functions are perhaps the most spectacular of the properties of complement, they are not essential in conferring resistance to invasive microorganisms. Thus, complement in some species, such as the horse, appears to be poorly lytic, and in species such as humans or rabbits the congenital absence of components from the terminal complement pathway has no apparent adverse effects on resistance to disease. The nature of the benefits conferred on an animal by the possession of a lytic complement are therefore quite unclear.

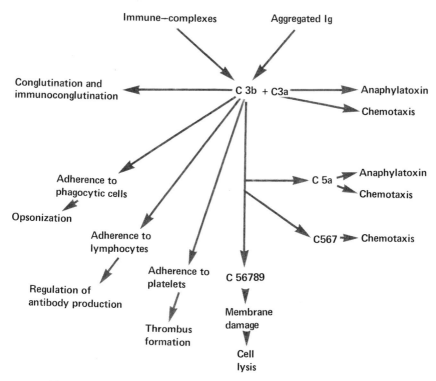

Figure 8–6 The biological consequences of complement activation.

Of all the complement components, the only one in which an absolute deficiency appears to be life-threatening is C3, and it is generally felt that the activation of C3 represents the single most important step in the complement system. Many cells, including B-lymphocytes, macrophages, neutrophils and non-primate platelets, carry receptors for C3b. By means of the receptors on macrophages and neutrophils, C3b can act as a powerful opsonin, ensuring the adherence of antigen to these cells. The presence of C3b receptors on B cells suggests that this molecule is also involved in the regulation of the immune response, whereas the receptor on platelets implies a possible role in the blood clotting process. B cells also have a receptor for factor H.

A feature of fixed C3b is the presence on this molecule of an antigenic site not normally recognized as "self" by the body. The generation of C3b therefore results in the formation of autoantibodies against this newly formed antigenic determinant. These autoantibodies are known as immunoconglutinins (Chapter 21). Immunoconglutinins will clump any particles with fixed C3 on their surface. In bovidae—i.e., cattle, buffalo, etc.—there also exists a serum protein (not an immunoglobulin) known as conglutinin, which can also bind to fixed C3b and, like immunoconglutinin, cause C3b-coated particles to clump (strictly speaking, conglutinate). The biological significance of conglutinin is not known.

Various polypeptide fragments, many of which have significant biological properties, are generated during the course of the classical complement pathway. The kinin generated from C42 by C1 has already been discussed as a mediator of hereditary angioedema. The peptides C3a and C5a are anaphylatoxic; that is, they will act on mast cells, causing them to release their contents of vasoactive factors (Chapter 17) and, as a result, provoke local increases in vascular permeability. While C3a and C5a appear to have very similar biological activities, they appear to act on either different receptors or different mast cell populations, since a tissue rendered unresponsive to one anaphylatoxin still reacts with the other. The peptides C5a and C3a and the trimolecular complex C567 are chemotactic for neutrophils, eosinophils and macrophages. Neutrophils, in particular, are strongly influenced by these factors and in consequence are readily attracted to the region of maximal chemotactic factor concentration, such as sites of immune-complex deposition or of bacterial invasion.

COMPLEMENT DEFICIENCIES

The effects of a congenital deficiency in individual complement components vary greatly. Thus, a deficiency in a component of the classical pathway may have little visible effect as a result of a compensatory increase in the activity of the alternate pathway.

The most severe consequences occur in humans or animals deficient in C3. Thus, some Brittany spaniels have been reported to have a congenital deficiency of C3 that is inherited as an autosomal recessive condition. Dogs that are homozygous for this deficiency have no detectable C3 (Figure 8–7), whereas heterozygous animals have C3 levels that are approximately half of normal. The homozygous animals suffer from recurrent sepsis and local bacterial infections.

Some Finnish-Landrace lambs have a very low serum C3 level associated with the presence of a mesangiocapillary glomerulonephritis (Chapter 19). However, crosses between this breed and Dorsets may also have a low serum C3 and yet be quite healthy.

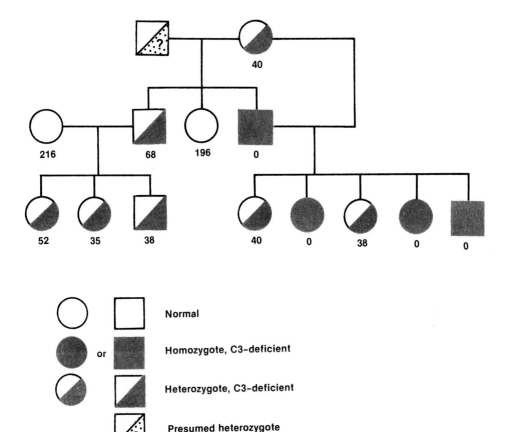

Figure 8–7 The inheritance of C3 deficiency in a colony of Brittany spaniels. The number below each circle or square represents the animal's C3 level as a percentage of a standard reference serum. The mean level in healthy spaniels was 126. (From Winkelstein JA, Cork LC, Griffin DE, et al. 1981. Genetically determined deficiency of the third component of complement in the dog. Science 212 1169–1170. Used with permission.)

THE COMPLEMENT SYSTEM, CLOTTING AND INFLAMMATION

The complement system is closely linked to both the clotting process and inflammation (Fig. 8–8). For example, activated complement generally promotes clotting. Not only do complement-lysed cells activate the clotting cascade through Hageman factor, but C3b directly promotes thrombus formation by causing platelet aggregation. Because of this, extensive cell lysis or immune-complex formation that occurs within the blood stream may provoke intravascular coagulation. This is commonly observed in acute graft rejection, where destruction of graft vascular endothelium by complement can cause intravascular thrombosis and graft destruction. In hemolytic disease of newborn calves (Chapter 18), massive complement-mediated destruction of erythrocytes can provoke disseminated intravascular coagulation and death.

The major contribution of the complement system to the inflammatory process is by chemotactically attracting leukocytes to sites of complement activation. However,

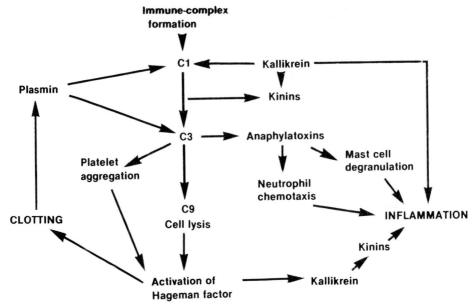

Figure 8–8 Some of the interactions between the clotting, complement and inflammatory systems.

proteolytic enzymes such as plasminogen released from neutrophils or macrophages as they ingest particles can also activate C1 or C3 and thus enhance the process significantly. The anaphylatoxins C3a and C5a enhance inflammation by promoting the release of mast-cell vasoactive factors. C3b-induced platelet aggregation also provides a source of inflammatory mediators. The role of complement-mediated inflammation is discussed further in Chapter 19.

INFLAMMATION AS A CONSEQUENCE OF IMMUNE REACTIONS

The major participants in the defense of the body against invading microorganisms—antibodies, lymphocytes and plasma cells—are found within the blood stream. If an organism or other foreign material penetrates the tissues, the body's defenses are mobilized and directed toward the site of invasion. This process of focusing the defenses at a specific site gives rise to inflammation.

The so-called cardinal signs of inflammation are redness, heat, swelling and pain. These arise as a result of a marked local increase in blood flow (redness and heat) and extravasation of plasma (swelling and pain). The increase in blood flow serves to bring more antibodies to the area, and the increase in vascular permeability permits these antibodies to permeate tissue spaces in high concentration.

Histologically, inflammatory sites are infiltrated by leukocytes, which migrate out of capillaries into these tissues. The specific types of leukocytes involved vary according to the nature of the inflammatory stimulus. Neutrophils usually function to destroy invading bacteria, eosinophils usually attack invading metazoan parasites, and lymphocytes attack virus-infected cells. Macrophages normally function in several roles, destroying bacteria or virus-infected cells or removing damaged tissue. The mechanisms involved in establishing specific inflammatory reactions are complex and are discussed in greater detail in Chapters 17 to 20. However, the reactions are introduced here to aid understanding of some aspects of resistance to infectious agents, since the development of an adequate and appropriate inflammatory response is, obviously, critical for the maintenance of the body's defenses.

Inflammatory responses of immunological origin are known as hypersensitivity reactions and may be classified into four basic types (Figs. 8–9 and 8–10) as suggested by Gell and Coombs.

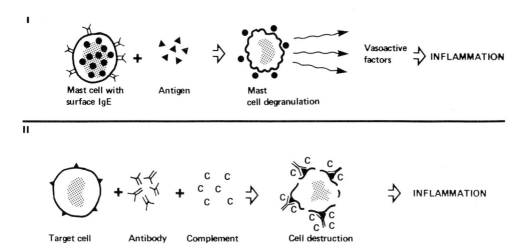

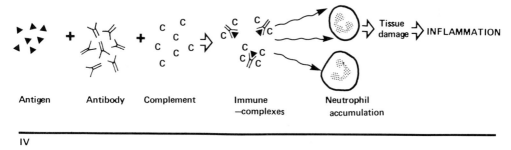

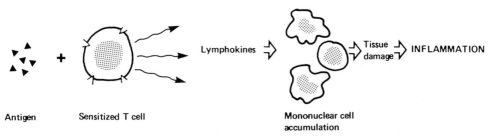

Figure 8–9 The four types of hypersensitivity reaction as classified by Gell and Coombs.

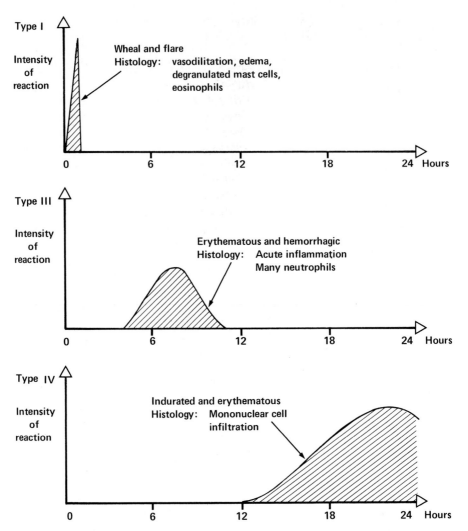

Figure 8–10 A schematic diagram showing the time-course, character and histology of inflammatory skin reactions resulting from intradermal injection of antigen and due to hypersensitivity types I, III and IV.

Type I or Immediate Hypersensitivity (Chapter 17).   IgE and some minor IgG subclasses can attach to mast cells or basophils through sites on their Fc region. If antigen binds to this cell-fixed antibody, then the mast cell or basophil will respond by releasing the vasoactive factors, especially histamine, contained within its granules. These factors are pharmacologically active and cause local acute inflammation within a few minutes. Mast cells will also release their granule contents on exposure to C3a and C5a—the anaphylatoxins.

Type II or Cytotoxic Hypersensitivity (Chapter 18).   Antibodies may participate in the destruction of cells either through complement or through the activities of cytotoxic cells. Cells such as neutrophils, eosinophils, macrophages and some lymphocytes possess receptors for the Fc portion of immunoglobulin. These cells may kill target cells coated with immune complexes by antibody-dependent cellular cytotoxicity (ADCC) (Chapter 6). Cells destroyed either in this way or through complement-mediated lysis may initiate an acute inflammatory reaction because of the release of biologically active cell breakdown products. This form of inflammation may be observed in graft rejection (Chapter 16).

Type III or Immune-Complex Hypersensitivity (Chapter 19).   Immune complexes may fix complement even if deposited in tissues. Activation of complement in this way will attract neutrophils through the production of chemotactic factors, and neutrophils will attempt to ingest the immune complexes. Unfortunately, under these circumstances neutrophils may release the proteolytic enzymes from their lysosomes into tissues, resulting in tissue destruction (see Fig. 19–2). Neutrophil-activated plasmin may in turn activate C1; C2 kinin may be produced; platelet aggregation may result in the release of more vasoactive amines; and mast cell degranulation may be mediated by anaphylatoxins. The total effect is therefore one of acute inflammation and tissue destruction.

Type IV or Delayed Hypersensitivity (Chapter 20).   Cell-mediated immune reactions may also participate in acute inflammatory reactions. Thus, if antigen is injected into an animal possessing appropriately sensitized T cells, then a local inflammatory reaction may result. This form of reaction is known as delayed hypersensitivity, since it generally takes at least 24 hours after administration of antigen for the response to reach maximal intensity. The inflammatory response results from the release of chemotactic and vasoactive lymphokines by sensitized T cells on encountering antigen (see Fig. 20–2). This type of reaction occurs in response to many bacterial antigens as well as in response to virus-infected cells and in graft rejection.

ANTIGEN-ANTIBODY INTERACTION AND MODULATION OF CELLULAR BEHAVIOR (Table 8–1)

Many cells possess surface receptors specific for C3b or for immunoglobulin Fc regions (see Table 6–2). These receptors presumably function as a means of transmitting some form of signal to the cell. Thus, immune complexes binding to macrophages or neutrophils initiate changes in cellular activity leading to phagocytosis of the inducing immune complexes. The precise mechanisms involved in the phagocytic process are not clear, but it appears that the immune complexes stimulate cell membrane activity. This increased activity may lead to complete enclosure of the complexes within the cell or, alternatively, if the amount of cell-bound immune complex is small, serve to move the cell toward the complexes in a form of chemotaxis.

Table 8–1 SOME OF THE CONSEQUENCES OF ANTIGEN-ANTIBODY INTERACTION ON CELL SURFACES

CELL TYPE	*CONSEQUENCE*
Macrophage	Phagocytosis, chemotaxis, cytotoxicity
Neutrophil	Phagocytosis, chemotaxis, cytotoxicity, degranulation
Eosinophil	Degranulation, helminthicidal activity
Platelet	Degranulation, clumping
Mast cell	Degranulation
B-Lymphocyte	Differentiation and division
Null-lymphocyte	Cytotoxicity

A second type of response seen following antigen–antibody–cell-membrane inter-action is degranulation, such as occurs in mast cells, platelets and, occasionally, neutrophils. For example, if antigen binds and "bridges" two mast cell–fixed IgE molecules, then intracellular enzymes are activated and cause the cell to release the contents of its granules into the extracellular fluid (Chapter 17). Platelets bound to immune complexes release not only vasoactive factors but also procoagulants and adenosine diphosphate, which potentiates the reaction. On occasion, neutrophils re-spond to immune complexes by releasing the contents of their lysosomes into extra-cellular fluid.

A third form of response to antigen-antibody interaction is the generation of cytotoxic activity (Chapter 6). Cells that can participate in this process and destroy foreign (allogeneic) cells include macrophages, neutrophils and null lymphocytes. All these cells may exert their cytotoxicity regardless of whether they first bind to antibody-coated target cells or if they bind antibody first and then bind to antigens on target cell surfaces (Table 6–5). A similar toxic effect may be mediated by eosinophils that bind to helminths, destroying them through IgG bound to the helminth surface (Chapter 15).

Most serum immunoglobulins cannot bind to cell Fc receptors unless they are first complexed with antigen. Nevertheless, some antibodies, known as cytophilic or cytotropic antibodies, may bind to Fc receptors even when uncomplexed. Examples of cytophilic antibodies include IgE antibodies, which are cytophilic for mast cells, and sheep IgG2, which is cytophilic for neutrophils and appears to act as a cell-bound opsonin, since it enhances the phagocytic ability of these cells.

ADDITIONAL SOURCES OF INFORMATION

Fearon DT, and Austin KF. 1980. Current concepts in immunology. The alternative pathway of comple-ment—A system for host resistance to microbial infection. N Engl J Med *303* 259–263.

Fearon DT, Ruddy S, Schur PH, and McCabe WR. 1975. Activation of the properdin pathway of complement in patients with gram-negative bacteremia. N Engl J Med *292* 937–940.

Gell PGH, Coombs RRA, and Lachmann PJ (eds). 1974. Clinical Aspects of Immunology. 3rd Ed. Blackwell Scientific Publications, Oxford.

Kolb WP, and Muller-Eberhard HJ. 1975. The membrane attack mechanisms of complement. Isolation and subunit composition of the C5b-9 complex. J Exp Med *141* 724–735.

Mayer MM. 1973. The complement system. Sci Am *229* 54–70.

Metzger H. 1974. Effects of antigen binding on the properties of antibody. Adv Immunol *18* 169–207.

Osler AG. 1976. Complement Mechanisms and Functions. Foundations of Immunology Series. Prentice-Hall, Inc., Englewood Cliffs, N.J.

Pangburn MK, Morrison DC, Schraber RD, and Muller-Eberhard HJ. 1980. Activation of the alternative complement pathway: recognition of surface structures on activators by bound C3b. J Immunol *124* 977–982.

Podack ER, Esser AF, Biesecker G, and Muller-Eberhard HJ. 1980. Membrane attack complex of comple-ment. A structural analysis. J Exp Med *151* 301–313.

Polley MJ, and Nachman R. 1978. The human complement system in thrombin-mediated platelet function. J Exp Med *147* 1713–1721.

Porter RR, and Reid KBM. 1978. The biochemistry of complement. Nature *275* 699–704.

Winkelstein JA, Cork LC, Griffin DE, et al. 1981. Genetically determined deficiency of the third component of complement in the dog. Science *212* 1169–1170.

9

Detection and Measurement of the Humoral Immune Response

The tests that measure the humoral immune response fall into three categories (Table 9–1). The most sensitive (in terms of the amount of antibody detectable are the primary binding tests, which directly measure interaction between antigen and antibody. In contrast, secondary binding tests measure the consequences of immune complex formation *in vitro*. Theoretically, these tests are, therefore, much less sensitive than the primary binding tests, but they are considerably simpler to perform. The consequences of antigen-antibody interaction include precipitation of soluble antigen, agglutination of particulate antigens and activation of the complement cascade. Tertiary tests measure the consequences of the immune response *in vivo*. In determining the protective effect of an antiserum in an animal, tertiary tests thus measure not only the combination between antigen and antibody but also the opsonizing capacity of these complexes as well as the phagocytic and destructive capacity of the cells of the mononuclear-phagocytic system. Tertiary tests are usually less sensitive than primary binding tests but reflect much more appropriately the practical consequences of the immune response.

Table 9–1 THE SMALLEST AMOUNT OF ANTIBODY PROTEIN DETECTABLE BY CERTAIN SELECTED IMMUNOLOGICAL TESTS

TESTS	μg PROTEIN/ml
PRIMARY BINDING TESTS	
ELISA	0.0005
Competitive radioimmunoassay	0.00005
SECONDARY BINDING TESTS	
Ring test	18
Gel precipitation	30
Bacterial agglutination	0.05
Passive hemagglutination	0.01
Hemagglutination inhibition	0.005
Complement fixation test	0.05
Virus neutralization	0.00005
Bactericidal activity	0.00005
Antitoxin neutralization	0.06
TERTIARY (IN VIVO) TESTS	
Passive cutaneous anaphylaxis	0.02

REAGENTS EMPLOYED IN IMMUNOLOGICAL TESTS

Serum. The most common source of antibody is serum obtained by allowing a blood sample to clot and the clot to retract. Serum may be stored frozen and used when required. If it is important that the serum be devoid of complement activity, then this may be accomplished by heating it to 56°C for 30 minutes. Complement is found in all fresh serum, but if hemolysis is to be measured, it is usual to employ unheated guinea pig serum as a source of this reagent. Serum used as a source of complement in this way should be stored frozen in aliquots and, once thawed, used promptly. It should not be repeatedly frozen and thawed.

Antiglobulins. As described in Chapter 4, because immunoglobulins are proteins they function as antigens when injected into an animal of a different species. For example, purified dog immunoglobulins can be inoculated into rabbits. The injected animals respond by making antibodies known as antiglobulins. Depending on the purity of the injected immunoglobulin, it is possible to make nonspecific antiglobulins against immunoglobulins of all classes or very specific antiglobulins directed against single classes or subclasses (or even against specific allotypes or idiotypes (Chapter 4)). Antiglobulins are essential reagents in many immunological tests.

Hybridomas. Plasma cells may become neoplastic and cause tumors known as myelomas (Chapter 22). Mouse myeloma cells can be grown in tissue culture, where they may secrete very large quantities of homogeneous (monoclonal) immunoglobulin. This immunoglobulin is of unknown antigen specificity and is thus of little practical use. It is possible, however, to fuse a myeloma cell together with a normal plasma cell that is actively producing specific antibody against a well-defined antigen. The resulting cell hybrids, or hybridomas, can be selected so that they will combine the most desirable qualities of both parent cells and produce very large quantities of absolutely homogeneous specific antibody when cultured (Fig. 9–1).

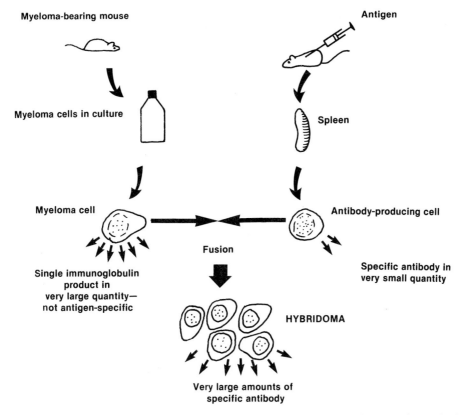

Figure 9–1 The production of hybridoma antibodies by fusion of a specific antibody-producing cell with a neoplastic plasma cell.

These hybridoma-derived monoclonal antibodies are pure and specific and can be used as standard chemical reagents. The antibodies can be obtained in almost unlimited amounts and are much cheaper than animal-derived antibodies. It is certain that hybridomas will be used increasingly in immunodiagnostic procedures within the next few years.

PRIMARY BINDING TESTS

Antigens and specific antibodies combine reversibly to form immune complexes. In general, primary binding tests are performed by allowing the reactants to combine and then measuring the amount of immune complex formed. It is usual to use radioisotope, fluorescent dye or enzyme-labeling in order to identify one of the reactants. After allowing the reaction to proceed, the immune complexes are separated from the uncombined material, and the amount of label in these immune complexes is then estimated.

Radioimmunoassays for Antibody. One widely employed primary binding test for antigen is called the RAST (Radio Allergo-Sorbent Test). In this technique, antigen-impregnated cellulose discs are immersed in test serum so that antibody binds to them. After washing, the disc is immersed in a radiolabeled antiglobulin solution.

The antiglobulin will bind to the disc only if antibodies have first bound to the antigen. By counting the radioactivity of the disc it is possible to measure the level of antibody in the serum. If antiglobulins specific for a particular immunoglobulin class or subclass are used, it is possible to measure the level of antibodies of that class or subclass in a serum. The RAST is most commonly used to measure levels of specific IgE in allergic animals.

Radioimmunoassays for Antigen. Competitive immunoassays are widely employed to detect antigen. They are based on the principle that unlabeled antigen may displace labeled antigen from immune complexes. The amount of labeled antigen displaced in this way is related in a simple fashion to the amount of unlabeled antigen added. Several different assays of this type have been developed. They differ in the way in which the antigen is labeled and measured. The most commonly used of these is the competitive radioimmunoassay in which antigen is labeled with an isotope such as ^3H, ^{14}C or ^{125}I. When labeled antigen is mixed with its specific antibody, they combine to form immune complexes that may be precipitated with ammonium sulfate. The radioactivity of the supernatant fluid provides an estimate of the proportion of antigen bound by antibody. If unlabeled antigen is added to a mixture of labeled antigen and antibody, it will compete with the labeled antigen for antibody-binding sites. As a result, some labeled antigen will be unable to bind antibody, and hence the amount of radioactivity in the supernatant will be increased. If a standard curve is first constructed by using known amounts of unlabeled antigen, then the amount of antigen in a test sample may be measured by reference to this standard curve (Fig. 9–2).

This type of test is extremely sensitive and is commonly used for detecting trace amounts of drugs. For example, morphine may be measured in urine at concentrations of 10^{-8} to 10^{-10} M by means of competitive radioimmunoassay.

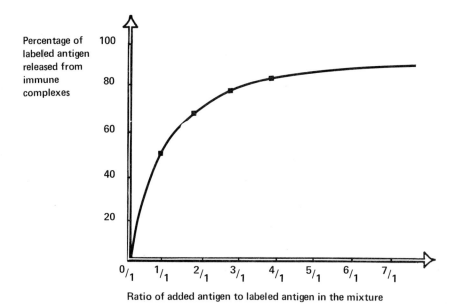

Figure 9–2 The principle of competitive radioimmunoassay. The proportion of isotope-labeled antigen released from immune complexes into supernatant fluid is related to the amount of unlabeled antigen added to the mixture.

Tests Involving Enzyme Labeling.   The most important of these techniques are the enzyme-linked–immunosorbent assays (ELISAs). As with other primary binding tests they may be used to detect and measure either antibody or antigen.

In the indirect ELISA for antibody, polystyrene surfaces are used to adsorb protein antigens. Polystyrene tubes are first coated with antigen by incubating the antigen solution in the tubes overnight (Fig. 9–3). After unbound antigen is removed by washing, test serum is added to the tubes so that any antibodies in the serum will bind to the antigen on the tube wall. After incubation and washing to remove unbound antibody, the presence of bound antibodies is detected by addition of an enzyme-linked antiglobulin. This binds to the antibody and, following incubation and washing, may be detected and measured by addition of the enzyme substrate. The enzyme and substrate are selected so that a colored product develops in the tube. The intensity of the color change is therefore proportional to the amount of enzyme-linked antiglobulin that is bound, which in turn is proportional to the amount of antibody present in the serum under test. The color that develops may be estimated visually or, preferably, read in a spectrophotometer.

A modification of this technique that is used to detect antigen involves first coating the wells with specific antibody. The antigen solution is then added, followed, after washing, by specific antibody, enzyme-labeled antiglobulin and substrate, as described for the indirect technique. In this test, the intensity of the color reaction is

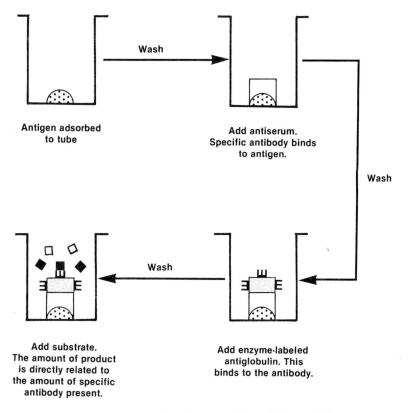

**Antigen adsorbed
to tube**

**Add antiserum.
Specific antibody binds
to antigen.**

Wash

**Add substrate.
The amount of product
is directly related to
the amount of specific
antibody present.**

**Add enzyme-labeled
antiglobulin. This
binds to the antibody.**

Figure 9–3   The procedure for the indirect ELISA technique.

related directly to the amount of bound antigen. A test of this type is used in the diagnosis of feline leukemia.

The enzymes used in the ELISA techniques are chosen primarily on the bases of cost and their ability to be easily assayed. They include alkaline phosphatase, lysozyme, horseradish peroxidase and β-galactosidase. Because of its relative simplicity, the indirect ELISA shows promise of becoming a useful aid in the immunodiagnosis of many bacterial, viral and parasitic infections.

Tests Involving Immunofluorescence. Fluorescent dyes are also very commonly employed as labels in primary binding tests, the most important being fluorescein isothiocyanate (FITC). FITC is a yellow compound that is readily conjugated to immunoglobulins without affecting their reactivity. When irradiated with invisible ultraviolet or blue light at 290 and 145 μm, it re-emits visible green light at about 525 μm. FITC-labeled immunoglobulins may be employed in a number of techniques, the most important of which are the direct and indirect fluorescent antibody tests (Table 9–2).

Table 9–2 COMPARISON OF TECHNIQUES INVOLVED IN DIRECT AND INDIRECT FLUORESCENT ANTIBODY TESTS

TEST	*DIRECT FLUORESCENT ANTIBODY TEST*	*INDIRECT FLUORESCENT ANTIBODY TEST*
Requirements	Antigen? Fluorescent-labeled antibody	Antigen Fluorescent-labeled antiglobulin Antibody?
Method	1. Put FITC-labeled antibody onto suspected antigen preparation 2. 3. Wash and examine	Put suspected antiserum onto known antigen preparation Wash, then cover with FITC-labeled antiglobulin Wash and examine
Detects	Fluorescence indicates presence of antigen	Fluorescence indicates presence of antibodies in serum

DIRECT FLUORESCENT ANTIBODY TEST (Fig. 9–4A). This test is used to identify the presence of antigen. Antibody directed against a specific antigen such as a bacterium or virus may be labeled with FITC. A tissue section or smear containing this organism may be incubated with the labeled antiserum and then washed to remove unbound antibody. If examined by dark field illumination under a microscope with an ultraviolet light source, then the antigenic particles that have bound the labeled antibody are seen to fluoresce brightly. This direct test can be used to identify bacteria when their numbers are very low. For example, it can be used when examining the feces of animals suspected of shedding *Mycobacterium paratuberculosis* or when examining smears from lesions for the presence of *Fusobacterium necrophorum, Listeria monocytogenes* or the clostridial organisms (Fig. 9–5). It may also be employed to detect viruses growing in tissue culture or in tissues from infected animals. It is thus possible to detect rabies virus in the brains of infected animals and antigens of the feline leukemia virus on the surface of infected cells by means of this technique (see Fig. 14–7).

DIRECT FLUORESCENT
ANTIBODY TEST

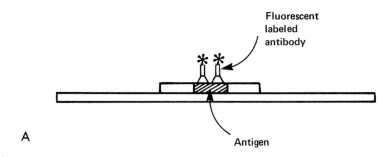

A

INDIRECT FLUORESCENT
ANTIBODY TEST

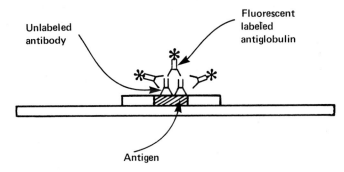

B

Figure 9–4 *A,* The direct fluorescent antibody test is employed to detect antigen by means of FITC-labeled antibody directed against that antigen. The labeled antibody will only bind to specific antigen, and therefore fluorescence seen under the ultraviolet microscope indicates that antigen is present in the material under examination. *B,* The indirect fluorescent antibody test is employed to detect and measure either antigen or specific antibody. Antigen present in a frozen section, smear or culture will bind antibody from serum. After washing, this antibody may be detected by using a FITC-labeled antiglobulin serum.

INDIRECT FLUORESCENT ANTIBODY TEST (IFA) (Fig. 9–4B). The indirect fluorescent antibody test may be used for the detection and measurement of antibodies in serum or for the demonstration and identification of antigens in tissues or cell cultures. When testing for antibody, antigen is employed as a tissue smear, section or cell culture. This is incubated in a serum suspected of containing antibodies to that antigen, and the serum is then washed off, leaving antibodies bound to the antigen. These bound antibodies may be visualized by incubating the smear in FITC-labeled antiglobulin serum. When this is removed by washing and the slide examined, fluorescence indicates that antibody was present in the test serum. The quantity of antibody in the test serum may be estimated by examining increasing dilutions of serum on a number of different antigen preparations.

The indirect fluorescent antibody test has a number of advantages over the direct technique. Since each antibody molecule binding to antigen will itself bind several labeled antiglobulin molecules, then fluorescence will be considerably brighter than in the direct test. Similarly, by using antiglobulin sera specific for each immunoglobulin class, the class of specific antibody present in the serum may also be determined.

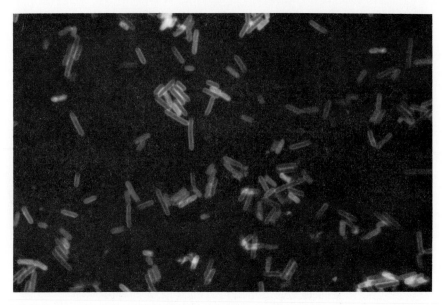

Figure 9–5 Direct immunofluorescence of a smear of *Clostridium chauveoi*. (Courtesy of Dr. C. L. Gyles.) (See also Figs. 19–7 and 21–6.)

Other Labels Used in Primary Binding Tests.   Several other labels have been employed as alternatives to radioisotopes, enzymes or fluorescent dyes in primary binding tests. For example, reagents linked to the iron-containing protein ferritin may be used to identify the location of antigens in tissues examined by electron microscopy. The ferritin molecule is a protein of 700,000 daltons containing 23 per cent iron as ferric hydroxide or phosphate. The iron is concentrated within the molecule and on electron microscopy can be detected as a characteristic electron-dense spot. Therefore, if ferritin is linked to an immunoglobulin, the location of antigen may be readily observed on electron micrographs. A similar technique has employed peroxidase conjugated to immunoglobulin, and the presence of the enzyme was then identified by histochemical techniques.

SECONDARY BINDING TESTS

Secondary binding tests are two-stage processes. The first stage is the interaction between antigen and antibody, a reaction that is not markedly affected by temperature but may be reversed by high ionic strength or low pH. The second stage is determined by the physical state of the antigen. Thus, if antibodies combine with soluble antigens in solution under appropriate conditions, the complexes precipitate. If the antigens are particulate—for example, bacteria or erythrocytes, then they agglutinate (clump). Under other circumstances, the combination of antigen and antibody may lead to activation of complement, which can also be measured.

PRECIPITATION

If a suitable amount of a clear solution of soluble antigen is mixed with its homologous antiserum and incubated at 37°C, the mixture becomes cloudy within a few minutes, then flocculent, and finally a precipitate settles to the bottom of the tube within an hour or so. If increasing amounts of soluble antigen are mixed with a constant amount of antibody, the results obtained are determined by the relative proportions of the reactants. No obvious precipitate is formed at low antigen concentrations. As the amount of antigen increases, larger quantities of precipitate result until the amount is maximal. With the addition of more antigen, the amount of precipitate gradually diminishes, until none is observed in tubes containing a large excess of antigen (Fig. 9–6).

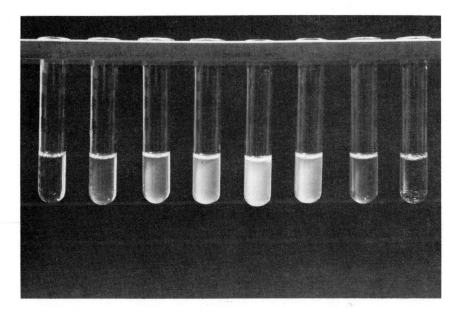

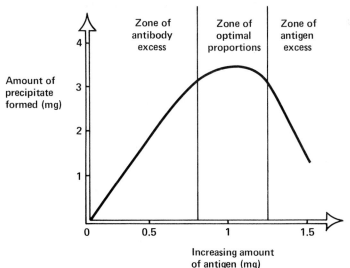

Figure 9–6 A photograph of the effect of mixing increasing amounts of bovine serum albumin with a constant amount of rabbit antiserum to that antigen. The tube with the greatest amount of precipitate is the one in which the ratio of antigen and antibody is considered to be in optimal proportions. A quantitative precipitation curve of this test graphically shows the effect of adding increasing amounts of antigen to a constant amount of antibody.

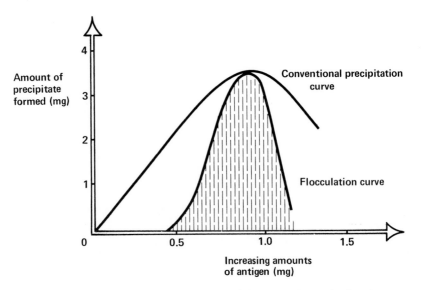

Figure 9–7 A quantitative precipitation curve of the type obtained when horse serum is used. Notice how flocculation occurs only over a narrow range of antigen-antibody mixtures.

Precipitating antibodies in horse serum behave in a somewhat different fashion, producing a distinct flocculation over a very narrow range of antigen concentrations. This appears to be a particular property of the IgG(T) antibody class (Fig. 9–7).

In the first stage of these reactions, only a little antigen is complexed to antibody, and since antibody is in excess, free antibody may be found in the supernatant and little precipitate is deposited. In the tubes where maximal precipitation occurs, both antigen and antibody are completely complexed and neither can be detected in the supernatant. This is known as the equivalence zone, and the ratio of antibody to antigen is here said to be in optimal proportions. When antigen is added to excess, then little precipitate is formed, although soluble immune complexes are present and free antigen may be found in the supernatant.

These results may be explained by the fact that antibodies are usually bivalent and therefore are able to cross-link only two antigenic determinants at a time, but protein antigens are generally multivalent, possessing a relatively large number of antigenic determinants. In the mixtures containing excess antibody, each antigen molecule is covered with antibody, preventing cross-linkage and thus precipitation. When the reactants are in optimal proportions, the ratio of antigen to antibody is such that extensive cross-linking and "lattice" formation occur. As this lattice grows in size it becomes insoluble and eventually precipitates (Fig. 9–8). In mixtures where antigen is in excess, each antibody molecule is bound to a pair of antigen molecules. Further cross-linkage is impossible in this case, and since these complexes are small and soluble, no precipitation occurs. The cells of the mononuclear-phagocytic system are most efficient at binding and removing complexes formed at optimal proportions and in antibody excess. Immune complexes formed in antigen excess are poorly removed by phagocytic cells but are deposited within vessel walls and in glomeruli, where they contribute to an acute inflammatory response classified as a type III hypersensitivity reaction (Chapter 19).

Antibody is bivalent

Antigen is multivalent

Antigen mixed with excess antibody

Antibody mixed with excess antigen

Antigen and antibody mixed in optimal proportions

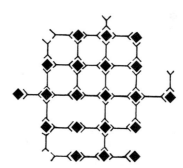

Figure 9–8 The mechanism of precipitation: In antibody excess and in antigen excess, only very small soluble immune complexes are produced. At optimal proportions, however, large insoluble complexes are generated.

If antigen and antibody solutions are layered, one on top of the other, without mixing, the components will diffuse into each other. Where the ratio of the reagents is in optimal proportions, a band of precipitate forms. A technique such as this, sometimes called an Ascoli test or a "ring" test, has been used to detect anthrax bacilli in hides. Antiserum against *Bacillus anthracis* is allowed to react in a capillary tube with an extract of hide suspected of being derived from an infected animal. A line of precipitate at the interface of the two fluids constitutes a positive reaction. Unfortunately, this technique requires a certain steadiness of hand, and the result is easily obscured if the two solutions are inadvertently mixed. The reaction, however, can be stabilized by conducting the test in gels.

Immunodiffusion. A simple technique is to cut two round wells 5 mm in diameter and about 1 cm apart in a layer of agar in a Petri dish. One well may be filled with antigen, the other with antiserum; the reactants will diffuse out radially. A circular concentration gradient therefore is established for each reactant, and these eventually overlap. Thus, optimal proportions for the occurrence of precipitation will occur in one zone of the superimposed gradients, and an opaque white line of precipitate will appear in this region (Fig. 9–9). This technique is known as the double diffusion test and, since it was first described by the Swedish immunologist O. Ouchterloney, is sometimes known as the Ouchterloney technique.

If several antigen-antibody mixtures are used, each component is unlikely to reach optimal proportions in exactly the same position. Consequently, a separate line of precipitation is produced for each interacting set of antigens and antibodies present. This test may also be used to determine the relationship between antigens. If two antigen wells and one antibody well are set up as in Figures 9–9 and 9–10, then lines will form between each antigen well and the antibody well. If these two lines are completely confluent, then the two antigens are considered to be identical. If the lines cross over, then the two antigens are different, whereas if the lines merge with spur formation, then a partial identity exists, with each antigen possessing antigenic determinants in common. The line that continues as a spur possesses antigenic determinants not present in the other. The double diffusion technique may be used to identify the presence of either antigen or antibodies in body fluids; for example, the Coggin's test is a double diffusion method of detecting the presence of antibodies against equine infectious anemia virus in horses. In this test an extract of infected horse spleen or a cell culture antigen is reacted with the serum of horses under test in agar gel, and the occurrence of a line of precipitate constitutes a positive reaction. A similar test may be employed to identify cattle infected with bovine leukemia virus. The antigen in this case is semipurified viral glycoprotein.

RADIAL IMMUNODIFFUSION (MANCINI TECHNIQUE) (Fig. 9–11). If antigen is allowed to diffuse into agar in which specific antiserum is incorporated, then a ring of

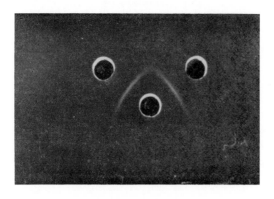

Figure 9–9 Precipitation in agar gel. Antigen and antibody diffusing from their respective wells precipitate in a region where optimal proportions are achieved. In this example, the antigen is identical in both of the top wells. As a result, the precipitation lines fuse to show a line of complete identity.

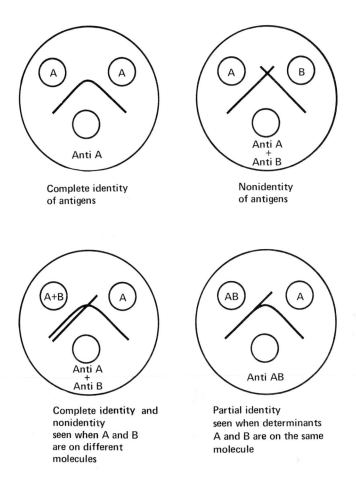

Figure 9–10 The use of the gel-diffusion technique in determining the relationships between two antigens.

precipitate indicating the zone of optimal proportions will form around the well. The area of this ring is directly related to the amount of antigen added to the well. If the technique is first standardized using known amounts of antigen, then a standard curve may be constructed and unknown solutions of antigen accurately assayed. A reversed radial immunodiffusion test employing antigen-impregnated agar has been used with success for the measurement of antibodies to *Mycoplasma mycoides* and some other organisms.

IMMUNOELECTROPHORESIS AND RELATED TECHNIQUES. While double diffusion techniques give a separate precipitation line for each antigen-antibody system in a mixture, it is often difficult to resolve all the components in a very complex mixture in this way. One technique that may be used to improve the resolution of the system is to separate the antigen mixture by electrophoresis prior to undertaking immunodiffusion. This technique is known as immunoelectrophoresis and is usually employed to identify proteins in body fluids.

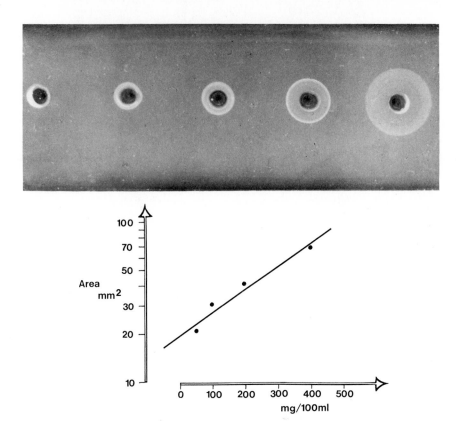

Figure 9–11 Radial immunodiffusion. In this case antiserum to bovine IgA is incorporated in the agar and is used to measure bovine serum IgA levels.

Immunoelectrophoresis involves the electrophoresis of the antigen mixture in agar gel in one direction. A trough is then cut in the agar just to one side and parallel to this line of separated proteins. Antiserum is placed in this trough and allowed to diffuse laterally. When the diffusing antibodies encounter antigen, curved lines of precipitate are formed. One arc of precipitation forms for each of the constituents in the antigen mixture (Fig. 9–12). This technique can be used to resolve the proteins of normal serum into between 25 and 40 distinct precipitation bands. The exact number depends upon the strength and specificity of the antiserum employed (Fig. 9–13). By means of this technique it is possible to identify the absence of a normal serum protein such as occurs in animals with a congenital deficiency of some complement components. It is also possible to detect the presence of excessive amounts of an individual component, as is found in animals with a myeloma (Chapter 22).

If, instead of permitting antigen to diffuse into agar-containing antiserum as in the radial immunodiffusion technique, the antigen is driven into the antiserum agar by electrophoresis, then the ring of precipitation around each well becomes deformed into a rocket shape. The length of the rockets is proportional to the amount of antigen placed in each well. This technique, known as electroimmunodiffusion, "rocket" electrophoresis or electroimmunoassay, may be employed to quantitate antigen (Fig. 9–14).

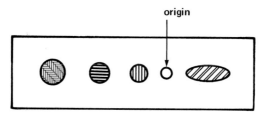

Stage 1.   Serum placed in a well on an
agar plate is electrophoresed

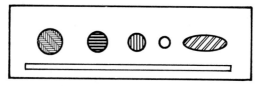

Stage 2.   Antiserum is placed in a trough
cut parallel to the electrophoretic run

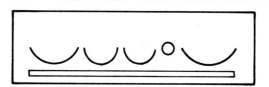

Arcs of precipitate form as each serum
protein meets its specific antibody

Figure 9–12   The principle of immunoelectrophoresis.

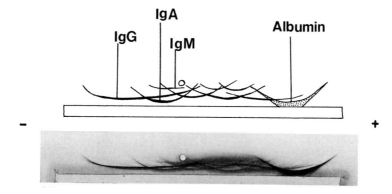

Figure 9–13   Immunoelectrophoresis of normal pig serum showing the precipitation lines produced by some of the major serum proteins.

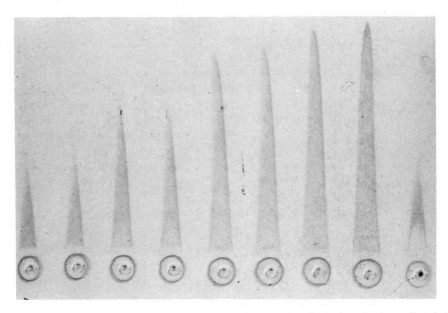

Figure 9–14 Electroimmunodiffusion. In this example, lactoferrin from bovine milk is being estimated. The height of each "rocket" is proportional to the amount of antigen placed in the wells at the bottom. (See page 133.) (Courtesy of Dr. R. Harmon.)

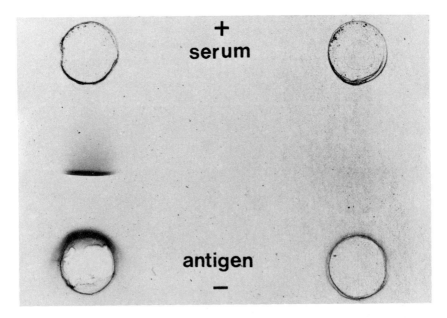

Figure 9–15 Counter-immunoelectrophoresis. In this example, serum antibody to the Aleutian disease virus is detected by its reaction with a preparation of viral antigen. *Left*, a positive reaction; *right*, a negative reaction. (Courtesy of Dr. S. H. An.)

When electrophoresed in agar gel, some antibodies move cathodally because of a flow of buffer through the agar toward the cathode. This phenomenon is called electroendosmosis. If an antigen is strongly negatively charged so that it moves toward the anode in spite of this flow, then it is possible by a suitable arrangement of wells in an agar plate to drive antigen and antibody together by electrophoresis. A precipitate may be produced in this way within a few minutes. This technique is known as "counter-immunoelectrophoresis" and may be used for the rapid identification of bacteria and mycoplasma and for the diagnosis of viral diseases such as Aleutian disease of mink (Fig. 9–15). In this case, solutions containing the Aleutian disease agent and antibody are electrophoresed in such a way that they are driven together. The development of a line of precipitate within 30 to 40 minutes indicates the presence of antibodies in the test serum and suggests that that mink is infected. By using large sheets of agar it is possible, by means of this technique, to test large numbers of sera within a few minutes.

TITRATION OF ANTIBODIES

Although the detection of antibodies or antigen is sufficient for many tests, it is usually desirable to arrive at some estimate of the amount of reactants present. In the case of tests designed to detect the presence of specific antibody, this quantitation is often accomplished by titration. Titration is a procedure in which the serum under test is made up in a series of increasing dilutions (Fig. 9–16). Each dilution is then tested for activity in the test system. The reciprocal of the highest dilution giving a positive reaction is known as the titer, or titre (depending on geographical location) and provides a measure of the amount of antibody in that serum.

AGGLUTINATION

In the same way that bivalent antibodies may link soluble antigens to form an insoluble complex that then precipitates, antibody may cross-link particulate antigens, resulting in their clumping or agglutination. Agglutination may be produced by mixing a suspension of antigenic particles, such as bacteria, with antiserum. Antibody combines rapidly with the particles—the primary interaction—but agglutination is a much slower process, since adherence between particles occurs only when they touch each other. Normally, these suspensions are stable, their constituent particles prevented from clumping by a net negative charge or "zeta potential" on their surface. However, immunoglobulins are relatively positively charged and on coating particles they tend to neutralize this zeta potential. As a result, the particles can approach closely and agglutination may occur.

Antibodies differ in their capacity to promote agglutination, IgM antibodies being considerably more efficient than IgG or IgA antibodies in producing this form of reaction (Table 9–3).

If excessive antibody is added to a suspension of antigenic particles, then, just as in the precipitation reaction, it is possible for each particle to be so coated by antibody that agglutination is inhibited. This lack of reactivity seen at high antibody concentrations is termed a prozone. Another possible cause of prozone formation is the presence of antibodies that do not cause agglutination even when bound to the particles. These

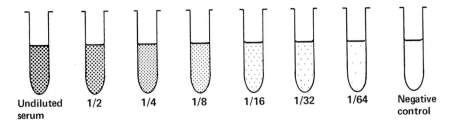

Undiluted serum   1/2   1/4   1/8   1/16   1/32   1/64   Negative control

A constant amount of antigen is added to each tube

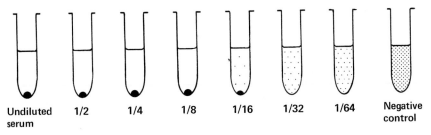

Undiluted serum   1/2   1/4   1/8   1/16   1/32   1/64   Negative control

Figure 9–16 The principle of antibody titration. Serum is first diluted in a series of tubes. A constant amount of antigen is then added to each tube and the tubes incubated. At the end of the incubation period, agglutination has occurred in all tubes up to a serum dilution of 1/16. The titer of the serum is therefore 1/16.

nonagglutinating antibodies are also known as incomplete antibodies. The reasons for their lack of agglutinating activity are not completely clear; one possible reason is that the antigenic determinants with which they react lie deep within the surface coat of the particle, so deep, in fact, that cross-linking cannot occur. An alternative suggestion is that they are capable of only restricted movement in their hinge region (Chapter 4), causing them to be functionally "monovalent."

Antiglobulin tests. If it is necessary to test for the presence of incomplete

Table 9–3 ROLE OF SPECIFIC IMMUNOGLOBULINS IN DIAGNOSTIC TESTS

*PROPERTY**	*IgG*	*IgM*	*IgA*	*IgG(T)*
Agglutinating	+	+++	+	−
Complement-fixing (heterologous guinea pig complement)	+	+++	−	−
Precipitating	+++	+	±	±
Neutralizing	+	++	+	+
Time of appearance after exposure to antigen	3–7 days	2–5 days	3–7 days	3–7 days
Time to reach peak titer	7–21 days	5–14 days	7–21 days	7–21 days

*The properties listed may vary somewhat between species.

antibodies on the surface of particles such as bacteria or erythrocytes then a direct antiglobulin test may be used (Figure 9–17). The washed particles are mixed with an antiglobulin serum and, if incomplete antibodies are present, agglutination will occur.

In order to test for the presence of incomplete antibodies in a serum, an indirect antiglobulin test is used. In this technique, the serum under test is first incubated with antigen particles, which adsorb the incomplete antibodies. After washing to remove unbound antibody, the coated particles are mixed with an antiglobulin serum. On reacting with bound antibody, the antiglobulin will cross-link the particles and cause agglutination.

Passive Agglutination. Since agglutination is a much more sensitive technique than precipitation, it is sometimes considered desirable to convert a precipitating system to an agglutinating one. One way this may be done is by chemically linking soluble antigen to inert particles such as erythrocytes, bacteria or latex, so that specific antibody will cause these sensitized particles to agglutinate. Erythrocytes appear to be among the best particles for this purpose, and tests that employ coated erythrocytes are termed passive hemagglutination tests. Some antigens such as the bacterial lipopolysaccharides adsorb naturally to erythrocytes, and it is possible to use this phenomenon to advantage in diagnostic tests. Unfortunately, these lipopolysaccharides are also adsorbed to erythrocytes *in vivo* so that the erythrocytes are destroyed by the antibacterial immune responses; as a consequence, anemia is a feature of many diseases caused by gram-negative organisms (Chapter 13).

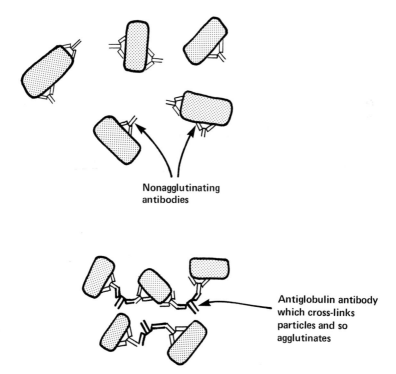

Nonagglutinating
antibodies

Antiglobulin antibody
which cross-links
particles and so
agglutinates

Figure 9–17 The principle of the direct antiglobulin test. The presence of an antiglobulin antibody is required to agglutinate erythrocytes coated with nonagglutinating antibody.

COMPLEMENT FIXATION

As discussed in Chapter 8, the activation of the complement system by immune complexes results in the generation of factors capable of disrupting cell membranes. If the immune complexes are generated on erythrocyte surfaces, then the erythrocyte membranes are lysed and hemolysis occurs. It is possible to use this reaction to measure serum antibody levels. The most important test of this type is the hemolytic complement fixation test (CFT). The CFT is one of the most widely applicable of all immunological techniques. Once the required reagents are prepared and standardized, the CFT may be used to detect many immune interactions. The end point is very easily read and, unlike the hemagglutination tests, does not depend upon the settling of the erythrocytes and is less affected by prozones. In addition, this test does not depend upon the availability of purified suspensions of antigens and is therefore commonly used in the diagnosis of viral diseases. The most important disadvantage of this test is its complexity, particularly with regard to the standardization and preparation of the required reagents.

The hemolytic complement fixation test is performed in two parts (Fig. 9–18). First, antigen and the serum under test (deprived of its complement by heating at 56°C) are incubated in the presence of normal guinea pig serum, which provides a source of complement. (Guinea pig serum is most commonly used because its complement has a high hemolytic activity—i.e., it lyses erythrocytes well.) After allowing the antigen–antibody–complement mixture to react for a short period, the amount of free complement remaining is measured by adding an "indicator system" consisting of antibody-coated sheep erythrocytes. Lysis of these erythrocytes, seen as the development of a transparent red solution, is a negative result, since it indicates that complement was not fixed and that antibody was therefore absent from the serum under test. Absence of lysis (seen as a cloudy red cell suspension) is a positive result. It is usual to titrate the serum being tested so that, if antibodies are present in that serum, as it is diluted the reaction in each tube will change from no-lysis (i.e., positive) to lysis (i.e., negative). The titer may be considered to be the highest dilution of serum in which no more than 50 per cent of the red cells are lysed.

Before a hemolytic complement fixation test is performed, all reagents, antigen, complement, sheep erythrocytes and antibody against the erythrocytes (hemolysin) must be carefully standardized. For example, addition of the correct amount of complement is critical, since too little complement results in incomplete lysis whereas excessive complement is not completely fixed by immune complexes and therefore will lead to false-negative results. Excessive antigen interferes with complement fixation, whereas insufficient antigen may fail to fix complement in demonstrable amounts. The hemolysin should be heated at 56°C for 30 minutes in order to destroy its content of complement.

ANTICOMPLEMENTARY EFFECTS.   One problem commonly encountered when performing complement fixation tests is the presence of anticomplementary activity in the serum under test. That is, the test serum appears to fix complement in the absence of antigen. There are several possible reasons for this occurrence. In serum taken from infected animals, any immune complexes present will effectively bind some complement. Similarly, the presence of bacterial contaminants in serum may activate complement through the alternate pathway.

Pig serum has the curious property of possessing procomplementary activity—that

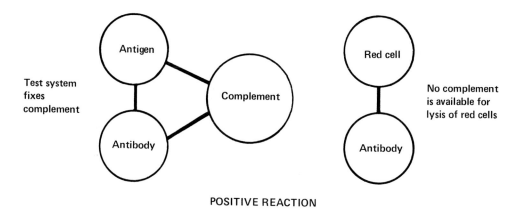

POSITIVE REACTION

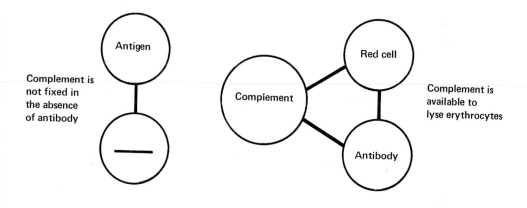

NEGATIVE REACTION

Figure 9–18 The principle of the complement fixation test. Complement, if fixed by antigen and antibody, is unavailable to lyse the indicator system. In the absence of antibody the complement will remain unfixed and available for lysis of the indicator system. (Modified from Roitt I. Essential Immunology. Blackwell Scientific Publications, Oxford.)

is, it accentuates the hemolytic activity of the added complement. As a result, it is difficult to perform complement fixation tests on pig serum.

   Modifications of Complement Fixation Tests.   Various modifications of the CFT have been devised to overcome some of its limitations. For example, avian antibodies cannot fix mammalian complement. This disadvantage may be overcome either by using avian complement or, alternatively, by adding to the usual CF test system a complement-fixing indicator antibody against the antigen (Fig. 9–19). If the test serum is from an infected bird (i.e., contains antibodies), then on mixing with antigen, immune-complex formation will occur, and as a result, when indicator antibody and

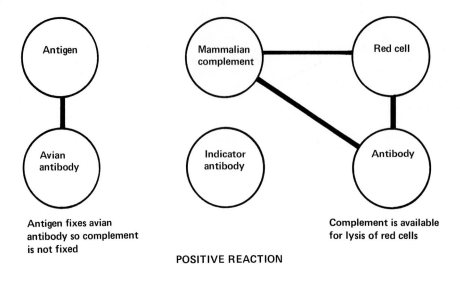

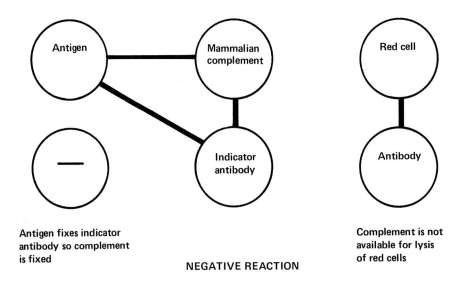

Figure 9–19 The principle of the indirect complement fixation test. In the presence of avian antibody, complement is not fixed and remains available to lyse the indicator system. In the absence of avian antibody, complement if fixed by indicator antibody and the indicator system is not lysed. Lysis is therefore evidence of a positive reaction, and the absence of lysis is a negative reaction.

complement are subsequently added, they will not be fixed. Addition of a second indicator system consisting of antibody-coated sheep erythrocytes consequently results in lysis. If, on the other hand, the test serum is negative, then the antigen remains free to bind to the indicator antibody and fix complement; as a consequence, the indicator system does not lyse. As can be imagined, because of its complexity this is not a widely employed test.

Some complements, such as that from the horse, are not hemolytic. The fixation of this type of complement, however, can be measured by estimating its ability to clump erythrocytes in the presence of immunoconglutinin. Immunoconglutinin is a natural antibody directed against antigenic determinants on fixed C3 (Chapter 8). The test is performed in the same way as the hemolytic complement fixation test except that the indicator system contains a source of immunoconglutinin in addition to antibody-coated erythrocytes. The test is read by measuring not hemolysis, but immunoconglutination—a very strong agglutination. This test has been used for the diagnosis of glanders in horses.

Complement fixation tests may also be modified by supplementing the guinea pig complement with homologous complement. Tests of this type have been employed successfully in detecting antibodies to vesicular stomatitis, bluetongue and other viruses in bovine and swine sera. The mechanism of this test is in some doubt, but it is possible that homologous Clq is required for activation of the guinea pig complement.

Cytotoxicity Tests. Complement may cause membrane damage, not only to erythrocytes but also to nucleated cells and to protozoa. Antibodies against cell surface antigens thus may be measured by reacting target cells with antibody in the presence of complement and estimating the resulting cell death. A simple method of doing this is to add a dye such as trypan blue or eosin-Y to the cell suspension. Living cells do not take up these dyes while dead ones stain intensely. This form of test is employed in the identification of class I histocompatibility antigens (Chapter 16). A modification of this technique, known as the Sabin-Feldman dye test after its originators, is used in the diagnosis of toxoplasmosis. Normally, living *Toxoplasma gondii* organisms stain deeply with methylene blue. In the presence of antibody and complement they lose this staining property. Antibody against *Toxoplasma* organisms may therefore be titrated using this technique.

TESTS INVOLVING VIRAL HEMAGGLUTINATION AND ITS INHIBITION

Certain organisms are capable of agglutinating mammalian and avian erythrocytes. Antibodies directed against these organisms may inhibit this hemagglutination. The detection of virus-induced hemagglutination may be used as a preliminary test when attempting to identify a virus, whereas inhibition of this phenomenon by antibody may be employed either as a method of identifying a specific virus or to measure antibody levels in serum. Hemagglutinating organisms include ortho- and paramyxoviruses, alpha-, flavi and bunyaviruses as well as some adeno-, reo-, parvo- and coronaviruses. They also include some mycoplasmata such as *Mycoplasma gallisepticum*.

Hemagglutination inhibition tests are performed in two general ways. In the first (sometimes called the α procedure), the amount of virus added to each tube is kept constant while the serum to be tested is serially diluted. (It is first necessary to titrate out the virus in order to determine its hemagglutinating activity, and it is common to employ four or eight times this minimal dose, i.e., four or eight hemagglutinating units, in a test.) After virus and antibody are mixed, they are allowed to stand for a standard period of time before a suspension of washed erythrocytes is added to each tube. The hemagglutination inhibition (HI) titer of the serum is obtained by multiplying the highest dilution of serum that just inhibits hemagglutination by the number of hemagglutinating units of virus involved.

An alternative method of estimating antibody levels by hemagglutination inhibition is to add a standard amount of antiserum to each tube while serial dilutions are made of a virus suspension of known hemagglutinating activity (the β procedure). This is a useful technique in laboratories where very large numbers of sera must be tested, since virus dilutions need be made only once, at the beginning of each day's testing, and there is no necessity to perform serial dilutions on each serum to be tested. By comparing the hemagglutinating titer of the virus in the presence of both a normal and a test serum, it is possible to arrive at an estimate of the inhibitory power of that test serum.

While hemagglutination inhibition tests are technically relatively simple, problems may be encountered as a result of the presence in test serum of nonantibody hemagglutination inhibitors. Some of these are carbohydrates that may be destroyed by treatment of the test serum with bacterial neuraminidase (receptor-destroying enzyme, RDE). Others are lipoproteins that may be removed either by absorption of serum with washed kaolin or destroyed by trypsin treatment. It is also generally necessary to absorb the test serum with erythrocytes in order to remove natural hemagglutinins.

Some myxoviruses possess their own RDE, permitting them to elute from red cells after incubation and also rendering these red cells inagglutinable. For this reason, a false-positive result may be obtained if there is excessive delay in reading some hemagglutination inhibition tests.

TESTS INVOLVING ASSAYS IN LIVING SYSTEMS

If an organism or antigen possesses biological activity, it is possible to assay antibody for its capacity to neutralize this activity. These reactions include hemolysis of erythrocytes, lysis of nucleated cells, and disease or death in animals. Unfortunately, reactions such as these are subject to a high degree of variability since, because of variations in the test system, the result tends to change gradually over a wide range of doses of organism or antigen. For example, 0.0030 mg of tetanus toxin may kill some mice in a test group, but about five times that dose is required to kill all mice in the same group. For this reason, results obtained from a single positive or negative test are meaningless. In addition, if an attempt is made to assess the lowest dose of tetanus toxin that will kill all the animals in a group (the minimum lethal dose, MLD) it is found to be extremely variable (Fig. 9–20). It is equally difficult to estimate with precision the highest dose of toxin that will just fail to kill all test animals. The most exact method of measuring the lethal effects of a toxin has been found to be an estimate of the dose that will just kill 50 per cent of a group of test animals. In practice, it is usually not possible to arrive at this 50 per cent end point by direct experimentation. For this reason, it is usually necessary to calculate it by plotting the results against the dose of toxin given and arriving at the 50 per cent end point by interpolation.

In the example cited in the previous paragraph, the lethality of the toxin was estimated by measuring the dose required to kill 50 per cent of a group of experimental animals. This is known as the LD_{50}. Similarly, the dose of complement that just lyses 50 per cent of a red cell suspension is known as the CH_{50}. The dose of organisms that infects 50 per cent of animals is the ID_{50}, the dose that just infects 50

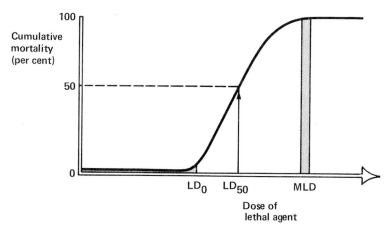

Figure 9–20 A cumulative mortality curve showing how the LD_{50} provides a relatively more accurate estimate of the lethal effects of a toxin than either the LD_0 or the MLD.

per cent of tissue cultures is the $TCID_{50}$, and the dose of antiserum or vaccine that protects 50 per cent of challenged animals is the PD_{50}.

Neutralization Tests. Neutralization tests are tests that estimate the capacity of antibody when mixed with antigen *in vitro* to neutralize its biological activity. These tests may be used to identify bacterial toxins. For example, *Clostridium perfringens* α toxin, which is a phospholipase, causes the development of an opaque white zone around colonies of this organism grown on agar containing either serum or egg yolk. Antiserum to the α toxin prevents the formation of this zone. This reaction, known as the Nagler reaction, therefore may be employed to identify organisms producing this toxin. A similar type of test may be used to identify the presence of staphylococcal α toxin by inhibiting its hemolytic activity with specific antiserum (Fig. 9–21).

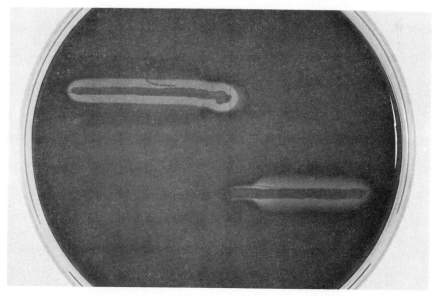

Figure 9–21 A blood agar plate, the center of which has been impregnated with antiserum to staphylococcal α toxin. The presence of this antiserum in the agar neutralizes the toxin produced by the staphylococcus and so inhibits hemolysis. (Courtesy of Mr. E. L. Thackeray.)

Viruses may be prevented from infecting cells after specific antibody has combined with and blocked critical sites. This reaction is the basis of the neutralization tests that are commonly employed in virology either for the identification of unknown viruses or for the measurement of specific antibody. Neutralization tests are highly specific and extremely sensitive. Thus, antiserum to coliphage T4 will neutralize phage-induced lysis of *Escherichia coli* because antibodies can block the receptor on the phage tail, thus preventing its attachment to a bacterium. A single antibody molecule is apparently sufficient to cause this blockage, and a phage neutralization test consequently may detect as little as 0.00005 μg of antibody.

All neutralization tests first require that the virus be titrated so that its infectivity is known. This may be done by measuring its ID_{50} in animals or embryonated eggs or its $TCID_{50}$ in cell cultures. Given a virus suspension of known infectivity, it is possible to measure the neutralizing activity of a serum by two methods. In one, the virus concentration is kept constant while antiserum is diluted. In this way it is possible to measure directly the neutralizing titer of an antiserum. Alternatively, the antiserum concentration may be kept constant and the virus diluted. This technique provides another measure of the neutralizing power of an antiserum, which can be expressed as a neutralization index. The neutralization index is the difference between the number of ID_{50}s or $TCID_{50}$s neutralized by the test serum and by a known negative serum. In general, an index of more than 50 is required before a serum is considered to be positive. Similarly, the difference between the indices of two viruses must be less than 20 when tested against a standard antiserum before they can be considered identical.

Neutralization tests in tissue cultures are particularly suitable for use with viruses that produce either readily identifiable cytopathic effects or hemadsorption of erythrocytes, since both of these reactions may be inhibited by prior exposure of the virus to antibody. In general, if a serum is to be titrated, increasing dilutions of antibody are mixed with a constant amount of virus (usually 100 $TCID_{50}$) for a specified period of time and then each virus-antiserum mixture is used to inoculate a set of culture tubes. After incubation, the dilution of antiserum at which 50 per cent of cultures show signs of infection, multiplied by the number of $TCID_{50}$ neutralized, is taken to be its titer.

While cytopathic effects may be observed microscopically, other alternative techniques for assessing infection are also available. In the metabolic inhibition technique, use is made of the change in pH that occurs when healthy cells are grown in tissue culture. For example, normal, actively metabolizing cells produce acid that turns phenol-red, the indicator dye, yellow. When cell metabolism ceases in infected cultures, this acid production does not occur. In consequence, either the phenol-red does not change color or, alternatively, the medium turns alkaline (red) as a result of the accumulation of cell breakdown products. This color change may be employed in determining the presence or absence of infected cells.

A second technique of identifying virus-infected cells makes use of the phenomenon of hemadsorption. Certain viruses are capable of inducing the development of "hemagglutinins" on the surface of infected tissue-culture cells. As a consequence, if a dilute suspension of washed erythrocytes is added to these cultures and examined 15 minutes later, the erythrocytes may be seen to be adherent to the infected cells. While many hemadsorbing viruses are also hemagglutinating, this is not an absolute relationship. For example, African swine fever virus is nonhemagglutinating but is hemadsorbing. The prevention of hemadsorption may be used as an indication of virus neutralization, especially with viruses that do not produce a significant cytopathic effect.

A third method of assessing virus cytopathogenicity is through inhibition of plaque formation. In this technique, a confluent cell monolayer is infected by a dilute suspension of virus before being covered by a layer of agar. Because of the presence of the agar, virus particles are not free to diffuse but are capable of infecting nearby cells only. As a result, localized areas of cytolysis, revealed as clear "plaques," develop in the monolayer. The number of plaques formed depends upon the number of infectious particles added to the culture. Antiserum that neutralizes the virus therefore reduces the number of plaques formed, and this activity may be detected in several ways. In the plaque neutralization test, the virus is incubated with antiserum before infecting the cell monolayer. In the plaque reduction test, antiserum is incorporated into the agar used to cover the infected monolayer. In the plaque suppression technique, the monolayer is covered with agar-containing antiserum and virus is placed on top of this in a second layer of agar. Only virus that is not neutralized by antibody succeeds in diffusing through the antiserum-agar layer to cause plaque formation.

Although virus neutralization tests utilizing cell cultures are perhaps the most widely applicable serological tests for virological work, it is also possible to assay antibody by measuring virus neutralization *in vivo*. For example, antiserum to pox viruses may be titrated by its capacity to inhibit pock formation on the chorioallantoic membrane of embryonated eggs, and antiserum to the equine encephalitis viruses may be titrated by its capacity to neutralize virus and so prevent death in mice injected intracerebrally with the virus-antibody mixture.

Protection Tests. Protection tests are a form of neutralization test carried out entirely *in vivo*. It is possible to measure the protective properties of a specific antiserum by administering it in increasing dilutions to a group of test animals, which may be challenged subsequently with a standard dose of pathogenic organisms or toxin. Protection tests may therefore be classified as tertiary tests, since they measure not only the interaction between antigen and antibody *in vivo* but also the practical consequences of this in relation to disease resistance. Whereas protection tests provide a direct measure of the therapeutic efficacy of an antiserum, they are also subject to great experimental variation because of the difference among animals in their susceptibility to infection and in a number of other factors, such as the rate of absorption of antiserum, the level of activity of the mononuclear-phagocytic system and the catabolic rate of the passively acquired immunoglobulin.

As in neutralization tests, meaningful results can be obtained only if relatively large numbers of animals are employed and if the challenge dose is carefully standardized. It is usual to use a dose of organisms or toxin containing a known number of $LD_{50}s$ or $ID_{50}s$. Similarly, the protective effect of an antiserum may be expressed in $PD_{50}s$, the dose required to protect 50 per cent of a group of animals.

DIAGNOSTIC APPLICATIONS OF IMMUNOLOGICAL TESTS

The immune responses of animals can be utilized in two general ways in the diagnostic laboratory. First, specific antibody may be used to detect or identify antigen. Second, by detecting specific antibody in serum, it is possible to determine whether an animal has been exposed to a particular antigen and therefore to assist in the establishment of a diagnosis or determine the degree of exposure of the population to that antigen.

Obviously, the presence of antibodies to a particular organism in an animal serum indicates previous exposure to an antigenic determinant present on that organism. It does not, however, automatically provide proof that infection exists or that any concurrent disease is actually caused by the organism. For example, although the sera of most healthy horses contain antibodies to *Salmonella typhimurium*, this does not prove that most horses have salmonellosis. Because of this fact, it generally may be stated that the presence of antibodies to an organism in a single serum sample is of little diagnostic significance. Only if at least two samples are taken one to three weeks

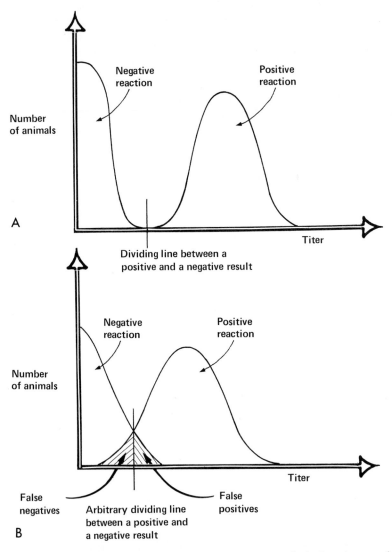

Figure 9–22 Schematic diagrams depicting an ideal test in which there is no ambiguity in interpreting test results (*A*) and a more typical test in which an arbitrary line must be used to separate positive from negative results (*B*). By moving this dividing line the relative proportions of false-positive and false-negative results may be changed.

apart and at least a fourfold rise in titer is shown can a diagnosis be made, and this should be done only in conjunction with careful analysis of clinical factors.

A second feature that must be considered in the interpretation of serological results is the possibility of errors. These may be of two types: false-positive reactions and false-negative reactions. A test in which a large proportion of the positive reactions are false is considered to be nonspecific, whereas one with a very high proportion of false-negative reactions is considered to be insensitive. In general, the level of such errors is set by the criteria used to differentiate positive from negative reactions. If these criteria are adjusted so that the number of false-positive reactions are reduced, then there will be an increasing proportion of false-negative reactions encountered, and vice versa (Fig. 9–22). Thus, highly sensitive tests tend to be relatively nonspecific and highly specific tests are generally insensitive. The establishment of criteria in reading tests and, from this, the sensitivity and specificity of a test are determined both by the requirements of the test procedure and by the consequences of false-positive and false-negative reactions. In ideal tests, it would be desirable for the criteria used in interpreting the test results to be so obvious and absolute that each test would be absolutely sensitive and specific. Unfortunately, such ideal tests are uncommon.

As has been evident from the discussions earlier in this chapter, the advantages and disadvantages of each immunodiagnostic test vary according to the specific requirements of the investigator, the nature of the antigen employed, and the complexity, sensitivity and specificity of each technique. In general, the selection of a diagnostic test represents a compromise between its sensitivity, its specificity and its complexity—that is, the number of steps involved, the degree of technical expertise required and the nature of the equipment needed to conduct the test. Although precise guidelines cannot be drawn up, it is usually most appropriate to use the most sensitive and specific test that can be satisfactorily performed with the available technical assistance and equipment.

TESTS USED IN THE DIAGNOSIS OF BACTERIAL INFECTIONS
(Table 9–4)

The agglutination test is widely employed in the diagnosis of bacterial infection, particularly those involving gram-negative organisms such as brucellae and salmonellae. The usual procedure in bacterial agglutination tests is to titrate serum (antibody) against a standard suspension of antigen. Bacteria are not, of course, antigenically homogeneous but are, in fact, covered by a mosaic of many different antigens. Thus, motile organisms will have flagellar (H) antigens, and agglutination by anti-H antibodies will produce fluffy cottonlike floccules as the flagellae stick together, leaving the bacterial bodies only loosely agglutinated. Agglutination of the somatic (O) antigens results in tight clumping of the bacterial bodies so that the agglutination is finely granular in character. Many organisms possess several O and H antigens as well as capsular (K) antigens. By means of a battery of specific antisera it is therefore possible to characterize the antigenic structure of an organism and consequently to classify it. It is, for instance, on this basis that the 1500 or so different species of salmonellae are classified.

O antigens are heat resistant and therefore remain intact on heat-killed organisms, whereas H antigens are heat labile. K antigens vary in their heat stability: the L

Table 9–4   SOME TESTS COMMONLY USED IN THE DIAGNOSIS OF SELECTED BACTERIAL INFECTIONS

DISEASE	TUBE AGGLU-TINATION	COMPLE-MENT FIXATION TEST	PASSIVE HEMAG-GLUTINA-TION	SKIN TEST	VAGINAL AGGLU-TINATION
Campylobacteriosis	+	−	−	−	+
Salmonellosis	+	−	−	−	−
Glanders	+	+	+	+	−
Erysipelas	+	+	+	−	−
Leptospirosis	+*	+	+	−	−
Listeriosis	+	−	−	−	−
Johne's disease	−	+	−	+	−
Tuberculosis	−	−	−	+	−
Contagious equine metritis	+	−	+	−	−

*A microagglutination test is probably the best of the available tests for leptospirosis.

antigen of *E. coli*, which is a capsular antigen, is heat labile, whereas another K antigen, antigen A, is heat stable. *Salmonella typhosa* possesses an antigen known as Vi, which although heat stable, is removed from the bacterial cells by heating. The presence of K or Vi antigens on an organism may render them O-inagglutinable and thus complicate agglutination tests. It should also be pointed out that rough variants of organisms (Chapter 13) do not form stable suspensions and therefore cannot be typed by means of an agglutination test.

Bacterial agglutination tests may be performed by mixing drops of reagents on glass slides or by titrating the reagents in test tubes or wells in plastic plates. Tube agglutination tests are commonly used for such diseases as salmonellosis, brucellosis, tularemia and campylobacteriosis. Slide agglutination tests are commonly used as screening tests. They include the brucella acid-antigen tests, in which organisms stained with the red dye rose-bengal are suspended in an acidic buffer (pH 3.6). There are several different tests of this type. The tests employed in the United Kingdom and Australia are considered to be relatively sensitive but of low specificity and as such may be used as screening tests to remove negative animals from further consideration. In contrast, the card test employed in the United States and Canada is considered to be of reduced sensitivity but is more specific than the other tests and consequently may be employed to eliminate positive animals.

One test for *Salmonella pullorum* in poultry is a slide agglutination test in which *S. pullorum* stained with gentian violet is mixed with whole chicken blood. Because of the stain, agglutination of the organisms is readily seen when the chicken carries antibodies to this organism. Leptospirosis is diagnosed by a "microscopic" agglutination test in which mixtures of living organisms and test serum are examined under the microscope for agglutination. This technique appears to detect IgM antibodies preferentially and is thus an excellent test for detecting recent outbreaks as well as for distinguishing between infected and vaccinated animals.

It is not mandatory that serum be used as the source of antibody for diagnostic tests. The presence of antibodies in body fluids other than serum, such as milk whey, vaginal mucus or nasal washings, may be of more significance, especially if the infection is of a local or superficial nature. One such test is the milk ring test used to

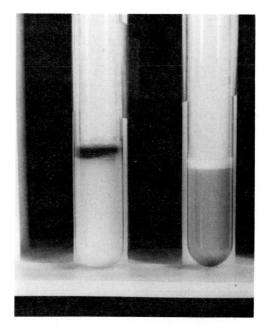

Figure 9–23 The milk ring test. Stained brucella remains suspended in the milk fraction in a negative test (*right*) but rises with the cream in a positive reaction (*left*). (Courtesy of Mr. E. L. Thackeray.)

detect the presence of antibodies to *B. abortus* in milk (Fig. 9–23). Fresh milk is shaken with organisms stained with hematoxylin or triphenyl tetrazolium and is allowed to stand. If antibodies, especially those of the IgM class, are present, then the organisms will clump and adhere to the fat globules of the milk and rise to the surface with the cream. If antibodies are absent, then the stained organisms will remain dispersed in the milk and the cream, on rising, will remain white.

The Serodiagnosis of Bovine Brucellosis (Table 9–5). In their attempts to eradicate brucellosis from their cattle, the countries of North America and Western Europe have employed vaccination of calves with strain 19 vaccine in conjunction with the serological detection and slaughter of infected animals. Unfortunately, since strain 19 of *Brucella abortus* is a living vaccine, the process of vaccination may be thought of as being nothing more than a controlled infection. It is therefore difficult to distinguish between the immune response to strain 19 and the response to natural infection. In order to assist in this differentiation, it has been usual to restrict the practice of vaccination to young animals so that their serum response will have declined to low levels by the time of serological testing as adults. Consequently, if antibodies are present in adult animals, they may be present in high levels as a result of infection or, alternatively, in low levels as a result either of very recent infection or of calfhood vaccination. In addition, some adult cattle possess a low level of anti-brucella antibodies in spite of a complete absence of infection. Therefore, the correct interpretation of the serological results from animals showing low levels of antibody is a matter of critical importance.

The most convenient of the serological tests available for the diagnosis of brucellosis is the serum agglutination test (SAT) performed in tubes. This test mainly detects strongly agglutinating antibodies of the IgM or IgG2 subclasses. Unfortunately, it has two major deficiencies. First, the major immunoglobulin produced in response to brucella infections is IgG1. IgG1 is not only a poor agglutinator but in excess is liable to block the agglutinating activity of IgM, resulting in false-negative reactions. Sec-

Table 9–5 SOME TESTS USED IN THE DIAGNOSIS OF BOVINE BRUCELLOSIS
AND IN THE DIFFERENTIATION BETWEEN VACCINATED AND
INFECTED CATTLE

TEST FOR BRUCELLOSIS	IMMUNOGLOBULIN CLASS DETECTED	ADVANTAGES OR DISADVANTAGES
ROUTINE TESTS		
Serum agglutination test (SAT)	IgM, IgG2, ³IgG1	Simple and standardized but fails to detect some nonagglutinating antibody and cannot differentiate vaccinated animals.
Complement fixation test (CFT)	IgG1 (IgM)	Complicated but detects nonagglutinating antibody and differentiates vaccinated animals.
OTHER ROUTINE TESTS		
Plate agglutination test	IgM, IgG2, IgG1	Simple but also fails to detect some non-agglutinating antibody.
Rose-bengal (acid-antigen) plate test	IgG1, IgM, (IgG2?)	Simple but sensitivity and specificity may vary.
Milk ring test	IgM, IgA, IgG	May be used in testing bulk milk.
SUPPLEMENTAL TESTS		
Heat inactivation test	IgG	IgM is destroyed reducing nonspecific reactions but also eliminating some specific reactions.
Rivanol precipitation agglutination test	IgG	
Mercaptoethanol agglutination test	IgG	

ond, false-positive reactions are associated with the SAT either because of residual antibodies produced following calfhood vaccination or as a result of ill-understood immunological reactions occurring in cattle unaffected by brucellosis.

The use of the complement fixation test (CFT) has largely overcome these problems, and the CFT has replaced the SAT in many countries in which eradication schemes are in progress. Since both IgG1 and IgM will fix guinea pig complement the CFT can be used on bovine serum, and is thus much less likely to produce false-negative reactions than the SAT. In addition, CFT titers do not persist in vaccinated cattle. This is probably because heating of the test serum to destroy complement also effectively destroys any residual IgM antibodies.

An alternative method of eliminating false-negative reactions in the SAT is to employ acid-antigen plate tests. These are plate agglutination tests carried out at low pH (3.6) buffer. At this pH, IgG1 becomes agglutinating, although the precise mechanisms involved are unclear. The indirect antiglobulin test may also be used to detect nonagglutinating antibodies.

To eliminate false-positive reactions in serum due to vaccination or non-brucella reactions, the IgM may be destroyed with mercaptoethanol. A positive agglutination reaction in the presence of this compound indicates the presence of IgG antibodies. Other techniques to reduce false-positive reactions involve precipitating out the IgM with Rivanol or heating the serum to 65°C for 15 minutes prior to testing. Either of these techniques selectively eliminates IgM antibodies while leaving IgG antibodies unaffected. The presence of a calcium chelating agent such as EDTA may also reduce some false-positive reactions. The simplest method of eliminating "nonspecific" antibodies is to sacrifice sensitivity for the sake of specificity and choose to ignore agglutination reactions occurring below an arbitrarily chosen titer. Consequently, for example, the SAT may be considered to be only unequivocally positive if a reaction is obtained at a titer of 1:100 in unvaccinated animals and at 1:200 in vaccinated ones.

Finally, it should be pointed out that infected cattle may occasionally have low antibody titers, and at times IgM may be the only class present. For this reason it is essential that the serological tests for brucellosis be interpreted with caution and in conjunction with careful analysis of the field situation.

TESTS USED IN THE DIAGNOSIS OF VIRAL DISEASES

Tests Used to Detect and Identify Viruses. Among the simplest and most widely employed tests for the detection of viruses are the direct and indirect fluorescent antibody techniques. These may be used to identify virus in the tissues of an infected animal as is done in rabies. If it is not possible to do this, it is usually necessary to grow the virus in experimental animals, chick embryos or tissue cultures in order to provide sufficient antigen for testing. Once sufficient virus has accumulated, it may be identified by its reaction with specific antiserum. The tests commonly employed for this purpose are fluorescent antibody tests, hemagglutination inhibition, virus neutralization, complement fixation and gel precipitation. The precise tests employed will depend on the nature of the unknown virus. Hemagglutination inhibition tests are technically simple and are preferred if the virus is a hemagglutinating one. They do, however, tend to be strain specific. The complement fixation test and gel precipitation test, as a broad generalization, tend to be largely group specific and thus lend themselves to attempts to identify the genus to which a virus belongs. In contrast, virus neutralization tests tend to be highly strain specific, so much so that they are perhaps best employed in the classification of a virus into its subtypes rather than in identifying the specific genus of a particular organism. There are, of course, exceptions to these generalizations: for example, the New Jersey and Indiana strains of vesicular stomatitis virus do not cross-react in the complement fixation test.

IMMUNOELECTRON MICROSCOPY. Specific antibodies may be employed to selectively enrich virus suspensions prior to electron microscopy. For example, a feces sample may be centrifuged, leaving a clear supernatant that contains a small number of many different viruses. After sonication to break up clumps, antibody specific for the virus of interest is added to the supernatant and, after a brief incubation, the fluid is centrifuged again. Virus particles clumped by antibody will be spun to the bottom, where they can be removed and examined by electron microscopy after negative staining (Fig. 9–24). The antibody, by clumping only the virus of interest, renders it much more visible in the electron microscope, and the presence of visible antibody within the virus-clumps provides direct confirmation of the identity of the virus.

Tests Used to Identify Antiviral Antibodies. In general, the most widely employed techniques for the identification of antibodies to viruses are hemagglutination inhibition, indirect ELISA, gel diffusion, complement fixation and virus neutralization. The first three of these are technically simple and are thus preferred. The complement fixation test and the virus neutralization tests are complex, thus restricting the circumstances in which they may be employed. The virus neutralization tests are also

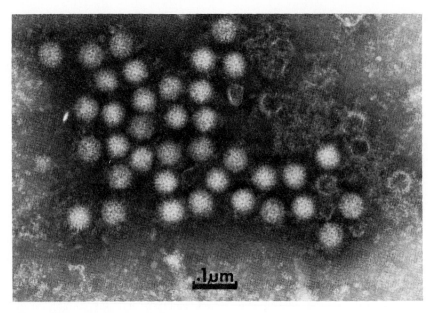

Figure 9–24 Immunoelectron microscopy of porcine rotavirus with convalescent antiserum. × 130,500. (Courtesy of Dr. L. Saif.)

extremely specific, which, as discussed earlier, tends to reduce their value as screening tests.

TESTS USED IN THE DIAGNOSIS OF PROTOZOAN INFECTIONS (Table 9–6)

In general, the tests used for the diagnosis of protozoan infections resemble those used in other situations. Thus, the complement fixation test, immunofluorescence techniques and passive agglutination are used in the diagnosis of toxoplasmosis, piroplasmosis and trichomoniasis. The Sabin-Feldman dye test was commonly used in toxoplasmosis but has now been largely replaced by the indirect fluorescent antibody test, which in turn is being replaced by the indirect ELISA.

Table 9–6 TESTS USED IN THE DIAGNOSIS OF SOME
SELECTED PROTOZOAN INFECTIONS

ORGANISM	DIRECT AGGLU-TINATION	PASSIVE HEMAG-GLUTINA-TION	COMPLE-MENT FIXATION	FLUO-RESCENT ANTIBODY TESTS	GEL DIFFUSION	SKIN TESTS
Coccidiosis	−	−	−	−	−	−
Toxoplasmosis	−	+	+	+	−	+
Babesiosis	+	+	+	+	+	−
Trichomoniasis	+	+	+	+	−	+
Trypanosomiasis	+	+	+	−	−	−

ADDITIONAL SOURCES OF INFORMATION

Journal

The Journal of Immunological Methods. Elsevier North-Holland (Biomedical Press), Amsterdam.

References

Delaat ANC. 1976. Primer of Serology. Harper & Row Pubs. Inc., New York.

Faulk WP. 1972. Recent developments in immunofluorescence. Prog. Allergy *16* 9–39.

Fernie DS, Cayzer I, and Chalmers SR. 1979. A passive hemagglutination test for the detection of antibodies to the contagious equine metritis organism. Vet Rec *104* 260–262.

Friedman H, Linna TJ, and Prier JE (eds). 1979. Immunoserology in the Diagnosis of Infectious Diseases. University Park Press, Baltimore.

Lennette EH, and Schmidt NJ (eds). 1979. Diagnostic Procedures for Viral Rickettsial and Chlamydial Infections. 5th Ed. American Public Health Association, Washington, DC.

Milstein C. 1980. Monoclonal antibodies. Sci Am *243* 66–74.

Pollack W, and Reckel RP. 1977. A reappraisal of forces involved in hemagglutination. Int Arch Allergy Appl Immunol *54* 29–42.

Rice CE. 1968. Comparative serology of domestic animals. Adv Vet Sci *12* 105–162.

Rose NR, and Friedman H (eds). 1980. Manual of Clinical Immunology, 2nd Ed. American Society of Microbiology, Washington, DC.

Schultz RD, and Adams LS. 1978. Immunologic methods for the detection of humoral and cellular immunity. Vet Clin North Am (Small Animal Practice) *8* 721–753.

Sutherland SS. 1980. Immunology of bovine brucellosis. Vet Bull *50* 359–368.

10

Immunity at Body Surfaces

Although animals possess an extensive array of defense mechanisms within the body, it is at the surface of an animal that invading microorganisms are first encountered and largely repelled or destroyed. The protective systems at body surfaces achieve this by establishing, through physical and chemical mechanisms, environments suitable for only the most adapted microorganisms. These surfaces are populated by an extensive microbial flora that, because it is well adapted, is also of low pathogenicity and effectively prevents the establishment of other, more poorly adapted and potentially pathogenic organisms. This environmental defense system is supplemented by immunological mechanisms in areas where the physical barriers to invasion are relatively weak.

NONIMMUNOLOGICAL SURFACE-PROTECTIVE MECHANISMS (Table 10–1)

That most obvious of the body surfaces, the skin, serves a number of functions, one of which is to present a barrier to invading microorganisms. The skin carries a dense and stable resident bacterial flora whose composition is regulated by a number of factors, including continuing desquamation, desiccation and a relatively low pH that is due, in part, to the presence of fatty acids in sebum. If any of these environmental factors is altered, then the composition of the skin flora is disturbed, its protective properties are reduced, and invasion may occur in consequence. Thus, skin infections tend to occur in areas such as the axilla or groin where both pH and humidity are relatively high. Similarly, animals forced to stand in water or mud show an increased frequency of foot infections as the skin becomes sodden, its structure breaks down, and its resident flora changes in response to alterations in the local environment.

The importance of the resident flora is seen to much greater effect in the digestive

Table 10–1 SOME NONIMMUNOLOGICAL PROTECTIVE MECHANISMS THAT ASSIST IN PREVENTING MICROBIAL INVASION AT BODY SURFACES

TYPE	*EXAMPLES*
Physical mechanisms	Desiccation
	pH extremes
	Desquamation
	Mucus barrier
	Fluid flow: e.g., saliva, urine, milk, vomiting, diarrhea
Chemical factors	Lysozyme
	Fatty acids
	Gastric acid
	Proteolytic enzymes
Biological factors	Competition with normal flora
	Antibiosis
	Generation of anaerobic or acidic conditions

tract, since it is essential not only for the control of potential pathogens but also for the digestion of some foods, such as cellulose in the diet of herbivores. In addition, the natural development of the immune system depends upon the continuous antigenic stimulation provided by intestinal flora. Because of the absence of a bacterial flora, gnotobiotic (germ-free) animals have hypoplastic secondary lymphoid organs that do not develop such features as secondary follicles. If the natural flora of the intestine is eliminated or its composition drastically altered (by aggressive antibiotic treatment, for example), then dietary disturbances result and the overgrowth of potential pathogens may occur. The flora of the digestive tract normally acts competitively against potential invaders through a number of mechanisms that supplement the other physical defenses of this system. Thus, in the mouth, the flushing activity of saliva is complemented by the generation of peroxidases from streptococci. In the stomach of some animals the gastric pH may be sufficiently low to have some bactericidal and viricidal effect, although this varies greatly between species and between meals. The dog, for instance, has a relatively low gastric pH relative to that of the pig. Similarly, the pH in the center of a mass of ingested food may not necessarily drop to low levels, and some foods such as milk are known to be potent buffers.

Farther down the intestine the resident bacterial flora tends to ensure that the pH is kept relatively low and the contents slightly anaerobic. The intestinal flora is also influenced indirectly by the diet; for instance, the intestine of milk-fed animals tends to be colonized largely by lactobacilli, which produce large quantities of bacteriostatic lactic and butyric acids. These acids inhibit colonization by potential pathogens such as *Escherichia coli*, so that young animals suckled naturally tend to have fewer digestive upsets than animals weaned early in life. In the large intestine the bacterial flora is composed largely of strict anaerobes.

Lysozyme (Chapter 13), the antibacterial and antiviral enzyme, is synthesized in the gastric mucosa and in macrophages within the intestinal mucosa. As a consequence, it is found in relatively large quantities in all the intestinal fluids. The role of phagocytic cells in the intestine is not clear, but macrophages do move out through the intestinal wall and may be active for a short time within the lumen.

In the urinary system, the flushing action and low pH of urine generally provide adequate protection; however, when urinary stasis occurs, urethritis resulting from the unhindered ascent of pathogenic bacteria is not uncommon. In adult female animals, the vagina is lined by a squamous epithelium composed of cells rich in glycogen. When these cells desquamate, they provide a substrate for lactobacilli that, in turn, generate large quantities of lactic acid, which protects the vagina against invasion. Glycogen storage in the vaginal epithelial cells is stimulated by estrogens and thus occurs only in sexually mature animals. Because of this, vaginal infections in humans tend to be commonest prior to puberty and after the menopause.

The protective mechanisms of the udder are, presumably, not of the most effective kind, at least in that biological anomaly the modern dairy cow. The flushing action of the milk serves to prevent invasion by some potential pathogens while milk itself contains bacterial inhibitors. A general term for these antibacterial substances in milk is lactenins. Lactenins include complement, lysozyme, the iron-binding protein lactoferrin and the enzyme lactoperoxidase. Lactoferrin competes with bacteria for iron and therefore renders it unavailable for their growth (see Chapter 13). Milk contains high concentrations of lactoperoxidase and thiocyanate (SCN^-) ions. In the presence of exogenous hydrogen peroxide the lactoperoxidase can oxidize the SCN^- to bacteriostatic products such as sulfur dicyanide. The hydrogen peroxide may be produced by bacteria such as streptococci or, alternatively, by the oxidation of ascorbic acid. Some strains of streptococci are resistant to this bacteriostatic pathway, since they possess an enzyme that reduces the SCN^-. The phagocytic cells released into the udder in response to irritation may also contribute to antimicrobial resistance not only through their phagocytic efforts but also by providing additional lactoferrin and lysosomal peroxidases.

The respiratory tract differs from the other body surfaces in that it is in intimate connection with the interior of the body and it is required by its very nature to allow unhindered access of air to the alveoli. The system obviously requires a filter. In fact, air entering the respiratory tract is largely deprived of any suspended particles by turbulence that directs particulate matter onto its mucus-covered walls, where it adheres. The turbulence is brought about by the conformation of the turbinate bones, the trachea and the bronchi. This "turbulence filter" serves to remove particles as small as 5 μm in size before they reach the alveoli (Fig. 10–1).

The walls of the upper respiratory tract are covered by a layer of mucus produced by goblet cells and provided with "antiseptic" properties through its content of lysozyme and IgA. This mucus layer is in continuous flow, being carried from the bronchioles up the bronchi and trachea by ciliary action or backward through the nasal cavity to the pharynx. Here the "dirty" mucus is swallowed and presumably digested in the intestinal tract. Particles smaller than 5 μm that can by-pass this "mucociliary escalator" and reach the alveoli are phagocytosed by alveolar macrophages. Once these cells have successfully ingested particles, they migrate to the mucus "escalator" and in this way are also carried to the pharynx and eliminated.

IMMUNOLOGICAL SURFACE-PROTECTIVE MECHANISMS

Immunoglobulins A and E.   In addition to the environmental and chemical factors that protect body surfaces, there are two immunoglobulin classes that tend to

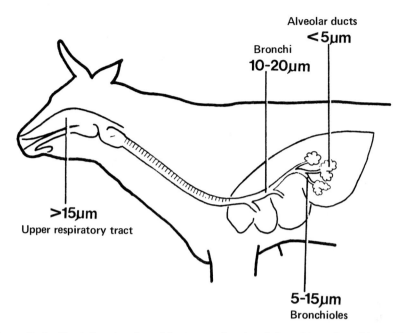

Figure 10–1 The influence of particle size on the site of deposition of particles within the respiratory tract.

be found in relatively high concentration in secretions such as saliva, intestinal fluid, nasal and tracheal secretions, tears, milk and colostrum, urine and the secretions of the urogenital tract (Table 10–2). Immunoglobulin E tends to be largely associated with immunity to helminths and type I hypersensitivities and so will be discussed in Chapters 15 and 17. Immunoglobulin A, however, appears to have evolved specifically for the purpose of protecting body surfaces.

The IgA monomer is a 6.8S molecule with a molecular weight of about 160,000 daltons having a typical four-chain Y-shaped structure and a somewhat elevated carbohydrate content relative to the other immunoglobulin classes. It tends to polymerize and is therefore usually found as a 9.3S dimer with the subunits bound together

Table 10–2 APPROXIMATE IgA LEVELS IN THE SERUM AND VARIOUS SECRETIONS OF THE DOMESTIC ANIMALS

ANIMAL	*SECRETION (mg/100 ml)*					
	SERUM	*COLOS-TRUM*	*MILK*	*NASAL SECRE-TIONS*	*SALIVA*	*TEARS*
Horse	170	1000	130	160	140	150
Cow	30	400	10	200	56	260
Sheep	30	400	10	50	90	160
Pig	200	1000	500	*	*	*
Dog	50	1500	400	*	*	*
Chicken	50			*	20	15

*Figures not currently available to the author.

through a J chain. IgA dimers can bind a protein with a molecular weight of 71,000 daltons synthesized by intestinal epithelial cells and hepatocytes and termed secretory component, to produce secretory IgA (SIgA), which is a 10.8S molecule with a molecular weight of about 400,000 daltons (Fig. 10–2). Secretory component renders IgA relatively resistant to proteolysis by digestive enzymes, although this resistance does vary between IgA subclasses. For example, porcine SIgA1 is more resistant than SIgA2 to pepsin digestion, but SIgA2 is more resistant than SIgA1 to some of the bacterial proteases found in the intestine. (It is of interest to note that pigs possess a subpopulation of circulating mononuclear cells with receptors for secretory component. The function of these cells or their receptor is unknown.)

Although it is apparent that IgA exerts a significant protective effect on mucosal surfaces, its mode of action is not completely clear. IgA, for instance, is not bactericidal, does not bind to macrophages or enhance phagocytosis, and fixes complement only by the alternate pathway. It does, however, have virus neutralizing activity, and it can also neutralize some viral and bacterial enzymes. Its most important mode

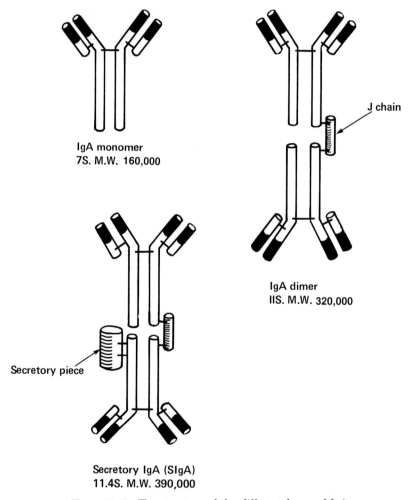

IgA monomer
7S. M.W. 160,000

J chain

IgA dimer
IIS. M.W. 320,000

Secretory piece

Secretory IgA (SIgA)
11.4S. M.W. 390,000

Figure 10–2 The structure of the different forms of IgA.

of action is to prevent adherence of bacteria and viruses to epithelial surfaces. The importance of this adherence may be seen, for example, in diseases of the intestinal tract caused by strains of *E. coli* possessing the K88 antigen. The K88 antigen is a pilus-like structure by which these organisms may bind to intestinal epithelial cells, so preventing their expulsion and promoting proliferation and enterotoxin production. Antibodies made specifically against the K88 antigen can inhibit this bacterial adherence and hence may protect animals against disease caused by these strains of *E. coli*.

IgA is synthesized by plasma cells in the gut-associated lymphoid tissue (GALT) in response to local antigenic stimulation. Much of this IgA diffuses directly into the intestinal lumen. As it diffuses, it combines with secretory component synthesized by intestinal epithelial cells. However, a significant proportion also diffuses into the portal circulation and is thus carried to the liver. Hepatocytes synthesize secretory component and incorporate it into their membrane, where it acts as an IgA receptor. The blood-borne IgA thus binds to hepatocytes, is absorbed into them and is carried across the hepatocyte cytoplasm to be released into the bile canaliculi. Bile is therefore extremely rich in IgA, and is a major route by which IgA reaches the intestinal lumen in nonruminants (Fig. 10–3). It is probably also a route by which foreign material bound to circulating IgA can be removed from the body.

The plasma cells in the GALT arise from precursor B cells. These B cells, upon encountering antigen, respond in a similar manner to lymphocytes elsewhere in the body—that is, they divide and some differentiate into plasma cells. However, some of these responding B cells are provoked into migrating into intestinal lymphatics, from which they reach the thoracic duct and the blood circulation. These recirculating cells have an affinity for body surfaces in general. As a result, they lodge throughout the intestinal tract, the respiratory tract, the urogenital tract and the mammary gland. The movement of IgA positive B cells to the mammary gland is of major importance in veterinary medicine, since it provides a route by which intestinal immunity can be

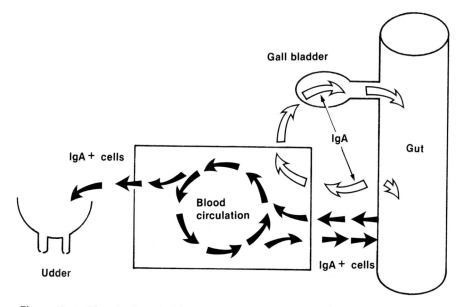

Figure 10–3 The circulation of IgA (white arrows) and of IgA-producing cells (black arrows). Both originate in the intestinal mucosa.

transferred to newborn animals via milk. Oral administration of antigen to a pregnant animal will result in the appearance of IgA antibodies in its milk. In this way the intestine of the newborn animal receives antibodies appropriate for any organisms it may encounter.

The ability to produce an anamnestic response appears to be relatively poorly developed in the surface immune systems. Multiple doses of antigen do not appear to increase the intensity or duration of the local immune response to any significant extent. The reasons for this are not clear but may relate to the structure of the intestinal lymphoid tissue, which, because it is not as formally organized as other lymphoid tissues with respect to the secondary follicles, cannot, perhaps, process antigen quite as efficiently for a secondary response.

Immunoglobulin G.   In ruminants, especially the bovine, IgG1 functions as the major secretory immunoglobulin and is the predominant immunoglobulin in milk, intestinal contents and nasal washings. The presence of IgG1 in bovine bile suggests that it may also be transported through hepatocytes in a manner similar to IgA. (In sheep, very little immunoglobulin of any class is found in bile. IgA and IgG1 presumably move directly into the intestinal lumen in this species.)

Immunoglobulin M.   IgM is only a minor component in secretions, although it may bind secretory component and therefore be protected against proteolytic digestion.

IMMUNITY IN THE GASTROINTESTINAL TRACT

The gastrointestinal tract is probably the major site of antigenic stimulation in animals. Antigenic particles such as bacteria can penetrate the intestinal mucosa relatively easily and in this way gain access to the lacteals and portal vessels. These organisms consequently are trapped in the mesenteric lymph nodes and liver, respectively. Other antigens may enter the body via the surface lymphoid tissues. For instance, the tonsils are particularly vulnerable to invasion by microorganisms. Tonsils possess a peculiar structural weakness in that their squamous epithelial covering is particularly thin at the bottom of the tonsillar crypts (Fig. 10–4). Viruses especially may enter the body by this route and multiply locally in the tonsil prior to the development of a viremia. The tonsils and Peyer's patches consist of relatively organized lymphoid tissues, possessing all the components required to mount an immune response—namely T cells, B cells and macrophages. Nevertheless, most IgA is formed in diffuse lymphoid nodules and in isolated plasma cells found in the walls of the intestine, in salivary glands and in the gall bladder. If bacteria succeed in penetrating the intestinal wall, then in the ensuing inflammatory response, capillary permeability will increase and IgG will be free to diffuse from the blood stream to the area of invasion. Thus, IgG may also act to protect body surfaces but usually only secondarily to an inflammatory reaction.

Because of the poor anamnestic response in the secretory immunoglobulin system, it is probably not possible to confer lifelong protection against intestinal infection using killed organisms as a vaccine. However, oral vaccination may be of some use in protecting against those diseases to which an animal is susceptible for only a short period. Diets containing killed *E. coli* given to calves and pigs have resulted in a reduced incidence of diarrhea, a better feedgain and an improvement in the overall health of the animals. Oral viable transmissible gastroenteritis vaccine may also be given to pregnant sows in order to stimulate an intestinal IgA response and seed

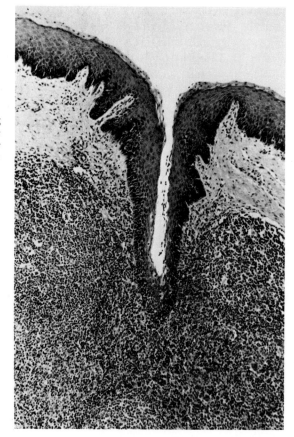

Figure 10–4 A section of pig tonsil showing a tonsillar crypt. Note how the epithelium thins out at the base of the crypt. × 150. (From a specimen kindly provided by Dr. S. Yamashiro.)

antibody-producing cells to the udder. This results in the appearance of specific antibodies in colostrum, and in the protection of suckling piglets.

IMMUNITY IN THE MAMMARY GLAND

The mammary gland is protected in nonspecific fashion by the physical barrier of the teat canal, by the flushing action of the milk and by the presence of lactenins of which the lactoperoxidase-thiocyanate system, lactoferrin and lysozyme are probably the most important. (It should be pointed out that lysozyme levels are very low in bovine milk.) In addition, milk also contains IgA and IgG1 in low concentrations. In simple-stomached animals, IgA predominates, whereas in ruminants the reverse is the case (see Chapter 11).

IgA is usually locally synthesized in the udder. Many of the IgA-producing cells in the mammary gland are derived from precursors originating in the intestinal tract. Once these cells colonize the gland they provide a local source of antibodies. IgG1, in contrast, is selectively transferred by an active transport mechanism from serum. If antigen is infused into a lactating mammary gland, it tends to be promptly flushed out again in the milk. If it is infused into a nonlactating gland, then a local immune response develops in which IgA and IgG1 predominate. Unfortunately, because of the continuous production of milk, antibody concentration in this fluid is liable to be relatively low even though, over a period of time, the amount of immunoglobulin secreted from the udder may be considerable. Because of this flushing action and dilution, milk antibodies do not normally give effective protection against bacterial invasion. In contrast, in cases of acute mastitis, the inflammatory response leads to the influx of actively phagocytic cells, especially neutrophils, and to the exudation of serum proteins. Only in this way may milk immunoglobulins rise to reach levels at which they can exert a protective influence.

Because the local immune response in the udder is relatively ineffective in preventing infection, attempts at vaccination against mastitis-causing organisms have been unsuccessful. The difficulties encountered in vaccination attempts are also accentuated by the wide variety of potential mammary pathogens. For example, there are five different antigenic types of *Streptococcus agalactiae* alone. In addition, there is some antigenic cross-reaction between this organism and bovine tissues. Because of these difficulties, if a vaccine is being considered for a mastitis problem, it should be autogenous and should be given either into the nonlactating gland toward the end of the dry period or into the supramammary lymph node. It may be anticipated that such a procedure will not totally prevent mastitis, but it may at least lessen the severity of acute infections.

IMMUNITY IN THE UROGENITAL TRACT

Antibodies of several classes, but particularly IgA, are found in cervico-vaginal mucus. In cows infected with *Campylobacter fetus*, these IgA antibodies may immobilize the organisms and clump them. As might be expected, IgG antibodies can also be found in these secretions, being derived by transudation from serum and rising considerably when inflammatory reactions occur. In addition, the presence of many mononuclear cells as well as the capacity of *C. fetus* to produce delayed skin reactions (type IV hypersensitivity) is compatible with the possibility that cell-mediated immunity is also involved in resistance to this local infection. Preputial washings of bulls infected with this organism may also contain agglutinins, but these are largely IgG1 with some IgM and IgA. A similar form of local immune response may also be directed against other organisms that cause infections of the cervix-vagina, and the presence of agglutinating antibodies in vaginal mucus may be used as a diagnostic test for brucellosis, campylobacteriosis and trichomoniasis. (The local immune response to trichomoniasis is largely mediated by IgE; see Chapter 15.)

IgA is present in small amounts in normal urine, produced presumably by lymphoid tissues in the walls of the urinary tract. If, however, a nephritis occurs, then IgG may also be found in relatively large amounts because of the breakdown in the glomerular barrier and defects in tubular reabsorption.

IMMUNITY IN THE RESPIRATORY TRACT

In addition to the tonsils, the respiratory tract possesses a considerable amount of lymphoid tissue in the form of nodules in the walls of the bronchi as well as lymphocytes distributed diffusely throughout the lung and the walls of the airways. The immunoglobulin synthesized in these tissues is mainly secretory IgA, particularly

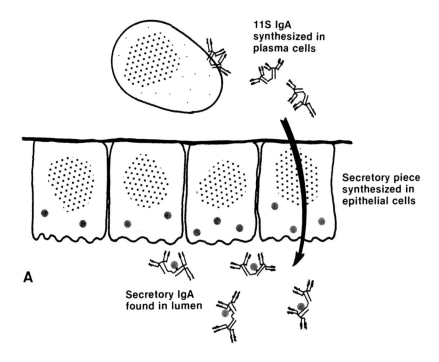

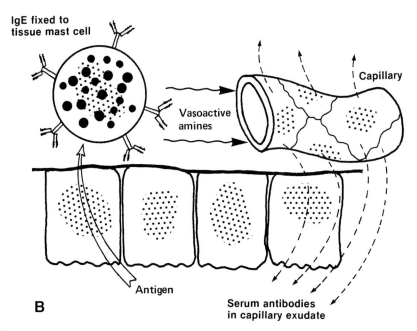

Figure 10–5 Two routes by which antibodies may reach and so protect mucosal surfaces. *A,* IgA antibodies diffuse through the mucosa and so bathe the surface in antibody. *B,* Antigen that penetrates the mucosa encounters mast cell–fixed IgE. The resulting release of vasoactive amines causes an increase in vascular permeability and exudation of large quantities of IgG.

in the upper regions of the respiratory tract. In the bronchioles and alveoli, however, the secretions contain a relatively large amount of IgG, the concentration of which is intermediate between the levels in the trachea and in serum. IgE is also synthesized in significant amounts in the lymphoid tissues of the upper respiratory tract. As on other body surfaces, IgA in the respiratory tract is thought to protect by preventing adherence of antigenic particles including microorganisms, whereas IgG is probably of major importance only when acute inflammation and transudation of serum protein occur. This situation will arise, for example, following a type I hypersensitivity reaction mediated by locally produced IgE, and it is tempting to suggest that the combination of IgA and IgE synthesis at mucosal surfaces is therefore not entirely fortuitous. It is possible that these immunoglobulins work in concert (Fig. 10–5), so that IgA produces a surface immunity serving to prevent antigen adherence and penetration. If, in spite of the presence of this IgA, antigen gains access to the tissues, then the subsequent IgE-mediated hypersensitivity reaction may serve to increase vascular permeability and make available large quantities of potent IgG in the resulting fluid exudate.

Large numbers of cells may be washed out of the lung by lavage with saline. These include alveolar macrophages and lymphocytes, and the lymphocytes are largely T cells. It is possible to demonstrate the production of macrophage migration inhibition factor by these cells under experimental situations and to show alveolar macrophage activation following infection with *Listeria monocytogenes*. It is likely, therefore, that cell-mediated immune reactions may be readily invoked among the cells that exist within the lower respiratory tract.

In attempting to vaccinate animals against diseases that cause local infections of the upper respiratory tract, such as bovine viral rhinotracheitis or parainfluenza 3, it would appear logical to apply antigen locally. In this way IgA production would be stimulated and invasion of the mucosa blocked. Systemic vaccination against these diseases gives a certain amount of immunity, since some IgG may be transferred from serum to the mucous surface; nevertheless, complete protection by IgG cannot be achieved in this way until invasion, inflammation and exudation have occurred.

ADDITIONAL SOURCES OF INFORMATION

Bienenstock J, and Befus AD. 1980. Mucosal immunology. Immunology *41* 249–270.
Bourne FJ. 1977. The mammary gland and neonatal immunity. Vet Sci Commun *1* 141–151.
Colloquium on selected diarrheal diseases of the young. 1978. JAVMA *173* 509–676.
Crago SS, Kulhary R, Prince SJ, and Mestecky J. 1978. Secretory component on epithelial cells is a surface receptor for polymeric immunoglobulin. J Exp Med *147* 1832–1837.
Guy-Grand D, Griscelli C, and Vassalli P. 1978. The mouse gut T lymphocyte, a novel type of cell. J Exp Med *148* 1661–1677.
Husband AJ, and Watson DL. 1978. Immunity in the intestine. Vet Bull *48* 911–924.
Kaltreider HB. 1976. Expression of immune mechanisms in the lung. Am Rev Resp Dis *113* 347–397.
Lamm ME. 1976. Cellular aspects of immunoglobulin A. Adv Immunol *22* 223–290.
Lascelles AK. 1979. The immune system of the ruminant mammary gland and its role in the control of mastitis. J Dairy Sci *62* 154–160.
Osborne CA, Klausner JS, and Lees GE. 1979. Urinary tract infections: normal and abnormal host defense mechanisms. Vet Clin North Am (Small Animal Practice) *9* 587–609.
Reiter B. 1978. Review of the progress of dairy science: antimicrobial systems in milk. J Dairy Res *45* 131–147.
Tomasi TB, Larson L, Challacombe S, and McNabb P. 1980. Mucosal immunity: the origin and migration patterns of cells in the secretory system. J Allergy Clin Immunol *65* 12–19.
Walker WA, and Isselbacher KJ. 1977. Intestinal antibodies. New Engl J Med *297* 767–773.
Wells PW, Dawson A McL, Smith WD, and Smith BSW. 1975. Transfer of IgG from plasma to nasal secretions in newborn lambs. Vet Rec *97* 455.

11

Immunity in the Fetus and Newborn Animal

Dizygotic cattle twins with anastomosing placental circulations are born with a mixture of blood cells. In spite of the fact that some of these cells are derived from the twin, they persist throughout each animal's life. Thus, exposure to foreign cells early in fetal life plus their persistence has led to the development of a state of tolerance. In the clonal selection theory, as first suggested by Burnet and Fenner, these "chimeras" were presented as evidence for the inability of the fetal animal to respond to antigen and to produce a "classic" immune response. Burnet and Fenner postulated that exposure of antigen-sensitive cells to potential antigens prior to birth resulted in tolerance and that this, therefore, accounted for the inability of the immune system to respond to self-antigens. Their theory seemed to be confirmed by the observation of Medawar that fetal mice exposed to foreign tissue cells while *in utero* became tolerant to them and so could retain skin grafts from the donor strain indefinitely. In contrast, mice exposed to the same cells after birth were capable of mounting an immune response as shown by prompt rejection of grafts from the donor strain.

In spite of the occurrence of calf chimeras, the young of the domestic animals differ markedly from the rodent models: their immune system is fully developed well before birth and considerable difficulty is encountered in producing tolerance by fetal immunization. Newborn domestic animals are therefore susceptible to infectious disease not because of any inherent incapacity to mount an immune response but because of the unprimed state of their immune system.

ONTOGENY OF THE IMMUNE SYSTEM

The development of the immune system appears to follow a consistent pattern. The thymus is the first lymphoid organ to develop and is followed closely by the secondary lymphoid organs. Immunoglobulin-containing cells are found almost immediately, but serum immunoglobulins are not usually found until some time later, if at all. The ability to respond to antigens may develop very rapidly after the lymphoid organs appear, but all antigens are not equally capable of stimulating fetal lymphoid tissue. It is possible to show a progressive increase in the number of antigens capable of provoking antibody formation in the fetus as development proceeds. The ability to mount cell-mediated immune responses develops at about the same time as antibody production.

Calf. The immune system of the calf develops very early in fetal life. Although the gestation period of the cow is 280 days, the fetal thymus is recognizable by 40 days postconception (Fig. 11–1). The bone marrow and spleen appear at 55 days. Lymph nodes are found at 60 days, but Peyer's patches do not appear until 75 days. The late development of the Peyer's patches suggests that they are probably not primary lymphoid tissues and therefore cannot be considered to be the mammalian bursal equivalent. Peripheral blood lymphocytes are seen in fetal calves by day 45, IgM-carrying cells by day 59, and IgG-carrying cells by day 135. The time of the earliest detection of serum antibodies depends on the sensitivity of the techniques used. It is, therefore, no accident that the earliest detectable immune responses are those directed against viruses, using exquisitely sensitive virus neutralization techniques. Calves have been reported to respond to rotavirus at 73 days and to parvovirus at 93 days. Calf peripheral blood lymphocytes can respond to pokeweed mitogen at

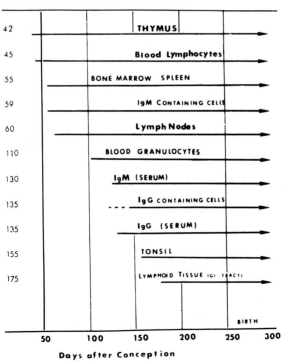

Figure 11–1 The ontogeny of the immune system in the bovine. (From Schultz RD. 1973. *Cornell Vet 63* 507–535. Used with permission.)

day 90, but this ability is temporarily lost around the time of birth as a result of elevated serum steroid levels.

Lamb. The gestation period of the ewe is about 145 days. The thymus and lymph nodes are recognizable by 35 and 50 days postconception respectively, but the Peyer's patches appear only at 80 to 90 days. Peripheral blood lymphocytes are seen in fetal lambs by day 35. They can produce antibodies to phage ϕx 174 at day 41 and reject allogeneic skin grafts by day 77. Antibodies to SV40 virus can be provoked by day 90, to T4 phage by day 105, to bluetongue by day 122 and to lymphocytic choriomeningitis virus by day 140.

Piglet. The gestation period of the sow is about 115 days. The porcine thymus develops by 40 days. Fetal piglets can produce antibodies to parvoviruses at 72 days and can reject allografts at approximately the same time. The number of circulating Ig-bearing cells rises dramatically between 70 and 80 days. The response to antigens in the fetus is essentially of the IgM type, but newborn and fetal piglets also produce a 4S immunoglobulin that may not have light chains.

Foal. The gestation period of the mare is about 340 days. Lymphoid cells are seen first in the thymus around 60 to 80 days postconception. They are found in the mesenteric lymph node and intestinal lamina propria at 90 days and in the spleen at 175 days. Peripheral blood lymphocytes appear at around 80 days. The equine fetus can respond to coliphage T2 at 200 days postconception and to Venezuelan equine encephalitis at 230 days. Normal newborn foals may have some serum IgM prior to suckling. In spite of this, it is claimed that plasma cells are not normally seen until about 240 days.

Puppy. The gestation period of the bitch is about 60 days. The thymus differentiates around day 28 and fetal puppies can respond to phage ϕx 174 on day 40. Peripheral blood lymphocytes will respond to phytohemagglutinin by 45 days postconception, and these cells can be detected in lymph nodes around 45 to 50 days and in the spleen by 50 to 55 days. The capacity to reject allografts also develops around day 45, although the rejection process is slow at this stage, and puppies may be made tolerant by intrauterine injection of antigen prior to day 42. Thymic seeding of T cells to the secondary lymphoid organs and the development of humoral immune responses therefore appears to be a relatively late phenomenon in the dog as compared with the other domestic animals.

Chick. Stem cells arise in the yolk sac membrane and migrate under chemotactic influences to the thymus and bursa between 5 and 7 days' incubation. These cells differentiate within the bursa, and follicles develop within this organ by 12 days. Lymphocytes with surface IgM that are able to bind antigen may be detected in the bursa by 14 days, and antibodies to keyhole limpet hemocyanin and to sheep erythrocytes may be produced by 16 and 18 days' incubation respectively. Lymphocytes with surface IgG develop on day 21 around the time of hatching, whereas IgA-positive cells first appear in the gut by three to seven days after hatching.

DEVELOPMENT OF PHAGOCYTIC CAPABILITY

In the fetal pig, peripheral blood leukocytes taken at 87 to 90 days postconception are fully capable of phagocytosing particles such as *S. aureus*. They are, however, deficient in bactericidal capacity, which only reaches adult levels by 100 days. Near the time of birth, the phagocytic and bactericidal capacity of these leukocytes declines as a result of an increase in fetal glucocorticoid synthesis. After birth, macrophages appear to have a depressed chemotactic responsiveness, and they are also able to support the growth of many viruses that macrophages from adult animals do not. Viricidal activity is gradually acquired, although this process appears to be under thymic influence, since the cells from neonatally thymectomized animals (mice) do not acquire this resistance, perhaps as a result of a deficiency of γ interferon. The serum of newborn animals is also deficient in some complement components, resulting in a poor opsonic activity that is reflected in an increased susceptibility to infection.

INFLUENCE OF THE ONTOGENY OF THE IMMUNE SYSTEM ON INTRAUTERINE INFECTION

Although the fetus is not totally defenseless, it is less capable than the adult of combating infection. It has been demonstrated that tissues taken from calves at 95 days post conception produce α and β interferon in amounts similar to those generated in adult tissues. It has also been shown, however, that the fetus is defective in production of γ interferon. Consequently, there are several diseases that may be mild or inapparent in the mother yet severe or lethal in the fetus. Examples of such diseases include bluetongue, infectious bovine rhinotracheitis (IBR), bovine virus diarrhea (BVD), rubella in humans and the protozoan infection toxoplasmosis.

In general, the response to these organisms is determined by the state of immunological development of the fetus. For example, if bluetongue vaccine, which is nonpathogenic for normal adult sheep, is given to pregnant ewes at 50 days postconception, it causes severe lesions in the nervous system of fetal lambs, including hydranencephaly and retinal dysplasia, whereas if it is given at 100 days or in newborn lambs, only a mild glial response is seen. Virus given to fetal lambs between 50 and 70 days postconception may be isolated from lamb tissues for several weeks, but if given after 100 days, reisolation is not usually possible.

Prenatal infection of calves with IBR virus produces an invariably fatal disease, in contrast to postnatal infection, which is relatively mild. The transition between these two types of infection occurs during the last month of pregnancy.

Infection of fetal calves with BVD prior to the development of their capacity to mount an immune response to this virus (day 200) leads to fetal death as a result of the development of severe malformations involving particularly the cerebellum and ocular tracts. Infections after this time lead to lymphoreticular hyperplasia and elevated immunoglobulin levels. This latter response is a common one; it is seen following many infections in which the fetus survives for a period. For this reason the presence of significant levels of immunoglobulins in a newborn, unsuckled animal is generally considered to be indicative of intrauterine antigenic stimulation.

IMMUNE RESPONSE OF NEWBORN ANIMALS

After developing in the essentially sterile environment of the uterus, newborn animals are launched into an environment rich in antigens. The young of the domestic animals are fully capable of mounting immune responses at birth. However, any immune response mounted by a newborn animal must of necessity be a primary response with both a relatively prolonged lag period and only low concentrations of antibodies produced. Therefore, unless immunological assistance is provided, newborn animals may succumb rapidly to organisms that present little threat to an adult. This "immunological assistance" is rendered in the form of passive immunity by means of antibody transferred from the mother through colostrum. Some evidence exists to suggest that maternal lymphoid cells may also be transferred to fetal lymphoid tissue via the placenta or to newborn animals through colostrum and transintestinal migration, but the biological significance of this is unclear.

TRANSFER OF IMMUNITY FROM MOTHER TO OFFSPRING

The route by which maternal antibodies reach the fetus is determined by the nature of the placental barrier (Table 11–1). In humans and other primates, the placenta is hemochorial—that is, the maternal blood is in direct contact with the trophoblast. This type of placentation allows IgG but not IgM, IgA or IgE to transfer to the fetus. In this way, maternal IgG may enter the fetal blood stream and the newborn human infant may have circulating IgG levels comparable to those of its mother. As a result of this IgG transfer, the infant is protected against septicemic infection. Nevertheless, the intestine of the human infant is not protected by this circulating IgG, and so the IgA required to protect the intestine from infection must be provided from maternal milk. Therefore, infants who are not breast-fed are more likely to suffer from digestive disturbances than those who are.

Dogs and cats possess an endotheliochorial placenta in which the chorionic epithelium is in contact with the endothelium of the maternal capillaries. In these species a small amount of IgG (5 to 10 per cent) may transfer from the mother to the puppy or kitten, but most is obtained through colostrum.

The placenta of ruminants is syndesmochorial—that is, the chorionic epithelium is in direct contact with uterine tissues, whereas the placenta of horses and pigs is

Table 11–1 RELATIONSHIP BETWEEN PLACENTAL TYPE AND TRANSFER OF IMMUNOGLOBULINS FROM MOTHER TO FETUS VIA PLACENTA OR COLOSTRUM

SPECIES	*TYPE OF PLACENTATION*	*TISSUE LAYERS INTERVENING BETWEEN MATERNAL AND FETAL CIRCULATION*	*PLACENTAL TRANSFER OF IMMUNOGLOBULIN*	*COLOSTRAL TRANSFER OF IMMUNOGLOBULIN*
Pig, horse, donkey	Epitheliochorial	6*	0	+++
Ruminants	Syndesmochorial	5	0	+++
Dog and cat	Endotheliochorial	4	+	+++
Primates	Hemochorial	3	++	+
Rodents	Hemendothelial	1	+++	+

*maternal capillary endothelium, uterine tissue, uterine epithelium, chorionic epithelium, fetal connective tissue and fetal capillary endothelium

epitheliochorial and the fetal chorionic epithelium is in contact with intact uterine epithelium. In animals with both of these types of placentation, the transplacental passage of immunoglobulin molecules is totally prevented, and the newborn of these species are thus entirely dependent on antibodies received through the colostrum.

SECRETION AND COMPOSITION OF COLOSTRUM AND MILK (Tables 11–2 and 11–3)

Colostrum represents the accumulated secretions of the mammary gland over the last few weeks of pregnancy together with proteins transferred from the blood stream under the influence of estrogens and progesterone. It is, therefore, rich in IgG and IgA but also contains some IgM and IgE. The predominant immunoglobulin in the colostrum of all the major domestic animals is IgG, which may account for 65 to 90 per cent of its total immunoglobulin content; IgA and the other immunoglobulins tend to be minor but significant components. As lactation progresses and colostrum changes to milk, differences emerge between species. In primates and humans, IgA predominates in both colostrum and milk. In nonruminant domestic animals, IgG predominates in colostrum but its concentration drops rapidly as lactation proceeds (Fig. 11–2) and IgA predominates in milk. In ruminants, IgG1 is the predominant immunoglobulin in both milk and colostrum.

All of the IgG, most of the IgM and about half of the IgA in bovine colostrum are derived from serum, but only 30 per cent of the IgG and 10 per cent of the IgA in milk are so derived, the rest being produced locally in the udder. Colostrum also contains secretory component both in the free form and bound to IgA.

Absorption of Colostrum.　Young animals that suckle soon after birth take colostrum into their intestinal tract. In these young animals, the level of proteolytic activity in the digestive tract is low, and is further minimized by trypsin inhibitors in

Table 11–2　COLOSTRAL IMMUNOGLOBULIN LEVELS IN DOMESTIC ANIMALS

| SPECIES | IMMUNOGLOBULIN (mg/100 ml) | | | | |
	IgA	IgM	IgG	IgG(T)	IgG(B)
Horse	500–1500	100–350	1500–5000	500–2500	50–150
Bovine	100–700	300–1300	3400–8000		
Sheep	100–700	400–1200	4000–6000		
Pig	950–1050	250–320	3000–7000		
Dog	500–2200	14–57	120–300		

Table 11–3　MILK IMMUNOGLOBULIN LEVELS IN DOMESTIC ANIMALS

| SPECIES | IMMUNOGLOBULIN (mg/100 ml) | | | | |
	IgA	IgM	IgG	IgG(T)	IgG(B)
Horse	50–100	5–10	20–50	5–20	0
Bovine	10–50	10–20	50–750		
Sheep	5–12	0–7	60–100		
Sow	300–700	30–90	100–300		
Dog	110–620	10–54	1–3		

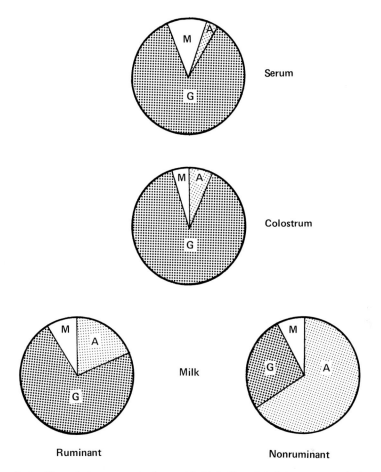

Figure 11–2   The relative concentrations of IgG, IgM and IgA in serum, colostrum and the milk of ruminants and nonruminants.

colostrum. Therefore, colostral proteins are not degraded and used as a food source but instead reach the small intestine, particularly the ileum, intact. Here they are actively taken up by epithelial cells through pinocytosis and passed through these cells into the lacteals and possibly the intestinal capillaries, eventually reaching the systemic circulation; in this way newborn animals obtain a massive transfusion of maternal immunoglobulin.

The domestic animals differ in the selectivity and duration of their intestinal permeability. In the horse and pig, protein absorption is somewhat selective, IgG and IgM being preferentially absorbed while SIgA is left in the intestine. In ruminants, the intestine is unselectively permeable and all immunoglobulins are absorbed, although IgA is gradually re-excreted. Young pigs and probably other young animals possess large amounts of free secretory component within their intestinal tract. Colostral IgA and, to a lesser extent, IgM can bind to the secretory component, which may serve to inhibit their absorption.

The period for which the intestine is permeable to proteins varies between species and, to a degree, between immunoglobulins. In general, permeability is highest immediately after birth and declines rapidly thereafter, perhaps because the intestinal cells that absorb immunoglobulins are replaced by a more mature cell population. The length of the absorptive period is a matter of debate among authorities. As a general rule, absorption of all immunoglobulin classes will have dropped to a relatively low level after approximately 24 hours.

Unsuckled animals normally possess extremely low levels of immunoglobulin in their serum. The successful absorption of colostral immunoglobulin immediately supplies them with serum immunoglobulins (particularly IgG) at a level approaching that found in adults (Fig. 11–3). Because of the nature of the absorptive process, peak serum immunoglobulin levels are normally reached between 12 and 24 hours after birth. After absorption ceases, these passively acquired antibodies will immediately commence to decline through normal catabolic processes. The rate of antibody decline depends upon the immunoglobulin class involved (Table 11–4), while the time taken for the immunoglobulins to decline to unprotective levels also depends on their initial concentration.

As intestinal absorption is taking place, a marked proteinuria is seen in young animals. This is largely due to the absorption from the intestine of proteins such as β-lactoglobulin and polypeptides that are sufficiently small to be excreted in the urine. In addition, the glomeruli of newborn animals are permeable to macromolecules so that the urine of neonatal ruminants also contains intact immunoglobulin molecules. The proteinuria ceases spontaneously with the termination of intestinal absorption.

The secretions of the mammary gland gradually change from colostrum to milk, which is rich in both IgG1 and IgA in ruminants and in IgA in nonruminants. For the first few weeks of life, while proteolytic digestion is poor, these immunoglobulins can be found throughout the length of the intestine and in the feces of young animals. As the digestive capacity of the intestine increases, eventually only IgA protected by secretory component is left intact. SIgA is therefore continuously present in the intestine of young animals and is the most important factor serving to protect them against enteric infection. The amount of IgA in the intestine can be relatively large; for instance, a three-week-old piglet may receive 1.6 g daily from the sow's milk.

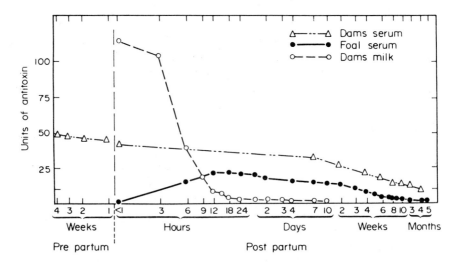

Figure 11–3 *Clostridium perfringens* antitoxin levels in serum, colostrum and milk of six pony mares and in the serum of their foals from birth to five months. (From Jeffcott LB. 1974. J Comp Pathol *84* 96. Used with permission.)

Table 11-4 METABOLIC HALF-LIVES OF SERUM IMMUNOGLOBULINS IN
DOMESTIC ANIMALS

| | HALF-LIFE (DAYS) | | | | |
SPECIES	IgG	IgA	IgM	IgG(T)	IgE
Horse	11.5 – 23	*	*	20	*
Bovine	17(G1) – 22(G2)	2.8	4.8		2.0
Sheep	14.5(G1) – 10.6(G2)	1.8	4.1		*
Sow	6.5 – 22.5	2.3	3.5–6.5		*
Chicken	4.1	1.7	*		*
Human	23	6.0	5.0		2.7

*Figures not currently available to the author.

The protective role of IgA has been discussed in the previous chapter. It should be pointed out, however, that IgA may also serve to control the absorption of intact antigen molecules by neonates. Children who lack IgA commonly develop IgE antibodies to cow's milk proteins. The deficiency in IgA may permit antigens to be absorbed and therefore encounter antigen-sensitive cells potentially capable of producing IgE. This is, perhaps, an example of IgA serving as a primary defensive mechanism while IgE serves a secondary role (see Fig. 10–5).

Consequences of the Transfer of Passive Immunity from Mother to Offspring. The initial transfusion of IgG from colostrum is required for the protection of young animals against septicemic disease. The continuous intake of IgA into the intestine is required for protection against enteric disease. Failure of either of these processes predisposes the young animal to infection.

Many reasons for the failure of adequate colostral transfer are possible. On occasion, colostrum may be abnormally low in IgG. This is sometimes associated with premature births. Since colostrum represents the accumulated secretion of the udder in late pregnancy, premature births result in an insufficient quantity of colostrum being available for the offspring. Much more commonly, failure in colostral transfer is the result of inadequate colostral intake by the newborn animal. This may be due to too many offspring, since the amount of colostrum produced does not rise in proportion to the number of young, or it may be due to poor mothering, a particular problem among young mothers. It also may be due to weakness in the newborn or to physical problems such as damaged teats or jaw defects. If a failure of immunoglobulin transfer has occurred, then these young animals will have low or insignificant serum immunoglobulin levels and as a consequence be at increased risk from colisepticemia, pneumonia and other infections. In addition, for reasons unknown, it has been shown that colostrum-deprived animals (lambs) are neutropenic and that their few remaining neutrophils are relatively inefficient at phagocytosis compared with neutrophils from colostrum-fed animals. The inflammatory responses of these animals are also depressed.

Animals with low immunoglobulin levels can be identified by means of tests that estimate serum immunoglobulin levels, such as the zinc sulfate turbidity test (Chapter 4), or by radial immunodiffusion. Suitable sources of supplemental immunoglobulin for such animals include stored, frozen colostrum, normal adult serum and immunoglobulin-rich fractions of serum or colostral whey. Although some of these are commercially available, it is perhaps more appropriate to employ colostrum or serum

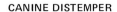

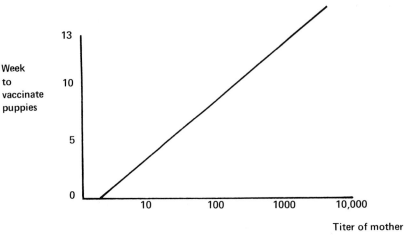

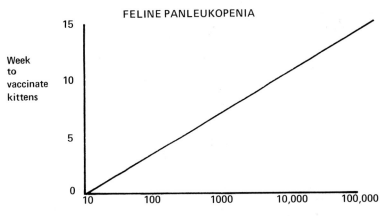

Figure 11–4 Nomographs showing the relationship between the antibody titer of the mother and the age at which to vaccinate her offspring with modified live virus vaccine. (The data used in these is taken from Scott et al. 1970. JAVMA *156* 439–453 [FPL] and from Baker et al. 1959. Cornell Vet *49* 158–167 [CD]. Used with permission.)

from another animal in the same environment, thus ensuring that the antibodies present in the transferred material correspond to the antigens likely to be encountered by the young animal.

Colostral transfer of immunity is essential for the welfare of young animals, but it may also cause problems. If, for instance, a mother becomes immunized against fetal red cells, colostral antibodies may cause massive erythrocyte destruction in the fetus, a condition known as hemolytic disease of the newborn, which is discussed at length in Chapter 18.

Transfer of Cell-Mediated Immunity by Milk. Bovine milk contains up to a million lymphocytes per milliliter, about half of which are T cells. These milk lymphocytes may survive for up to 36 hours in the intestine of newborn animals, and it is possible that they penetrate the intestinal wall and reach the liver. There is evidence that cell-mediated immunity may be transferred to newborn animals in this way. Thus, tuberculin sensitivity, a cell-mediated hypersensitivity reaction, may be transferred to calves by tuberculin-positive cows, and it has been shown that the ability to reject skin grafts or induce tolerance may be transferred to newborn rats through the milk of sensitized mothers. Perhaps more importantly, these transferred cells may be vectors for the transmission of some viruses to the newborn.

DEVELOPMENT OF THE IMMUNE RESPONSE IN NEONATAL ANIMALS

Local Immune Response.   By the time colostrum has converted to milk, the lymphoid tissues of the intestine of neonatal animals have become fully responsive to ingested antigen. For example, calves orally vaccinated with coronavirus vaccine at birth are resistant to virulent coronavirus by three to nine days, while piglets vaccinated orally three days after birth with transmissible gastroenteritis virus (TGE) vaccine develop neutralizing antibodies in the intestine 5 to 14 days later. Much of this early resistance is attributable to interferon, but there is an early intestinal IgM response that switches to IgA by about two weeks. In the growing animal, the SIgA response appears earlier and reaches adult levels well in advance of the other immunoglobulins. This capacity of the unprimed intestinal tract to respond rapidly to antigens is also seen in germ-free pigs. In these animals, antibody synthesis in the intestinal tract can be detected by 4 days, and the intestine appears to become immunologically "normal" by 10 days after infection with *E. coli*.

Systemic Immune Response.   As described in Chapter 7, the level of the immune response is controlled in part by a negative feedback whereby specific antibody inhibits further production of more antibody of the same specificity. The passive immunization of the newborn animal by maternal antibody also inhibits the immune response of the young animal. The precise mechanisms of this suppression are not clear, but it is probably due both to central suppression and to antigen masking and sequestration. If calves fail to suckle and are therefore hypogammaglobulinemic, they will commence to synthesize their own immunoglobulin by about one week of age. In calves that have suckled and thus have serum immunoglobulins, immunoglobulin synthesis does not commence until about four weeks of age. Colostrum-deprived piglets respond well to pseudorabies (Aujesky's disease) virus by two days after birth, but if they are suckled, immunoglobulin synthesis does not commence until they are five to six weeks old. Colostrum-deprived lambs synthesize IgG1 at one week and IgG2 by three to four weeks; if colostrum-fed, however, IgG2 synthesis does not occur until five to six weeks.

Not only does passively derived maternal antibody inhibit neonatal immunoglobulin synthesis, it also prevents the successful vaccination of young animals. This refractory period may persist for many months, its length depending on the amount of antibody transferred to the neonate and the half-life of the immunoglobulins involved.

This problem can be illustrated using the example of vaccination of puppies against canine distemper, but it must be emphasized that the same problems arise in the employment of all vaccines in young animals, including birds that receive antibodies from their mothers through the yolk.

Maternal antibodies absorbed from the puppy's intestine on suckling reach maximal levels in serum by 12 to 24 hours after birth. Thereafter as homologous immunoglobulins, their levels will decline through catabolism. The catabolic rate of proteins is exponential and can therefore be expressed as a half-life. Thus, the half-life of antibodies to distemper and canine infectious hepatitis is 8.4 days, and the half-life of antibodies to feline panleukopenia is 9.5 days (Fig. 11–4). On the average, the level of passively acquired antibodies to distemper in puppies will have declined to insignificant levels by about 10 to 12 weeks, although in extreme cases they may persist for as long as 16 weeks. In a population of puppies, it is apparent that the proportion of susceptible animals increases gradually from a very few or none at birth, to almost all at 10 to 12 weeks. Puppies that are susceptible to the disease are also able to be vaccinated. Immediately after birth few puppies can be successfully vaccinated but by 10 to 12 weeks almost all can. If canine distemper were not enzootic in Western Europe and North America, it would be sufficient to delay vaccination until the puppies were 12 weeks old, thus ensuring that all puppies were capable of being successfully vaccinated. Unfortunately, a delay of this type would mean that an increasing proportion of puppies, fully susceptible to disease, would be without immune protection. Although this is unacceptable, it is not economically feasible to vaccinate puppies at short intervals from birth to 12 weeks, a procedure that would ensure protection; a compromise must therefore be reached.

One possible protocol is to vaccinate puppies at 9 to 10 weeks when about 30 per cent of puppies are susceptible and capable of being effectively vaccinated, and then give a second dose at 16 weeks in order to boost the successfully vaccinated puppies and to protect those not protected by the first dose. A simpler procedure is to vaccinate all puppies when presented and then revaccinate at 12 to 16 weeks. There are many similar alternative procedures, all aimed at conferring early protection while leaving as few puppies as possible unprotected. In any case, puppies should be revaccinated every one or two years depending on the type of vaccine employed. Colostrum-deprived orphan pups may be vaccinated at two weeks of age. Similar considerations apply in the case of cats being vaccinated with feline panleukopenia vaccine (Fig. 11–4).

An alternative method of overcoming the problems caused by maternal immunity to canine distemper is by the use of measles vaccine. Measles is closely related to distemper virus; the viruses share common surface antigens but possess different cell-binding antigens. Maternal antidistemper antibodies are therefore unable to prevent measles infection of cells and, as a result, cannot prevent the development of an antimeasles cell-mediated immune response. This antimeasles response is, however, capable of protecting dogs against distemper. Measles vaccine given to puppies at six weeks of age can therefore protect against distemper in spite of the presence of a high level of antidistemper antibody. Calves and foals vaccinated under six months of age should always be revaccinated at six months or after weaning, although maternally derived antibodies to bovine virus diarrhea may persist for up to nine months in calves.

Antiserum may be used in circumstances of doubtful immunity when there is a necessity for immediate protection. This form of treatment tends to complicate analysis of these situations, since it prolongs the time required before passive immunity wanes and active immunization can be successfully initiated.

Passive Immunity in the Chick. Chicks acquire IgG antibody from the yolk. This immunoglobulin is readily transfered from hen serum to the yolk while the egg is still in the ovary. In the fluid phase of the yolk, IgG is therefore found at levels equal to those in maternal serum. In addition, as the egg passes down the oviduct, IgM and IgA from oviduct secretions are acquired with the albumin. As the chick embryo develops it absorbs some of the yolk IgG, which then appears in its circulation. The maternal IgM and IgA in the albumin appear in the amniotic fluid and are swallowed by the embryo, so that when the chick hatches it possesses IgG in its serum and IgM and IgA in its gut. The newly hatched chick does not absorb all the yolk sac antibody until about 24 hours after hatching. These maternal antibodies effectively prevent successful vaccination until they disappear at between 10 and 20 days after hatching.

ADDITIONAL SOURCES OF INFORMATION

Campbell SG, Siegel MJ, and Knowlton BJ. 1977. Sheep immunoglobulins and their transmission to the neonatal lamb. NZ Vet J 25 361–365.

Cole GJ, and Morris B. 1973. The lymphoid apparatus of sheep: its growth, development and significance in immunologic reactions. Adv Vet Sci 17 225–263.

Crawford TB, and Perryman LE. 1980. Diagnosis and treatment of failure of passive transfer in the foal. Equine Practice 2 17–23.

Fahey KJ, and Morris B. 1978. Humoral immune responses in fetal sheep. Immunology 35 651–661.

Halliday R. 1978. Immunity and health in young lambs. Vet Rec 103 489–492.

Jeffcott LB. 1972. Passive immunity and its transfer with special reference to the horse. Biol. Rev. 47 439–464.

Perryman LE, McGuire TC, and Torbeck RL. 1980. Ontogeny of lymphocyte function in the equine fetus. Am J Vet Res 41 1197–1200.

Schultz RD, Wang TJ, and Dunne HW. 1974. Development of the humoral immune response in the pig. Am J Vet Res 32 1331–1336.

Solomon JB. 1971. Fetal and Neonatal Immunology. Frontiers of Biology series, Vol 20. Elsevier North-Holland, New York.

Toivanen P, Asantila T, Granberg C, Leino A, and Hirvonen T. 1978. Development of T cell repertoire in the human and sheep fetus. Immunol Rev 42 185–201.

12

Immunoprophylaxis: General Principles of Vaccination and Vaccines

The observation that individuals who had recovered from an infectious disease were resistant to subsequent reinfection long preceded the development of immunology and our understanding of the immune response. In fact, the attempts to reproduce this phenomenon in a controlled fashion by Jenner and Pasteur provided the impetus for the early development of immunology. Their efforts to produce immunity by artificial exposure to infectious agents were so successful that many diseases, which had long been major scourges of mankind, were rapidly controlled. Vaccines were successfully developed against smallpox, rabies, tetanus, anthrax, cholera and diphtheria as well as against other diseases, and their success has been responsible, in part, for the recent phenomenal increase in the world's population. Fortunately, the successes in the development of human vaccines have been matched by similar improvements in the control of animal diseases, thus expanding the food supply and at least delaying the widening of the gap between food supplies and demand.

In general, vaccination involves giving antigen derived from an infectious agent to an animal so that an immune response is mounted and resistance to that infectious agent is achieved. Several criteria first must be satisfied in determining whether vaccination is either possible or desirable in controlling a specific disease. The first is the absolute identification of the causal organism. Although this appears to be an obvious requirement, it has not always been followed in practice. For instance, in the pneumonic disease of cattle known as shipping fever, it is possible to consistently isolate *Pasteurella multocida* or *P. hemolytica* from the lungs of cattle at autopsy. However, it is not possible to reproduce the shipping fever syndrome by the use of these organisms alone, and evidence suggests that the disease process owes much to virus infection and immunopathological mechanisms. Nevertheless, pasteurella vaccines have been used in large quantities for many years in attempts to control this condition, despite their ineffectiveness.

Secondly, it must be established that an immune response can in fact protect against the disease in question. In some diseases, such as equine infectious anemia and Aleutian disease in mink, the immune response appears to be responsible for many of the disease processes. In other infections, such as foot-and-mouth disease in pigs and African swine fever, very poor or no protective immunity can be induced. In African swine fever, antibodies, in spite of being produced in large quantities and being capable of fixing complement or inhibiting viral hemadsorption *in vitro*, are unable to cause virus neutralization. In foot-and-mouth disease in pigs, the immune response is transient and relatively ineffective, so that animals that have been clinically infected become fully susceptible to reinfection as soon as three months later. Thus, for a vaccine to produce prolonged effective immunity against foot-and-mouth disease in pigs, it must induce an immune response superior to that produced by natural infection.

Finally, before using a vaccine we must be sure that the risks of vaccination do not exceed those associated with the chance of contracting the disease itself. A good example of this is pneumonic pasteurellosis of cattle, in which excellent experimental and epidemiological data show that pasteurella bacterins may increase, not reduce, the severity of the lung lesions. In addition, because the detection of antibodies is a common diagnostic procedure, unnecessary use of vaccines may complicate diagnosis based on serological techniques and perhaps make final eradication of a disease difficult, if not impossible. Because of this, the decision to use vaccines for the control of any disease must be based on considerations not only of the severity of the problem but also of the prospects for its control by other techniques.

When vaccines are used to control disease in a population of animals rather than in individuals, the concept of herd immunity should also be considered. This herd immunity is the resistance of an entire group of animals to disease conferred by the presence in that group of a proportion of immune animals. Herd immunity presumably acts by reducing the probability of a susceptible animal meeting an infected one so that the spread of disease is slowed or terminated. If it is acceptable to lose individual animals from disease while preventing epizootics, it may be possible to do this by selective vaccination.

TYPES OF IMMUNIZATION PROCEDURES
(Fig. 12–1)

There are two methods by which an animal may be rendered immune to infectious disease. One method, termed passive immunization, produces a temporary resistance by transferring antibodies from a resistant to a susceptible animal. These passively transferred antibodies give immediate protection, but, since they are gradually catabolized, this protection wanes and the recipient eventually becomes susceptible to reinfection once again.

As an alternative procedure to passive immunization, active immunization has much to commend it. This technique involves administering antigen to an animal so that it responds by mounting a protective immune response that may be either antibody- or cell-mediated or both. Reimmunization or exposure to infection will result in a secondary immune response. The disadvantage of this form of immunization is that protection is not conferred immediately. However, once established it is long-lasting and capable of restimulation (Fig. 12–2).

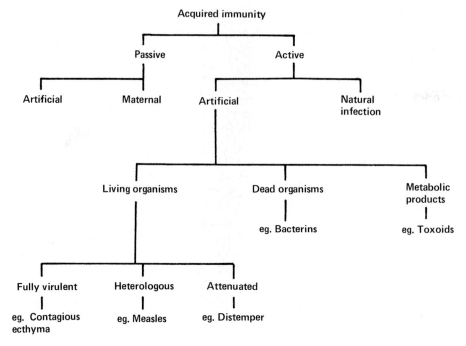

Figure 12–1 A classification of the types of acquired immunity and of the methods employed to induce protection.

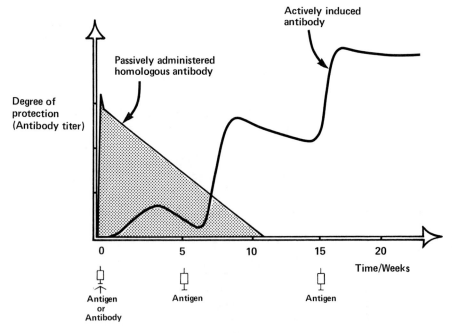

Figure 12–2 The levels of serum antibody (and hence the degree of protection) conferred by active and passive methods of immunization.

PASSIVE IMMUNIZATION

Passive immunization requires that antibodies be produced in a donor animal by active immunization, and that these antibodies, after partial purification, be given to susceptible animals in order to confer immediate protection. These antisera may be raised against a wide variety of pathogens. For instance, they can be produced in cattle against anthrax, in dogs against distemper, in cats against panleukopenia and in humans against measles. Their most important role is in protection against toxigenic organisms such as *Clostridium tetani* or *Cl. perfringens*, using antisera raised in horses. Antisera made in this way are known as antitoxins and are generally produced in young horses by a series of immunizing inoculations. The toxins of the clostridia are proteins and can be made nontoxic by treatment with formaldehyde. Formaldehyde-treated toxins are known as toxoids. Initially, the horses are given toxoids, but once antibodies are produced, subsequent injections may contain purified toxin. The responses of these animals are monitored, and once their antibody levels are sufficiently high, the horses are bled. Bleeding is undertaken at regular intervals until the titer drops, when the animals are again "boosted" with antigen. Plasma is separated from the horse blood and treated with 48 per cent saturated ammonium sulfate in order to concentrate and purify the globulin fraction. The purified globulin fraction, rich in antibodies to the toxin, is then dialyzed, filtered, titrated and dispensed.

In order to check the potency of preparations of antitoxin, comparison must be made with an international biological standard. In the case of tetanus antitoxin, this is done by comparing the dose necessary to protect guinea pigs against a fixed dose of tetanus toxin with the dose of the standard preparation of antitoxin required to do the same. An alternative method of checking the potency of antitoxin preparations is to compare the ability of the test and standard antisera to flocculate a fixed amount of toxin. This method measures the power of the antitoxin to combine with toxin and has certain advantages, since toxins are relatively unstable and their toxicity may fluctuate while their antigenicity remains constant. The international standard antiserum for tetanus toxin is a quantity held at the Statens Serum-Institute, Copenhagen; an International Unit (I.U.) of tetanus antitoxin is the specific neutralizing activity contained in 0.03384 mg of the international standard. The U.S. Standard Unit (A.U.) is twice the International Unit.

Tetanus antitoxin is given to animals in order to confer immediate protection against tetanus. At least 1500 I.U. of antitoxin should be given to horses and cattle; at least 500 I.U. to calves, sheep, goats and swine; and at least 250 I.U. to dogs. The exact amount should vary with the amount of tissue damage, the degree of wound contamination and the time elapsed since injury. Tetanus antitoxin is of little use once clinical signs appear, although massive doses of up to 5000 I.U. may be of some assistance.

Although antisera give prompt immunity, certain problems are associated with their use. For instance, horse tetanus antitoxin may be given safely to horses, in which it is not generally regarded as foreign, and it will persist for a relatively long period of time, being removed only by catabolism. If, however, horse tetanus antitoxin is given to an animal of another species such as a cow or dog, then it is regarded as foreign, an immune response is mounted against it, and it is rapidly eliminated. In order to reduce their antigenicity for other species of animals, antitoxins are usually treated with pepsin so as to destroy the immunoglobulin Fc region and leave intact only the portion of the immunoglobulin molecule required for toxin neutralization—the F(ab)'2 fragment.

If the amount of circulating horse immunoglobulin is relatively large at the time an immune response is mounted by the immunized host, the immune complexes formed may participate in the type III hypersensitivity reaction known as serum sickness (Chapter 19). If repeated doses of horse antitoxin are given to an animal, there also exists the possibility of IgE production and the occurrence of a type I hypersensitivity reaction such as anaphylaxis (Chapter 17). Finally, the presence of high levels of circulating antibody may interfere with active immunization against the same antigen. This is a phenomenon similar to that seen in newborn animals passively protected by maternal antibodies.

ACTIVE IMMUNIZATION

The most important advantages of active immunization compared with passive protection are the prolonged period of protection achieved and the recall and boosting of this protective response by repeated injections of antigen or by exposure to infection. An ideal vaccine for active immunization (vaccination) should, therefore, give prolonged strong immunity. This immunity should be conferred on both the animal vaccinated and any fetus carried by it. In obtaining this strong immunity, the vaccine should be free of adverse side effects. The ideal vaccine should be cheap, stable, adaptable to mass vaccination and, ideally, should stimulate an immune response distinguishable from that due to natural infection so that vaccination and eradication may proceed simultaneously.

Living and "Dead" Vaccines. Unfortunately, two of the prerequisites of an ideal vaccine, high antigenicity and absence of adverse side effects, tend to be mutually incompatible. In particular, living organisms stimulate the best immune response but may present hazards as a result of residual virulence, whereas "dead" organisms are relatively poor immunogens but are usually much safer (Table 12–1).

The relative advantages and disadvantages of vaccines containing living or "dead" organisms may be seen, for example, in the vaccines available against *Brucella abortus* in cattle. *B. abortus* is the cause of contagious abortion in cattle, and in the absence of an effective eradication scheme, vaccination is required to control the disease. The organism, however, is a facultative intracellular parasite that is capable of living within macrophages and that must be controlled by a cell-mediated immune response, although antibodies also contribute to resistance. As a broad generalization, living organisms are much more capable of stimulating cell-mediated immunity than

Table 12–1   COMPARISON OF THE RELATIVE MERITS OF LIVING
AND "DEAD" VACCINES

ADVANTAGES OF LIVING VACCINES	ADVANTAGES OF "DEAD" VACCINES
Strong, long-lasting immunity	Unlikely to cause disease due to residual
Few inoculating doses required	virulence or reversion
Adjuvants unnecessary	Stable on storage
Less chance of hypersensitivity	
Virus vaccines may stimulate interferon	
production	

are "dead" organisms. For these reasons, a vaccine containing a living but avirulent strain of *B. abortus* is required for the control of this infection. The vaccine strain of *B. abortus* (strain 19) gives rise to an excellent life-long immunity in cows and successfully prevents abortion, although it may not completely prevent infection (particularly in the udder). Strain 19 is "never" transmitted between cattle and is very stable, its biological properties not having changed since it was first isolated in 1930. In general, it may be regarded as an excellent vaccine.

However, strain 19 may cause systemic reactions, particularly in adult Jersey cows; local swelling at the injection site, high fever, anorexia, listlessness and a drop in milk yield have all been reported to occur following vaccination. Strain 19 may also cause abortion in pregnant cows and, while avirulent for heifers, can cause orchitis in bulls and undulant fever in humans. In addition, a small proportion of vaccinated cattle may remain persistently infected with strain 19 for many months. In order to eradicate brucellosis, it is necessary to employ serological tests to identify infected animals, and strain 19 gives rise to an antibody response that is only with difficulty distinguished from that seen in response to natural infection. One method used to assist in this differentiation is to ensure that strain 19 is given only to heifer calves between 2 and 10 months of age (3 to 6 months in the United Kingdom, 3 to 9 months in Canada, 2 to 6 months for dairy calves in the United States, and 2 to 10 months for beef calves in the United States), in the hope that the serum antibody response will have declined to low levels by the time the animal reaches breeding age and is tested for brucellosis. In areas where there is extensive brucellosis, it may be economically beneficial to use a reduced dosage of strain 19 vaccine in adult cattle. In this procedure, adult cattle are given one twentieth of the standard dose of strain 19. This confers resistance to brucellosis while the antibodies provoked decline rapidly. This technique reduces the losses due to the presence of positive serological reactors as well as hastening the elimination of brucellosis from the herds. Its disadvantages include the occurrence of occasional persistent titers (reduced considerably by the use of the Rivanol precipitation test and the complement fixation test—Chapter 9), a consistently positive milk ring test and, occasionally, persistent strain 19 infection. (For further details of the techniques available for distinguishing between *B. abortus* vaccinated and infected cattle, see Chapter 9.)

Because of the disadvantages associated with the use of strain 19, a dead vaccine utilizing a formolized rough strain of *B. abortus* has been developed. This organism (strain 45/20), which is administered in a water-in-oil adjuvant emulsion in two doses, will only protect cattle for less than a year. The immune response to this vaccine is readily distinguishable from that due to an infection, since it is devoid of antigens present on smooth virulent strains (Chapter 13). This vaccine is not permitted in North America but was used with some success in heavily infected herds in the United Kingdom, where slaughter would have been uneconomical. Uninfected animals were vaccinated with 45/20 while the infected animals were removed as soon as economics allowed.

The advantages of vaccines that contain dead organisms, such as 45/20, are that they are safe with respect to residual virulence and are relatively easy to store, since the organisms are already dead. These advantages of dead vaccines correspond to the disadvantages of live vaccines such as strain 19. That is, some live vaccines may possess residual virulence, not only for the animal for whom the vaccine is made but also for other animals. They may possibly revert to a fully virulent type or spread to unvaccinated animals—a feature not seen when strain 19 is used. The capacity of a vaccine to spread can, in some circumstances, be advantageous. For example, the widespread use of living polio virus vaccine in humans in the developed countries has resulted in a replacement of the original virulent wild strain in the population by vaccine strains. Live vaccines always run the risk of contamination with unwanted organisms; for instance, outbreaks of reticuloendotheliosis in chickens in Japan and Australia have been traced to contaminated Marek's disease vaccine. It has been suggested, but is as yet unproven, that the adenovirus of poultry EDS 76 (egg drop syndrome 1976) and canine parvovirus may also have been distributed in contaminated vaccines. Contaminating mycoplasma may also be present in some vaccines. Finally, vaccines containing living attenuated organisms require care in their preparation, storage and handling in order to avoid killing the organisms.

Similarly, the disadvantages of "dead" vaccines correspond to the advantages of living vaccines. Thus, the use of adjuvants to increase effective antigenicity can cause severe local reactions, while multiple dosing or high individual doses of antigen increase the risks of producing hypersensitivity reactions as well as adversely affecting cost. Most important, however, vaccines containing living organisms commonly give a much better immunity than vaccines containing inactivated or "dead" organisms. One reason for this is that the living vaccine virus may invade host cells and induce interferon production, thus conferring early protection on susceptible animals. The increased efficacy of live vaccines is probably also due to the particular distribution of living organisms within the body as well as to the biochemical changes brought about by the killing process.

Inactivation and Attenuation of Organisms Used in Vaccines.   If organisms are to be inactivated for use in vaccines, it is desirable that the "dead" organisms be as antigenically similar to the living organisms as possible. Therefore, a crude method of killing organisms such as heating, which causes extensive protein denaturation, is usually unsatisfactory. If chemicals are to be used, it is essential that they produce very little change in the antigens responsible for stimulating protective immunity. One compound used in this way is formaldehyde, which acts on amino and amide groups in proteins and on non–hydrogen-bonded amino groups in the purine and pyrimidine bases of nucleic acids to form cross-links and so confer structural rigidity. Proteins can also be mildly denatured by acetone or alcohol treatment. In the case of louping-ill vaccine, alcohol treatment of the virus increases the antigenicity of the vaccine, although the mechanism involved is unknown. Alkylating agents that cross-link nucleic acid chains are also suitable for killing organisms, since by leaving the surface proteins of organisms unmodified, they do not interfere with antigenicity. Examples of these include ethylene oxide, ethyleneimine, acetylethyleneimine and β-propiolactone, all of which have been used in veterinary vaccines.

Although the difference between living and "dead" organisms is, in the final analysis, only biochemical, it has profound influence on the effectiveness of vaccines. As a compromise, therefore, it is possible to reduce the virulence of an organism until, although living, it is not capable of causing disease. This process of reduction of virulence is known as attenuation. Simple methods of attenuation include heating organisms to just below their thermal death point or exposing organisms to marginally sublethal concentrations of inactivating chemicals. Presumably, organisms injured by these processes are at a disadvantage when inoculated into an animal and, instead of multiplying rapidly and causing disease, may be phagocytosed and processed for the immune response.

The commonly used methods of attenuation involve adapting organisms to un-usual conditions so that they lose their adaptation to their usual host. These techniques include culturing in unfavorable media or at an unfavorable temperature. For example, the BCG (bacille Calmette-Guérin) strain of *Mycobacterium bovis* was rendered avir-ulent by being grown for 13 years on bile-saturated medium. The strain of anthrax currently used in vaccines was rendered avirulent by growth in 50 per cent serum agar under an atmosphere rich in CO_2 so that it lost its capacity to form a capsule. Pasteur's fowl cholera *(Pasteurella multocida)* vaccine was grown under conditions in which there was a shortage of nutrients.

Whereas bacteria can be rendered avirulent by culture under abnormal conditions, viruses may be attenuated by growth in species to which they are not naturally adapted. For example, rinderpest virus, which is normally a pathogen of cattle, was first attenuated by growth in goats, but this caprinized virus retained its virulence for some breeds of cattle. In an attempt to solve this problem, a rabbit-adapted (lapinized) vaccine was introduced, which had less residual virulence. In the course of further attempts to obtain a rinderpest vaccine devoid of residual virulence, a tissue culture–adapted vaccine was developed, which has proved extremely successful in controlling this disease in Africa. Similar examples include the adaptation of African horse sickness virus to mice and of canine distemper virus to ferrets.

As an alternative method of attenuation, mammalian viruses may be grown in eggs. This has been done for canine distemper, bluetongue and rabies vaccines. The Flury strain of rabies vaccine has been attenuated by repeated passage through eggs. Although used for many years, the low egg passage (LEP) strain (passaged 40 to 50 times) has been shown to cause disease in dogs and has therefore been withdrawn. The high egg passage vaccine (HEP) has been attenuated by 178 passages in eggs and appears to be completely safe for dogs and cats. In the case of some avian viruses, attenuation may be brought about by growth in eggs of another species; for instance, the virus of fowl influenza can be attenuated in pigeon eggs. At present, the most commonly employed method of attenuation is by prolonged tissue culture, and most veterinary vaccines are now attenuated in this way. Although the tissue culture can be derived from many species, it is common to employ cultures of cells from the species to be vaccinated in order to reduce the possibilities of side effects resulting from the administration of foreign tissues. In these cases virus attenuation may be accomplished by culturing the organism in cells to which they are not adapted. For example, virulent canine distemper virus preferentially attacks lymphoid cells. For vaccine purposes, therefore, this organism is cultured repeatedly in canine kidney cells, as a result of which its virulence is lost.

An example of attenuation by growth in unusual species is the SAD (Street-Alabama-Dufferin) strain of attenuated rabies vaccine. This virus, originally isolated from a rabid dog in Alabama, was passaged through mice, hamster kidney tissue culture, chick embryos, porcine kidney tissue culture and, finally, canine kidney tissue culture. When grown on porcine tissue culture, the SAD strain can be used to vaccinate all species of domestic animals, a single dose providing protection for several years. When grown in canine tissue culture, it is used to vaccinate dogs. Unfortunately, SAD rabies vaccine may cause clinical rabies in cats and therefore cannot be used in that species.

Some vaccination processes use, instead of artificially attenuated organisms, related organisms normally adapted to another species. For example, just as Jenner used cowpox as a vaccine in humans, so measles virus can be used to protect dogs against distemper and bovine virus diarrhea virus can protect against hog cholera, since these organisms are antigenically related.

Finally, under some circumstances it is possible to use fully virulent organisms in vaccination procedures just as the Chinese did with smallpox, although this is generally done only if a better technique is not available. Vaccination against contagious ecthyma of sheep is of this type. Contagious ecthyma (orf) is a disease of lambs that, by causing massive scab formation around the mouth, prevents feeding and thus results in a failure to thrive. The disease has little systemic effect, and lambs recover completely within a few weeks and are immune thereafter. It is usual to vaccinate lambs by rubbing dried, infected scab material into scratches made in the inner aspect of the thigh. The local infection at this site has no untoward effect on the lambs, and they become solidly immune. Because the vaccinated animals may spread the disease, however, it is necessary to separate them from unvaccinated stock for a few weeks.

SUBUNIT VACCINES. Because of the adverse side effects associated with the presence of extraneous material in vaccines, much attention has been given to the elimination of unwanted antigens. The inevitable end-point of this process is the purification of the individual proteins that give rise to protective antibodies. Such subunit vaccines are, theoretically, much more efficient than other types of inactivated vaccines, although they may not be as potent as vaccines containing living organisms.

Unfortunately, the production of large quantities of purified virus proteins is difficult and costly. One solution to this problem may be the use of recombinant DNA technology. For example, in the case of both rabies and foot-and-mouth disease viruses, the protective antigens and their genes are well described. It is possible to incorporate these viral genes into bacteria so that they synthesize large quantities of viral antigen, which may then be used in vaccines.

Subunit vaccines may also be prepared by means of purified bacterial antigens. Attachment pili of enteropathogenic *E. coli*—for example, K88 or K99—can be incorporated into bacterins. The antipilus antibodies thus provoked will protect animals by preventing bacterial attachment to the intestinal wall. Vaccines consisting of purified ribosomal fractions of pathogenic bacteria have also been used to provoke protective cell-mediated immunity with encouraging results.

ADMINISTRATION OF VACCINES

Immunization by subcutaneous or intramuscular injection is the simplest and most usual method of administration of vaccines. This approach is obviously excellent for relatively small numbers of animals and for diseases in which systemic immunity is important. However, in some conditions, systemic immunity is not as important as local immunity, and it is perhaps more appropriate to administer the vaccine at the site of potential invasion. Therefore, intranasal vaccines are available for infectious bovine rhinotracheitis of cattle, for feline rhinotracheitis and calicivirus infections, and for infectious bronchitis and Newcastle disease in poultry. All these techniques require that each animal be dealt with on an individual basis; when numbers are very large, other methods must be employed. Aerosolization of vaccines enables them to be inhaled by all the animals in a flock. This technique is employed in vaccinating against canine distemper and mink enteritis on mink ranches, and against Newcastle disease in poultry. Alternatively, the vaccine may be put in the feed or drinking water; this is done with *Erysipelothrix rhusiopathiae* vaccines in pigs and against Newcastle disease, infectious laryngotracheitis and avian encephalomyelitis in poultry. Fish may be vaccinated by adding antigen to the water in which they live.

Adjuvants. In Chapter 4, adjuvants were discussed in relation to their function. In veterinary medicine, adjuvants are usually required to potentiate the immunogenicity of dead vaccines and toxoids (Table 12–2). One exception to this is the use of saponin in anthrax vaccines, where it is required to modify conditions at the site of injection so that the anthrax spores may germinate. Saponin is also employed as an adjuvant for foot-and-mouth disease vaccines. Oil-based adjuvants are not usually appropriate for use in animals intended for human consumption, since the oil may track through fascial planes and spoil the meat. Freund's complete adjuvant is quite unacceptable in food animals, not only because of the mineral oil, but also because the mycobacteria in the adjuvant will render animals positive to tuberculin, a critical drawback in any area where tuberculosis is under control. There is also evidence to suggest that Freund's complete adjuvant may be carcinogenic. By far the most widely employed adjuvants in commercial veterinary vaccines are those that employ mineral gels such as aluminum hydroxide, aluminum phosphate or aluminum potassium sulfate (alum). These adjuvants are produced in the form of a colloidal suspension to which the antigenic material is adsorbed. They are stable on storage, a feature not generally found in the oil-based adjuvants, and while they produce a small local granuloma on inoculation, they do not track nor make large parts of the carcass unsuitable for consumption. This type of adjuvant may therefore be considered to be the most suitable type for animals at present.

Mixed Vaccines. It has become commonplace to employ mixtures of several organisms as vaccines. For respiratory diseases of cattle, for example, vaccines are available that contain infectious bovine rhinotracheitis (IBR) virus, bovine virus diarrhea (BVD) virus, parainfluenza 3 (PI3) virus and even *P. multocida*. Such a mixture may be of use in outbreaks of respiratory disease when exact diagnosis is not possible, and may protect animals against several diseases with economy of effort. However, it can also be considered extremely wasteful to use vaccines against organisms that may not be causing problems.

Table 12–2 SOME EXAMPLES OF ADJUVANTS EMPLOYED IN VETERINARY MEDICINE

ADJUVANT	*VACCINE*
Aluminum hydroxide	Leptospira Campylobacter Pasteurella Erysipelas Clostridia Anaplasma
Aluminum phosphate	Fusobacterium
Water-in-oil	Foot-and-mouth disease Brucella 45/20
Saponin	Foot-and-mouth disease Anthrax
DEAE dextran	Foot-and-mouth disease

Dogs may be given vaccine mixtures containing up to six of the following organisms—canine distemper virus, canine adenovirus 1, canine adenovirus 2, canine parvovirus, canine parainfluenza virus, leptospira bacterin and rabies vaccine—with a considerable saving in time and effort. Nevertheless, the production of balanced vaccine mixtures such as these is relatively complex, and many of their advantages may be offset by greater production costs.

When different antigens in a mixture are inoculated simultaneously, competition occurs between antigens. Manufacturers of mixed vaccines take this into account and modify their mixtures accordingly. However, vaccines should never be mixed indiscriminately, since one component may dominate the mixture and interfere with the response to the other components.

Vaccination Schedules. Although it is not possible to give appropriate schedules for each of the veterinary vaccines available, certain principles are common to all methods of active immunization.

Since newborn animals are passively protected by maternal antibodies, it is not usually possible to vaccinate animals successfully early in life. If stimulation of immunity is deemed necessary at this stage, the mother can be vaccinated during the later stages of pregnancy, the vaccinations being timed so that peak antibody levels are achieved at the time of colostrum formation.

Once an animal is born, successful active vaccination is usually possible only when passive immunity is waning. Since it is rarely possible to put an exact date to the loss of maternal immunity, it is therefore necessary to vaccinate at least twice. The second injection is given about 15 weeks after birth in small animals and at six months in larger animals to ensure successful vaccination.

The interval between booster doses of vaccines varies; "dead" vaccines, which produce weak immunity, may require frequent boosters, perhaps as often as every six months, whereas living vaccines, which produce a long-lasting immunity, may require boosting only once every two to three years. The interval between boosters is determined also by the disease. Some diseases are seasonal and vaccination may be required only prior to the time disease outbreaks can be expected. Examples of these include the vaccine against the lungworm *Dictyocaulus viviparus* given in early summer just prior to the anticipated lungworm season, the vaccine against anthrax given in spring and the vaccine against *Clostridium chauvoei* given to sheep before turning them out to pasture. Bluetongue of lambs is spread by midges *(Culicoides varipennis)* and is thus a disease of midsummer and early fall. Vaccination in spring will therefore protect lambs during the susceptible period.

Failures in Vaccination (Fig. 12–3). The immune response, being a biological process, never confers absolute protection and is never equal in all members of a vaccinated population. Since the immune response is influenced by a large number of genetic and environmental factors, the range of immune responses in a large random population of animals tends to follow a normal distribution (Fig. 12–4). This means that, whereas most animals tend to respond to antigens by mounting an average immune response, a small proportion will mount a very poor immune response. This latter group of animals may not be protected against infection in spite of vaccination. Therefore, it is improbable that 100 per cent of a random population of animals will be protected by vaccination. The size of this unreactive portion of the population will vary with the nature of the antigen employed, and its significance will depend on the nature of the disease. Thus, for highly infectious diseases against which herd immunity is poor and in which infection is rapidly and efficiently transmitted, such as foot-and-

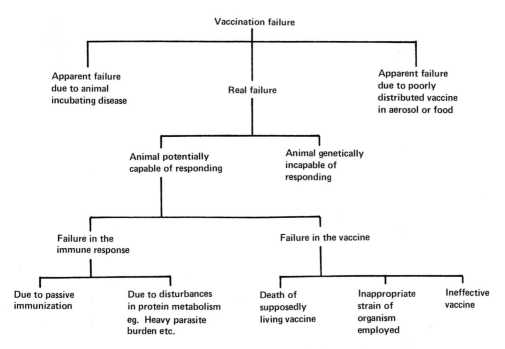

Figure 12–3 A classification of possible reasons for the failure of a vaccine to protect an animal.

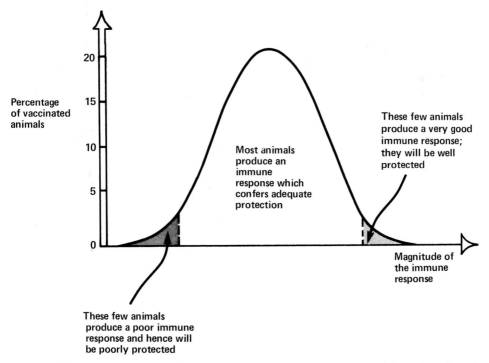

Figure 12–4 The normal distribution of immune responses in a population of vaccinated animals.

mouth disease, the presence of unprotected animals would permit the spread of disease and would thus disrupt control programs. Similarly, problems can arise if animals are individually important, for example domestic pets. In contrast, for diseases that are inefficiently spread, such as rabies, 60 to 70 per cent protection may be sufficient to effectively block disease transmission within a population and may therefore be quite satisfactory.

The second group of vaccine failures are due to circumstances in which the normal immune response is suppressed. For example, heavily parasitized or malnourished animals should not be vaccinated. Stress in general, including pregnancy, extremes of cold and heat, fatigue or malnourishment, will inhibit the normal immune response, probably because of increased steroid production. The most important cause of vaccine failure of this type is due to the presence of passively derived maternal immunity in young animals.

A third group of apparent vaccine failures are due to defects in vaccine administration. When large flocks of poultry or mink are to be vaccinated, it is common to administer the vaccine either as an aerosol or in drinking water. If the aerosol is not evenly distributed throughout a building, or if some animals do not drink, they may receive insufficient vaccine. Animals that subsequently suffer from disease may be interpreted as cases of vaccine failure. Other possible causes of apparent vaccine failure may be that the vaccinated animal was incubating the disease prior to inoculation or that supposedly live vaccine had "died" owing to poor storage, the use of antibiotics in conjunction with live bacterial vaccines, the use of chemicals to sterilize syringes or the excessive use of alcohol while swabbing the skin—procedures that may inactivate a virus vaccine.

Adverse Consequences of Vaccination. Residual virulence and toxicity are perhaps the most significant risks associated with the use of vaccines. For example, mild lesions of mucosal disease may be seen in calves vaccinated against bovine virus diarrhea (BVD). Vaccines containing killed gram-negative organisms may be intrinsically toxic owing to the presence of endotoxins, which can cause a "shock" with pyrexia and leukopenia. Although such a reaction is commonly only a temporary inconvenience to male animals, it may be sufficient to provoke abortion in pregnant females. The stress from this type of toxic reaction may also be sufficient to reactivate latent infections; for example, activation of equine herpesvirus has been demonstrated following vaccination against African horse sickness. One other form of toxicity is the "sting" produced by some inactivating agents such as formaldehyde. This can present problems not only to the animal being vaccinated but also to the vaccinator.

In addition to the difficulties associated with virulence and toxicity, vaccines, like any antigen, may provoke hypersensitivity reactions. For example, type I hypersensitivity can occur in response not only to the immunizing antigen, but also to other antigens found in vaccines, such as egg antigens or antigens derived from tissue culture cells. All forms of hypersensitivity are more commonly associated with multiple injections of antigen and are therefore associated with the use of "dead" vaccines.

Type III hypersensitivity reactions are also potential hazards. The clinical signs may include an intense local inflammatory reaction, or they may present as a generalized vascular disturbance such as purpura. A type III reaction can occur in the eyes of dogs vaccinated against infectious canine hepatitis (Chapter 14).

Type IV hypersensitivity reactions may occur in response to vaccination, but a much more common reaction is granuloma formation at the site of inoculation in response to the use of depot adjuvants. Some vaccines, however, are effective only by virtue of these local tissue reactions. For instance, Vallée's vaccine for Johne's disease involves the administration of the living organism in a mixture of oil and pumice dust. This mixture, not surprisingly, is highly irritating and on injection produces a large granuloma that eventually opens to the surface and discharges its oily contents. The effect of this vaccine is to protect cattle against clinical Johne's disease, although it does not prevent infection. Because it makes an animal both tuberculin and johnin positive, the use of this vaccine is prohibited in many countries (Chapter 20).

One other problem, which is seen in horses used for antiserum production, is amyloidosis associated with excessive stimulation of the antibody-forming system (Chapter 22). Although amyloidosis is not uncommon in domestic animals, it does not usually occur as a result of normal vaccination procedures.

Under some circumstances autoimmune disorders may be provoked by vaccination. For example, an allergic encephalitis may be provoked by the use of vaccines, such as some of the rabies vaccines, that contain central nervous tissue. An idiopathic polyneuritis (Guillain-Barré syndrome—Chapter 21) has been associated with the use of certain virus vaccines (most notably "swine" influenza) in humans. The precise pathogenesis of this syndrome is unclear.

PRODUCTION, PRESENTATION AND CONTROL OF VACCINES

The production of veterinary biologicals is controlled by the Animal and Plant Health Inspection Service of the U.S.D.A. in the United States, by the Health of Animals Branch of the Canada Department of Agriculture in Canada and by the Ministry of Agriculture in the United Kingdom. In general, regulatory authorities have the right to license establishments where vaccines are produced and to inspect these premises to ensure that the facilities are appropriate and that the methods employed are satisfactory. All vaccines have to be checked for safety and potency. Safety tests include a confirmation of the identity of the organism used and of the freedom of the vaccine from extraneous organisms (i.e., purity) as well as tests for toxicity and sterility. Because the living organisms found in vaccines normally die over a period of time, it is necessary to ensure that they will be effective even after storage. It is usual, therefore, to use an amount of microorganisms in generous excess of the dose required to protect animals under laboratory conditions, and potency is tested both before and after accelerated aging. Vaccines that contain inactivated organisms, although much more stable than living ones, also contain an excess of organisms for the same reason. Vaccines usually have a designated shelf life, and although properly stored vaccines may still be potent after the expiration of this shelf life, this should never be assumed and all expired vaccines should be discarded.

"Dead" vaccines are commonly available in liquid form and usually contain suspended adjuvant. These should not be frozen, and they should be shaken well before use. The presence of preservatives such as phenol or merthiolate in these will not control massive bacterial contamination, and multidose containers should be discarded after partial use. Many living vaccines are available freeze-dried in sealed vials. These store well but should be kept cool and away from light and should only be reconstituted with the fluid provided by the manufacturer.

ADDITIONAL SOURCES OF INFORMATION

Beard CW. 1979. Avian immunoprophylaxis. Avian Dis *23* 327–335.

Davidson I. 1975. Testing veterinary vaccines. Vet Rec *97* 389–392.

Fox JP, Elveback L, Scott W, Gatewood L, and Ackerman E. 1971. Herd immunity: basic concept and relevance to public health immunization practices. Am J Epidemiol *94* 179–189.

Hennessen W, and Huygelen C (eds). 1979. Immunization: benefits versus risk factors. Dev Biol Stand *43* 1–476.

Pharmaceutical Society of Great Britain. 1965 (Supplement 1970). British Veterinary Codex. Pharmaceutical Press, London.

Schultz RD, and Scott FW. 1978. Canine and feline immunization. Vet Clin North Am (Small Animal Practice) *8* 755–768.

Symposium. 1978. Advances in the applications of attenuated and killed vaccines. Am J Clin Path *70* 113–196.

Webster AC. 1975. The adverse effect of environment in the response to distemper vaccination. Aust Vet J *51* 488–490.

13

Resistance to Bacteria and
Related Organisms

Although animals live in an environment densely populated with bacteria, the vast majority of these organisms are capable neither of invading animal tissues nor of causing disease. Indeed, many of these bacteria are essential for the animal's well being, since they maintain an environment on body surfaces that is inimical to potential invaders, and assist in the digestion of foods, particularly celluloses. Nevertheless, many of these "commensal" organisms are also potential pathogens. For example, both *Clostridium tetani* and *Cl. perfringens* are commonly found among the intestinal flora, while *Bordetella bronchiseptica* is found in the nasopharynx of many healthy swine. It is apparent, therefore, that bacterial disease is not an inevitable consequence of the presence on body surfaces cf pathogenic organisms. It is, in fact, related to a number of other factors including the resistance of the host, the presence of damaged tissues, the exact location of the organism within the body and the disease-producing power (or virulence) of the organism. Only when the balance between host resistance and bacterial virulence is upset will disease or death result.

BACTERIAL STRUCTURE AND ANTIGENS

Bacteria are ovoid or spherical organisms consisting of a cytoplasm containing the essential elements of cell structure surrounded by a cell membrane. The cell membrane is in turn covered by a cell wall that in some bacteria is enclosed by a capsule. From the cell there may extend flagella and pili (Fig. 13–1). The bacterial cytoplasm contains

193

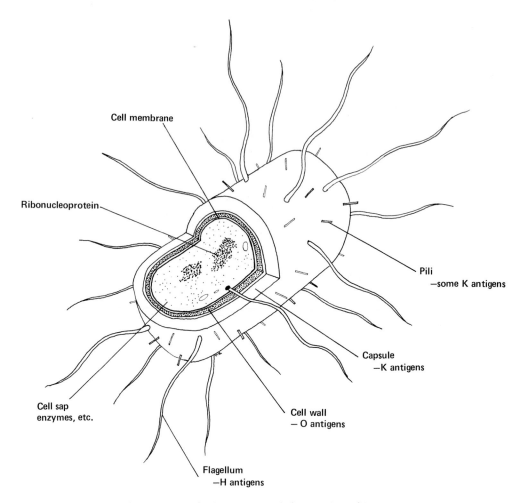

Figure 13-1 The structure of a bacterium and the position of its important antigens.

a complex mixture of enzymes and nucleoproteins, many of which are potentially antigenic. Since, however, these are confined to the interior of the organism, they are usually less important than the surface antigens in stimulating a protective immune response. The three major antigenic structures of the bacterial surface are the cell wall, the capsule and the flagella. The cell wall of gram-positive organisms is largely protein, whereas that of gram-negative organisms is a polysaccharide-lipid-protein structure. The cell wall antigens of gram-negative organisms are toxic (they are called endotoxins) and are collectively classified as O antigens. Bacterial capsules may be polysaccharide or protein in nature. Because of their hydrophilic properties, capsules render organisms resistant to phagocytosis; therefore, encapsulated organisms such as those of the *Klebsiella* species or *Streptococcus pneumoniae* are usually very poorly cleared from the blood stream unless antibody is present. For this reason, antibodies directed against these capsular or K antigens are essential for protection, and vaccines that do not contain K antigens tend to be relatively ineffective. Bacterial flagella consist of protein and so are fully antigenic. Their antigens are known as H antigens. One other significant group of bacterial antigens are the exotoxins, proteins secreted by or derived from the cytoplasm of gram-positive bacteria and responsible for some bacterial diseases. Exotoxins are highly immunogenic and are readily neutralized by antibodies (antitoxins).

PATHOGENESIS OF BACTERIAL INFECTIONS

Bacteria may cause disease by many different mechanisms but in general they may either release toxins or by invasion and multiplication cause physical destruction of host cells. The toxins of bacteria may be divided into two groups: (1) toxins derived from the interior of organisms such as the clostridia and loosely called exotoxins, and (2) endotoxins derived from the cell walls of gram-negative organisms such as the salmonellae. The differences between these two types of toxin are great (Table 13–1), and consequently the nature and significance of the immune response against toxigenic organisms varies according to the source of the toxin.

PATHOGENESIS OF DISEASE DUE TO EXOTOXIGENIC ORGANISMS

Exotoxins are produced within bacterial cytoplasm. Some are secreted through the living cell wall and so are considered to be extracellular toxins, whereas others are released only by lysis of bacteria and so are termed protoplasmic toxins. One of the most significant diseases caused by an exotoxin is tetanus, which occurs as a result of the release from *Cl. tetani* of a powerful protoplasmic neurotoxin. *Cl. tetani* is strictly anaerobic and will, therefore, grow only in areas where oxygen tension is low, usually as a result of tissue destruction. The tetanus toxin, also known as tetanospasmin, is released from the bacteria as a prototoxin and is activated by proteolytic enzymes. It travels from the site of bacterial growth along nerve trunks to the spinal ganglia, where it interferes with the passage of the inhibitory transmitter and so blocks inhibitory synapses. As a result of this interference, tetanic spasm of voluntary

Table 13–1 COMPARISON OF THE GENERAL PROPERTIES OF EXOTOXINS AND ENDOTOXINS

	EXOTOXINS	*ENDOTOXINS*
Source	Secreted by living, usually gram-positive organisms or re-leased from their cytoplasm on autolysis	Autolytic products from the cell walls of (usually gram-negative) bacteria
Chemical composition	Protein	Lipopolysaccharide-protein complexes
Lethality	Powerful toxins	Weak toxins
Stability	Heat labile	Heat stable
Activity	Each toxin has a specific pharmacological activity on a specific target	A nonspecific effect on a number of body systems
Antigenicity	Highly antigenic and readily neutralized by antibody	Weak antigen and poorly neutralized by antibody
Effect of formaldehyde	Forms toxoid	No effect

muscles and, eventually, nerve block and paralysis occur. The capacity to induce nerve blockage is also a property of the protoplasmic toxins of *Clostridium botulinum*. These toxins are absorbed intact following ingestion of contaminated food and cause death as a result of respiratory paralysis. The dose of botulinum toxin needed to block nervous activity is extremely small, only about eight molecules being required to block transmission by a neuron completely. A rather different type of exotoxin is the α toxin of *Cl. perfringens*, which is an extracellular phospholipase capable of causing hemolysis and tissue necrosis and in this way facilitating bacterial growth and invasion.

PATHOGENESIS OF DISEASE DUE TO ENDOTOXIGENIC ORGANISMS

The walls of gram-negative bacteria are complicated structures consisting of a complex of polysaccharides, lipids and proteins. These complexes, known as endotoxins, possess a number of important biological properties (Table 13–2). Most of these activities are associated with the polysaccharide-lipid portions of the complex. The toxic properties, for example, are due to the lipid component known as lipid A. The polysaccharide component, however, is responsible for the characteristic antigenicity of O antigens. It consists of an oligosaccharide attached to the lipid A (which is itself part of the cell membrane), and on the outer side of this complex are found a series of

Table 13–2   BIOLOGICAL PROPERTIES OF ENDOTOXINS

TARGET SYSTEM	EFFECT
Mononuclear phagocyte system	Stimulates macrophage activity and clearance of particles from the blood stream and causes elevations in serum lysozyme
Neutrophils	Impairs leukocyte migration, causes granulocytopenia, releases leukocyte pyrogens
Complement	Activates the alternate patnway, causes release of anaphylatoxins, which results in hypotension and shock, and causes platelet activation, which initiates the clotting system
Clotting	In addition to its effect on complement, endotoxin is also capable of activating the Hageman factor
Lymphocytes	B cell mitogen; stimulates B cells to release lymphokines
Antibody production	Stimulates Ab production, with earlier appearance and higher and more sustained levels of antibody in the 1° response; endotoxin also stimulates the release of antibody from plasma cells
Interferon production	Stimulates the release of preformed interferon within 2 to 4 hours
All cells	Stimulates glycolysis and in high doses is toxic

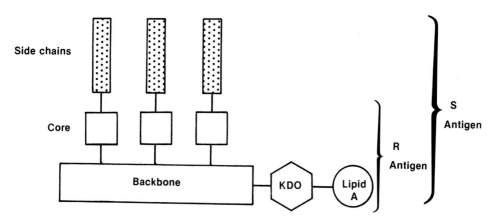

Figure 13–2 The basic structure of the lipopolysaccharide component of the cell wall of gram-negative bacteria such as the salmonellae. KDO is ketodeoxyoctonic acid. The backbone consists of repeating heptose-phosphate units. The core structure consists of glucose and galactose attached to N-acetyl glucosamine.

repeating trisaccharides (Fig. 13–2). The exact composition of these trisaccharides determines the surface antigenicity of the bacteria and many organisms are classified according to this antigenic structure. For example, the salmonellae are a group of bacteria that have been classified into about 1500 "species" through the use of O and H antigens. Thus, O antigen number 1 is a trisaccharide with glucose as its terminal sugar, O antigen number 2 has paratose, O antigen number 3 has mannose, etc. The terminal sugar that confers the antigenic specificity is said to be immunodominant.

Gram-negative bacteria may be found in two forms: One of these, known as the "smooth" form from the nature of its colonies, is fully virulent and possesses the entire surface structure described above. The other is known as the "rough" form. Rough colonies grown on agar possess a matt rather than a shiny surface, and the organisms agglutinate spontaneously when suspended in saline. These rough variants lack the outer trisaccharides and part of the oligosaccharides. Rough variants tend to be avirulent organisms, and several have therefore been employed in vaccines. Examples of these variants include strain 45/20 of *Brucella abortus* and strain 51 of *Salmonella dublin*.

Endotoxins possess a wide range of biological activities that do not depend on their source. When injected into animals they cause malaise, lethargy and temperature changes as well as a variety of other unpleasant effects that may contribute to the disease process. One of the most significant of these effects is the initiation of the complement cascade through the alternate pathway. The activated complement, particularly C3b, mediates extensive platelet aggregation and release of procoagulants. These procoagulants accelerate the coagulation cascade and thrombus formation while the endotoxin itself activates Hageman factor directly. If two spaced doses of endotoxin are given to a rabbit, one intradermally and the second intravenously but several hours later, a violent hemorrhagic necrotic reaction will occur at the site of the first injection within two to three hours. This reaction is due to local thrombosis and infarction at the intradermal injection site and is known as the local Shwartzman reaction. If both doses of endotoxin are given intravenously several hours apart, then disseminated intravascular coagulation and bilateral renal cortical necrosis may result. This tends to be lethal and is known as the generalized Shwartzman or the Shwartzman-Sanarelli reaction. It is probable that reactions of this type may contribute significantly to the destructive effect of infections caused by gram-negative organisms.

PATHOGENESIS OF INFECTION DUE TO INVASIVE ORGANISMS

Disease can be produced by bacterial invasion and subsequent destruction of tissues. This tissue destruction may be due to vascular damage resulting in thrombosis and infarction, to the release of destructive bacterial enzymes or to local metabolic depletion. Some organisms, for example, may secrete hyaluronidase, which, by splitting hyaluronic acid in connective tissue, opens up intercellular spaces and so allows bacteria to spread through tissues. Others secrete fibrinolytic enzymes (for example, streptokinases), which cause clot disruption, and collagenases and elastases, which through destruction of collagen and elastic fibers serve to disrupt the structure of connective tissues. Some of these bacterial proteases may also digest immunoglobulins or complement components. Other organisms, particularly staphylococci, release coagulases, which by causing clot formation may establish a substrate for bacterial growth.

Whereas some bacteria invade intercellular tissue through the use of proteolytic enzymes, others are intracellular parasites. The most notable bacterial examples of these include *B. abortus, Mycobacterium tuberculosis, Listeria monocytogenes* and the *Salmonellae*. Although readily phagocytosed by macrophages, these organisms apear to be resistant to bacteriolysis either by preventing lysosome-phagosome fusion or by being able to withstand the enzymic activities of the contents of normal macrophage lysosomes. For this reason, these organisms may multiply within macrophages and be distributed throughout the body within these cells. Cell death in these cases is caused by the expanding physical bulk of the growing organisms, which leads to cell rupture.

MECHANISMS OF ANTIBACTERIAL RESISTANCE

Although immunologists tend to be preoccupied with the specific immune responses, it must be pointed out that these responses represent only a portion of the defenses available to the animal body. Three general types of protection can, in fact, be identified. The first type is resistance as a result of species insusceptibility. An example of this is *B. abortus*, which is unable to infect chickens. The second type of protection is due to the presence of nonimmunological inhibitory substances, and the third type is mediated by specific immune responses. The specific immune responses are probably the most important of these protective mechanisms, as demonstrated by the inevitably fatal consequences of the failure of an animal to develop a functioning immune system (Chapter 22).

General Factors Influencing Resistance. The most important general factors that influence disease resistance are genetic. Under natural conditions, disease is but one of the selective pressures that act on an animal population. The spread of disease through a population may initially eliminate all susceptible animals but leave a resistant residue to multiply and make use of the newly available resources such as food. By appropriate breeding programs it is therefore possible to develop strains of animals that are either highly resistant or susceptible to a specific disease. (Much of this resistance is due to specific immune-response genes (Chapter 7)).

A second group of nonspecific factors that influence disease resistance are hormones. Age-related resistance is in many cases under hormonal influence. Thus, thyroxine, low doses of steroids, and estrogens may stimulate the immune response, whereas high doses of steroids, testosterone and progesterone are immunosuppressive. In stressed animals, increased steroid production may be immunosuppressive and so help precipitate disease. One example of this stress effect is seen when cattle are subjected to prolonged transportation under suboptimal conditions, as a consequence of which these animals are liable to contract virus infection. This infection results in the development of a pneumonia characterized by secondary invasion with pasteurella organisms and known as shipping fever. A second example is colitis X in horses, a disease associated with salmonella infections and apparently precipitated by stress such as surgery.

The last group of major nonspecific factors that influence disease resistance are nutritional. Malnutrition, specifically protein deficiency, may impair immunoglobulin production (perhaps through a stress mechanism). The negative protein balance incurred in heavily parasitized animals may also have an adverse effect on the immune response, so much so that as far as possible such animals should not be vaccinated until after their parasite burden is reduced. The stressful effect of surgery may also be magnified by the increase in protein catabolism that occurs following surgical intervention and results in a temporary immunosuppression (see also Chapter 22).

Specific Chemical Factors Contributing to Resistance. Convincing evidence of the ability of animal tissues to discourage bacterial invasion is apparent in the relative infrequency of bacterial infections as a consequence of minor skin wounds. Some of this resistance is due to the presence of potent antibacterial factors in tissues (Table 13–3), the most important of which is, perhaps, lysozyme, a bactericidal enzyme first recognized by Sir Alexander Fleming, the discoverer of penicillin. Lysozyme is found in tissues and in all body fluids except cerebrospinal fluid, sweat and urine; it is said to be absent from bovine neutrophils. It is found in particularly high concentrations in

Table 13–3 SOME NONIMMUNOLOGICAL PROTECTIVE FACTORS FOUND IN BODY TISSUES AND FLUIDS

GROUP	*NAME*	*MAJOR SOURCES*	*ACTIVITY AGAINST*
Enzymes	Lysozyme	Serum; leukocytes	Gram-positive and -negative bacteria; some viruses
Basic peptides and proteins	β-Lysin Phagocytin Leukin Plakin	Platelets Neutrophils Neutrophils Platelets	Gram-positive bacteria
Iron binding proteins	Transferrin Lactoferrin	Serum Leukocytes; milk	Gram-positive and -negative bacteria
Basic amines	Spermine; spermidine	Pancreas; kidney; prostate	Gram-positive bacteria
Complement components	—	Serum	Bacteria; viruses; protozoa
Peroxide splitting mechanisms	Myeloperoxidase; xanthine oxidase	Neutrophils; milk	Bacteria; viruses; protozoa
Interferon	—	Most cells but not neutrophils	Viruses; some intra-cellular protozoa

tears and egg white. Lysozyme splits the acylaminopolysaccharides of the capsules of some gram-positive bacteria, thus killing them. It is also capable of participating in the destruction of some gram-negative organisms in conjunction with complement. Although many of the bacteria killed by lysozyme are considered to be nonpathogenic, it might reasonably be pointed out that this susceptibility could account for their lack of pathogenicity. Lysozyme is found in very high concentrations in the lysosomes of neutrophils and so tends to accumulate in areas of acute inflammation, including sites of bacterial invasion. The pH optimum for lysozyme activity, although somewhat low (pH 3 to pH 6), is easily achieved in inflammatory sites as well as within phagosomes, and as a consequence it is here that its antibacterial activity is largely exerted. Finally, lysozyme may also act as a potent opsonin, facilitating phagocytosis in the absence of specific antibodies and under conditions in which its enzymatic activity may be ineffective.

The observation that kidneys remain relatively unaffected in miliary tuberculosis led to the isolation of two tetra-amines called spermine and spermidine, which, in conjunction with a serum α globulin, form a bactericidal complex active against acid-fast organisms, cocci and *Bacillus anthracis*.

Free fatty acids are also inhibitory to bacterial growth under some circumstances. In general, unsaturated fatty acids such as oleic acid tend to be bactericidal for gram-positive organisms, whereas saturated fatty acids are fungicidal. Because of this, scalp ringworm of children, which is somewhat refractory to conventional medical treatment, may resolve spontaneously at puberty when the amount of saturated fatty acids in sebum increases.

A number of peptides and proteins rich in basic amino acids (lysine and arginine) and with potent antibacterial properties have been isolated from mammalian cells and tissues. They are commonly derived from proteins digested as a result of the release of proteolytic enzymes from neutrophils or platelets. β-Lysin, a polypeptide active against *B. anthracis* and the clostridia, is released from platelets as a result of their interaction with immune complexes (Chapter 8).

One of the most important factors that influence the success or failure of bacterial invasion is the level of iron in body fluids. Most bacteria such as *Staphylococcus aureus, Escherichia coli, Pasteurella multocida* and *Mycobacterium tuberculosis* require iron for growth. However, within the body, iron is largely associated with the iron-binding proteins transferrin, lactoferrin and ferritin. In addition, serum iron levels tend to drop following bacterial invasion as a result of cessation of intestinal iron absorption and increased incorporation of iron into the liver. The effect of this action is to effectively hinder bacterial invasion. A similar situation occurs in the udder when, in response to bacterial invasion, neutrophils release their stores of lactoferrin and so enhance the bactericidal power of milk. In spite of this sequestration of iron, some bacteria such as *M. tuberculosis* and *E. coli* succeed in invading the body because they can release potent iron-chelating compounds (mycobactin and enterochelin). These compounds may withdraw iron from serum proteins and render it available to the organisms. In conditions in which serum iron levels are elevated, such as the hemolytic anemias, animals may become extremely susceptible to bacterial infection.

The production of reactive oxygen metabolites, which are important in neutrophils, has been discussed in Chapter 2. Similarly, interferon is discussed in Chapter 14 and the alternate complement pathway in Chapter 8.

SPECIFIC RESISTANCE TO BACTERIAL DISEASE MEDIATED BY THE IMMUNE SYSTEM

There are four basic mechanisms by which the specific immune responses combat bacterial infections (Table 13–4). These are (1) the neutralization of toxins or enzymes by antibody, (2) the killing of bacteria by antibodies, complement and lysozyme, (3) the opsonization of bacteria by antibody (and complement), which results in phagocytosis and destruction of bacteria, and (4) the phagocytosis and intracellular destruction of bacteria by activated macrophages. The relative importance of each of these processes depends upon the organisms involved and on the mechanisms by which they cause disease.

Immunity to Exotoxigenic Organisms. In disease caused by exotoxigenic organisms such as the clostridia or *B. anthracis*, the function of the immune response must be not only to eliminate the invading organisms but also to neutralize any toxin produced by them. Unfortunately, destruction of these bacteria may be quite difficult, especially if they are embedded in a mass of necrotic tissue. On the other hand, antibodies can readily neutralize bacterial exotoxins. It is thought that neutralization occurs as a result of steric hindrance of the combination between the toxin and its receptor on a host cell. The neutralization process therefore involves competition between receptor and antibody for the toxin molecule, and it is apparent that once the toxin has combined with the receptor, antibody will be relatively ineffective in reversing this combination. This result is observed in practice when the dose of antitoxin required to produce clinical improvement in a disease such as tetanus is greatly in excess of that required to prevent the development of clinical disease.

Immunity to Systemically Invasive Organisms. Protection against invasive bacteria is generally mediated by antibodies directed against the surface antigens of the bacteria. Antibodies against antigens in the interior of these organisms, such as ribonucleoprotein or enzymes, are consequently only of limited usefulness in protection (although bacterial ribonucleoprotein may have a significant role in the development of cell-mediated immunity).

Antibody directed against capsular (K) antigens may serve to neutralize the antiphagocytic properties of the capsule, thus opsonizing the organism and permitting bacterial destruction by phagocytic cells to take place. A more subtle protective effect has been reported to occur when antibodies are produced against strains of *E. coli* carrying the adherence antigens K88 or K99. In this case, the antibodies interfere with

Table 13–4 A CLASSIFICATION OF THE IMMUNOLOGICAL MECHANISMS OF ANTIBACTERIAL IMMUNITY

COMPONENTS OF THE IMMUNE SYSTEMS EMPLOYED	BACTERIAL ANTIGEN	RESULT
Antibody with complement (and lysozyme)	Bacterial surface antigens	1. Bacteriolysis 2. Phagocytosis
Antibody (alone)	Protein toxins or enzymes	Toxin or enzyme neutralization
Activated macrophages	Possibly bacterial ribonucleoprotein	Intracellular destruction of organism

the expression of the antigen, and it has been claimed that they are eventually able to cause deletion of the genetic material (plasmid) that codes for these antigens. Once the antigens are deleted, these strains of *E. coli* cannot adhere to the intestinal wall and are thus no longer pathogenic.

In organisms lacking capsules, antibodies directed against O antigens also function as opsonins. An example of the importance of bacterial capsules in the pathogenesis of disease is seen in anthrax. *B. anthracis* is an organism that possesses both a capsule and an exotoxin. Antitoxic immunity is protective in this disease but is slow to develop. In addition, toxin production tends to be prolonged, since the organism is encapsulated and phagocytic cells are therefore unable to eliminate the source of the toxin. As a result, death is usually inevitable in unvaccinated animals. The vaccine commonly employed against anthrax contains an unencapsulated but toxigenic strain of the organism. Given in the form of spores that can germinate, the unencapsulated organisms are eliminated by phagocytic cells before dangerous amounts of toxin are synthesized but not before antitoxic immunity is stimulated.

Whereas some bacteria are phagocytosed and destroyed by neutrophils or macrophages, or both, others are killed when free in the circulation. In sensitized animals, bacteria are destroyed by the actions of specific antibody and complement activated by the classical pathway. In unsensitized animals, the bacteria are destroyed by complement acting through the alternate pathway. Bacterial cell walls, lacking sialic acid, are capable of inactivating factor H and thus promoting the activation of C3. As a result, they are either opsonized or lysed. The importance of this pathway is apparent in bovine mycoplasma infections, in which pathogenic and nonpathogenic organisms may be differentiated on the basis of their ability to activate the alternate pathway. Nonpathogenic mycoplasmas activate the pathway; pathogenic ones do not.

Activation of the terminal complement pathway leads to the development of cell wall lesions similar to those seen by electron microscopy of complement-lysed red cells. The cell wall lesions alone are, however, insufficient to kill many gram-negative bacteria, but they reveal a substrate for the enzyme lysozyme. Lysozyme therefore acts on bacteria subsequent to complement to cause bacteriolysis (Fig. 13–3).

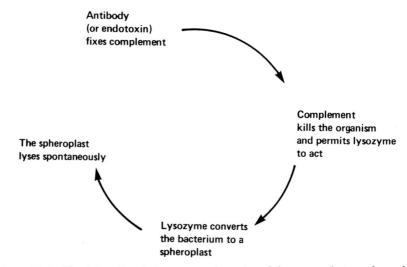

Figure 13–3 The interaction between complement and lysozyme that produces lysis of gram-negative organisms.

On a molar basis, IgM is about 500 to 1000 times more efficient than IgG in opsonization and about 100 times more potent than IgG in sensitizing bacteria for complement-mediated lysis. Therefore, during a primary immune response the quantitative deficiency of the IgM response is compensated for by its quality, thus ensuring early and efficient protection.

Immunity to Facultative Intracellular Parasites. Certain organisms of major veterinary importance, particularly *B. abortus, M. tuberculosis, L. monocytogenes, Corynebacterium ovis* and the salmonellae, are engulfed by macrophages but are resistant to subsequent intracellular destruction. These organisms (which are, therefore, facultative intracellular parasites) can replicate within macrophages in an environment free of antibody; as a consequence, the normal humoral immune response is relatively ineffective. Passively transferred antiserum will not confer protection against these bacteria, although passively transferred lymphocytes will. Therefore, protection against this type of organism is cell-mediated. Although macrophages from unimmunized animals are normally incapable of destroying these organisms, this ability is acquired by the macrophages about ten days after onset of infection. These changes that occur in these macrophages include increases in cell size, in metabolic activity and in the size and number of their lysosomes (see Fig. 6–11). These changes are associated with a significant increase in the bactericidal capacity of the cells (see Fig. 6–12). The changes themselves are a reflection of a form of "acquired cell-mediated immunity," which is mediated through lymphokines released by sensitized T cells on exposure to bacterial ribonucleoprotein (Fig. 13–4). The response of activated macrophages tends

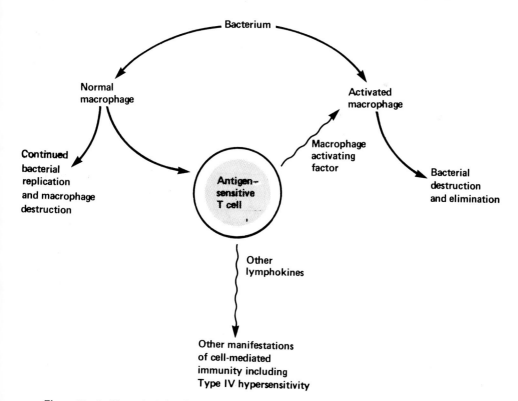

Figure 13–4 The principle of acquired cellular immunity to facultative intracellular parasites. Macrophages activated by T cells acquire the capacity to destroy otherwise resistant bacteria.

to be nonspecific, particulaly in listerial infections, and these cells are therefore capable of destroying a wide range of normally resistant bacteria. Thus, an animal recovering from an infection with *L. monocytogenes* shows increased resistance to infection by *M. tuberculosis*. The development of these activated macrophages often coincides with the appearance of delayed (type IV) hypersensitivity to intradermally administered antigen. It has also been noted that protective immunity against these bacteria cannot be induced by the use of vaccines containing killed organisms, although vaccines containing living bacteria are protective.

If, in a bacterial disease, it is observed that dead vaccines do not give good protection, that serum cannot confer protection, that antibody titers do not appear to relate to resistance and that delayed hypersensitivity reactions can be elicited to the bacterial antigens, then the possibility that cell-mediated immunity may play an important role in resistance to the causative organism should be considered and the use of vaccines containing living organisms should be contemplated.

METHODS EMPLOYED BY BACTERIA IN EVADING THE IMMUNE RESPONSES

Bacteria, like all parasites, are not well served either by the death of their chosen host or by their immune elimination. Mechanisms have thus evolved by which the consequences of the immune responses may be evaded. We have already discussed such features as the use of antiphagocytic capsules and facultative intracellular parasitism, both of which tend to delay bacterial destruction. Some organisms such as *E. coli, M. tuberculosis* and *Pseudomonas aeruginosa* secrete factors that can depress phagocytosis by neutrophils. The most extreme form of this is shown by *Pasteurella haemolytica*, which secretes factors that kill ruminant alveolar macrophages but not macrophages from swine, horses or humans. *Hemophilus pleuropneumoniae* will kill porcine macrophages.

Other organisms can inhibit the bactericidal activities of cells in a more subtle fashion. For example, the carotenoid pigments responsible for the color of *S. aureus* can quench singlet oxygen and so survive the respiratory burst. *P. multocida* is also capable of inhibiting the respiratory burst, whereas strains of *E. coli* may carry a plasmid that confers resistance to complement-mediated lysis. Other protective devices employed by pathogenic bacteria include the production of proteolytic enzymes specific for IgA produced by *Streptococcus gonorrhoeae* and *S. pneumoniae*.

Campylobacter fetus, an organism that normally colonizes the male and female genital tracts in cattle, shows cyclical antigenic variation. The successful destruction of a major portion of this bacterial population by a local immune response leaves a residual population of organisms that possess antigenic determinants differing from those of the original population. This residual population may multiply and be largely eliminated in turn by a second immune response, leaving a residual population of a third antigenic type. This process may be repeated for a prolonged period, and, because of the poor memory in the IgA-producing system (Chapter 10), the organisms may reutilize antigens without stimulating a secondary immune response.

Mycoplasma mycoides evades the immune response in a different fashion by exerting a toxic effect on T cells. The mechanism of this effect is not clear but may involve competition with these cells for essential nutrients. Whatever the cause, the result is a depression of the immune response. The fungal toxin aflatoxin is also immunosuppressive, reducing the resistance of poultry to *P. multocida* and salmonellosis. Finally, the release of cyclic AMP by some organisms may permit them to survive in intracellular locations by preventing the fusion of lysosomes with the phagosome (see Table 7–1).

ADVERSE CONSEQUENCES OF THE IMMUNE RESPONSES TO BACTERIA

Although the immune responses are generally considered to be beneficial in that they serve to eliminate invading bacteria, this is not necessarily always the case. The immune responses are capable of influencing the course of bacterial diseases without producing a cure and in some situations appear to result in an increase in the severity of the pathological lesions. An example of the modulating influence of the immune responses is observed in human leprosy, in which two very different forms of disease occur, both due to the same organism, *Mycobacterium leprae*. In the tuberculoid form of the disease, the immune response appears to be primarily cell-mediated and serum antibodies are low. The lesions, although almost devoid of organisms, consist of typical tubercle-like granulomas. In the lepromatous form of the disease, organisms are present in large numbers within invasive lesions and little cellular response occurs. The affected individual has high serum antibody levels but no detectable cell-mediated response. A similar variation in disease types occurs in brucellosis, in which some species such as guinea pig and swine tend to show localized granulomatous lesions, whereas in cattle the disease is of a more invasive type.

The adverse consequences of the immune responses correspond in their mechanisms to the hypersensitivity types described in Chapter 8. Thus, it has been suggested that in chickens suffering from fowl typhoid (salmonellosis) and in pigs with edema disease (caused by *E. coli*) (Chapter 17), death may be associated with a type I (anaphylactic) hypersensitivity reaction against bacterial products. A local type I hypersensitivity reaction is sometimes seen in sheep vaccinated against foot-rot by means of *Fusobacterium necrophorum* vaccine, but in this case it is felt that the hypersensitivity may assist in preventing reinfection.

Type II (cytotoxic) reactions may account for the anemia occurring in animals with salmonellosis. In these infections, bacterial lipopolysaccharides released from disrupted bacteria are readily adsorbed onto erythrocytes, and the subsequent immune response against the bacterium and its products therefore results in erythrocyte destruction. Although a similar anemia is observed in leptospirosis, its mechanism is unknown, since antibodies produced by infected animals may agglutinate normal red cells taken from the same animal prior to infection (Chapter 21).

Type III (immune complex) reactions may contribute to the development of arthritis in *Erysipelothrix rhusiopathiae (E. insidiosa)* infections in pigs or to the development of intestinal lesions in Johne's disease due to *Mycobacterium paratuberculosis*. In the former case, bacterial antigen tends to localize in joint tissues where local immune complex formation then results in inflammation and arthritis. Passively administered antiserum may therefore exacerbate the arthritis in these infected animals. In Johne's disease, type I or type III reactions occurring in the intestinal mucosa may result in an increased outflow of fluid and diarrhea. It is probable, however, that the intestinal lesions in this disease are etiologically complex, since diarrhea can be transferred to normal calves by either plasma or leukocytes, and antihistamines may reduce the diarrhea. The immune response to *M. paratuberculosis* is also known to be, in large part, cell-mediated. Type III hypersensitivity reactions may be involved in equine periodic ophthalmia as a result of the development of antileptospiral antibodies and also in purpura hemorrhagica of horses, in which a serum sickness–type of lesion may result from the immune response to *Streptococcus equi*.

Although cell-mediated immune responses are, in general, manifestly beneficial, they do contribute to the development of granulomatous lesions in some chronic infections (Chapter 20). The development of large granulomata, while serving to "wall off" invading organisms and so prevent their spread, may also involve uninfected tissues. If these granulomata involve essential structures such as airways in the lungs or large blood vessels, severe damage may occur.

ADDITIONAL COMMENTS ON ANTIBACTERIAL VACCINES USED IN ANIMALS

Toxoids. The immunoprophylaxis of tetanus is essentially restricted to toxin neutralization. Tetanus toxoid in an aluminum hydroxide suspension is normally given for routine prophylaxis, and a single injection of this material will induce protective immunity in 10 to 14 days. Conventional immunological wisdom would suggest that the previous use of antitoxin should interfere with the immune response to toxoid and must therefore be avoided. This is not true in practice, and both may be successfully administered simultaneously without problems. This may be because of the relatively small amount of antitoxin usually employed to protect animals.

Some other veterinary vaccines combine both toxoid and killed bacteria in a single dose by the simple expedient of formolizing a whole culture. These vaccines are sometimes called anacultures. Anacultures are used to vaccinate against *Clostridium haemolyticum* and *Cl. perfringens*. In vaccination against *Cl. perfringens*, trypsinization of the anaculture is commonly performed since this renders it more immunogenic. Toxoids, usually incorporated with an alum adjuvant, are available for most clostridial diseases and for diseases due to toxigenic staphylococci.

Bacterins. Bacterin is the term used to describe vaccines containing killed bacteria. It is usual to kill the organisms with formaldehyde and to incorporate them with alum or aluminum hydroxide adjuvants. Apart from the bacterins against pasteurellosis (shipping fever) and salmonellosis, which are of doubtful efficacy, most other bacterins are effective but somewhat limited in their usage. As with other dead vaccines, the immunity produced is relatively short-lived, usually lasting for not longer than a year and sometimes for a considerably shorter period. Thus, formolized swine erysipelas *(E. rhusiopathiae)* vaccine protects for only four to five months, and *S. equi* bacterins give immunity for less than a year, even though recovery from a natural case of strangles confers a lifelong immunity in horses.

Bacterins may be improved by adding purified immunogenic antigens to the killed bacteria. Thus, *E. coli* bacterins against enteric colibacillosis may be enriched and made much more effective by the addition of K88 or K99 antigens to the mixture. Antibodies to these antigens effectively block binding of *E. coli* to the intestinal wall and thus contribute significantly to the protective immune response.

One problem encountered when using coliform and campylobacter bacterins particularly is strain specificity. Several different antigenic types of each organism commonly occur, and successful vaccination requires immunization with appropriate bacterial strains. This is sometimes not possible if a commercial bacterin must be employed. One method of overcoming this difficulty is to use autogenous vaccines. These are vaccines that contain either organisms obtained from infected animals on the farm where the disease problem is occurring or from the infected animal itself. These can be very successful if carefully prepared, since the vaccine will contain all the antigens required for protection in that particular location. As an alternative to the use of autogenous vaccines, some manufacturers produce polyvalent vaccines containing a mixture of antigenic types. For example, leptospirosis vaccines commonly contain up to five different serovars. This practice, although effective, is inefficient, since only a few of the antigenic types employed may be appropriate in any given situation.

As pointed out earlier, the use of bovine respiratory disease vaccines containing killed *Pasteurella* organisms together with viral components has been shown to be associated with increased mortality due to respiratory disease. The reasons for this are unclear.

Living Bacterial Vaccines. Perhaps the most successful of the living bacterial vaccines in current practice is strain 19 of *B. abortus* (see page 183). Another successful living vaccine is the BCG (bacille Calmette-Guérin) strain of *M. bovis*. However, although this vaccine has been used with success in Europe, it has failed to protect against African and Asian strains of *M. tuberculosis*.

Another group of living vaccines are those employed for the prevention of anthrax. Older anthrax vaccines utilized Pasteur's technique of culturing the organisms at a relatively high temperature (42 to 43° C) so that their virulence is reduced. The anthrax vaccines currently available contain capsule-less mutants, which remain capable of forming spores. The vaccine is prepared as a spore suspension and is administered with saponin. A live avirulent vaccine is also employed against swine erysipelas, for which it has some decided advantages over the dead vaccines. In particular, it can be given in food, its efficiency is unaffected by antibiotic treatment, there seems to be no adverse effect of overdosing and it protects against arthritis, a feature not found in dead vaccines. Unfortunately, the avirulence of this strain is not fully fixed and there is some difficulty in preventing its reconversion to the virulent form. A rough strain of *S. dublin* (strain 51) is used in Europe to give good protection to calves when administered at two to four weeks of age. As discussed earlier, immunity to salmonellosis is cell-mediated and thus relatively nonspecific. For this reason, strain 51 may also give good protection against *Salmonella typhimurium*.

Vaccines against contagious bovine pleuropneumonia (CBPP) usually contain living organisms of reduced virulence. The organisms are cultured in eggs, and good protection used to be obtained by injecting this avianized vaccine into the tip of the tail of cattle. Unfortunately, the reaction of cattle to this organism, even in vaccine form, can be extremely violent and the tail usually dropped off! However, the severity of this toxic reaction tends to relate positively to the degree of immunity produced, weakly toxic vaccines giving poor immunity and strongly toxic vaccines giving good immunity. For this reason excellent immunity is now produced by giving the vaccine subcutaneously and, if necessary, controlling the subsequent reaction with tylosin.

CONCLUDING REMARKS

When antibiotics were first introduced, the stimulus for much research into antibacterial immunity was removed. As a result of the ready availability of antibiotics, the development of new vaccines against bacterial diseases slowed down so that they are now only a little more advanced than they were 35 years ago.

This situation is rapidly changing as the development of antibiotic resistance and alterations in agricultural economics increase the demand for efficient, cheap antibacterial vaccines. Many problems remain to be solved, however. These include the significance and role of cell-mediated immunity in bacterial disease and the relationship of this type of immunity to an apparent mandatory requirement for living organisms. In addition, a rapid expansion of the antigenic spectrum of many vaccines is urgently required in order to confer protection against a much wider range of different antigenic types of many organisms.

ADDITIONAL SOURCES OF INFORMATION

Adegboye DS. 1978. A review of mycoplasma-induced immunosuppression. Br Vet J *134* 556–560.
Alton GG. 1978. Recent developments in vaccination against bovine brucellosis. Aust Vet J *54* 551–557.
Barton CE, and Lomme JR. 1980. Reduced-dose whole-herd vaccination against bovine brucellosis: a review of recent experience. JAVMA *177* 1281–1220.
Liefman CE. 1980. Combined active-passive immunization of horses against tetanus. Aust Vet J *56* 119–122.
Kramer TT. 1978. Immunity to bacterial infections. Vet Clin North Am (Small Animal Practice) *8* 683–695.
Mims CA. 1976. The Pathogenesis of Infectious Disease. Grune and Stratton, New York.
Morrison DC, and Ryan JL. 1979. Bacterial endotoxins and host immune responses. Adv Immunol *28* 293–450.
Morrison WI, and Wright NG. 1976. Canine leptospirosis: an immunopathological study of interstitial nephritis due to *Leptospira canicola*. J Pathol *120* 83–89.
Reiter B. 1978. Antimicrobial systems in milk. J Dairy Res *45* 131–147.
Schwab JH. 1975. Immunosuppression by bacteria. *In* Hobart MS, and Neter E. (eds). The Immune System and Infectious Diseases (Fourth International Convocation on Immunology, June 1974). S. Karger, Basel, pp 64–65.
Wells PW, Evans HB, Burrells C, *et al.* 1979. Inability of passively acquired antibody to protect lambs against experimental pasteurellosis. Infect Immun *26* 25–29.
Winter AJ. 1979. Mechanisms of immunity in bacterial infections. Adv Vet Sci Comp Med *23* 53–69.
Woolcock JB. 1979. Bacterial Infection and Immunity in Domestic Animals. Developments in Animal and Veterinary Science series. Elsevier North-Holland, New York.

14

Resistance to Viruses and Related Organisms

This chapter discusses the nature of the immune responses to animal viruses. Since these organisms are obligate intracellular parasites, their very existence is threatened if they are completely eliminated from the body by the immune responses. Similarly, viruses are not well-served by the death of their host as a result of virus-mediated disease. As a consequence of these opposing factors, both viruses and their hosts must be amenable to a process of adaptation and selection. The viruses are selected for their ability to evade the hosts' immune responses, and host animals are selected for resistance to virus-induced disease. It is possible, therefore, to loosely classify viruses on the basis of their ability to evade the hosts' immune responses, a property that shows an inverse relationship to their virulence. For example, in infections where virus-host adaptation is poor, diseases tend to be acute and severe, but no detectable virus can be found in survivors. Diseases of this type include feline panleukopenia, canine distemper and the acute forms of Newcastle disease. Vaccination tends to be relatively successful in this type of infection. In a more adapted situation, although the viral disease may be relatively acute, mortality may not necessarily be high and the virus may be persistent. In addition, further attacks can occur as a result of infection by antigenic variants of the same species of virus. Examples of this type of virus infection include foot-and-mouth disease and influenza. Vaccination against diseases of this type tends to be difficult because of this antigenic variability. In an even more adapted state, some viruses cause persistent infection and the immune systems appear to be incapable of causing viral elimination. Diseases of this type include equine infectious anemia and Aleutian disease of mink. Vaccination against these diseases is essentially unsuccessful.

In studying the nature of the host responses to viruses, it is perhaps well to recognize that this continuing selective pressure on both host and virus exists and profoundly influences the outcome of all host-virus interactions.

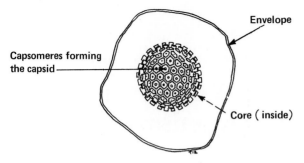

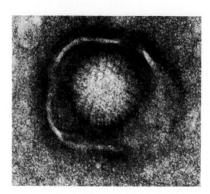

Figure 14−1 The structure of a virus (Equine herpesvirus type I) (× 184,000) and the position of important viral antigens. (Courtesy of Dr. J. Thorsen.)

VIRUS STRUCTURE AND ANTIGENS (Fig. 14–1)

Viruses are very small particles that consist of a nucleic acid core surrounded by a layer of repeating protein subunits. This protein layer is termed the capsid, and the constituent subunits are termed the capsomeres. Viruses may also be surrounded by an envelope containing lipoprotein and derived in part from the host cell. The complexity of viral antigens varies with the species; some such as pox viruses are complex whereas others such as foot-and-mouth disease virus are relatively simple. Antibodies can be produced against all the proteins situated both inside and on the surface of the virus. Antibodies against the nucleoprotein components are not usually considered to be highly significant from a protective point of view, but they may be of some assistance in diagnostic procedures.

PATHOGENESIS OF VIRUS INFECTIONS

Viruses are obligate intracellular parasites that invade and alter the properties of cells. The alterations in infected cells may be minimal, perhaps only detectable by the development of new antigens on the cell surface, or the changes may be extensive and result in either cell lysis or malignant transformation and the development of a tumor. In general, the severity of a virus disease in an animal is related to the magnitude of these cellular changes.

Of particular interest to immunologists are the virus diseases in which the cells of lymphoid tissues are infected primarily (Table 14–1). In some of these diseases the

Table 14–1 VIRUSES THAT AFFECT LYMPHOID TISSUES

VIRUSES THAT DESTROY LYMPHOID TISSUES
    Canine distemper
    Infectious bursal disease
    Newcastle disease
    Mouse thymus herpesvirus
    Feline panleukopenia
    African swine fever
    Bovine virus diarrhea

VIRUSES THAT STIMULATE LYMPHOID TISSUE ACTIVITY TO AN UNUSUAL EXTENT
    Visna
    Aleutian disease

VIRUSES THAT CAUSE LYMPHOID NEOPLASIA
    Marek's disease
    Feline leukemia
    Bovine leukemia
    Mouse leukemia

---

primary lymphoid organs may be specifically involved. For example, mice can be infected by a herpesvirus that causes massive necrosis of the cortex of the thymus. This "viral thymectomy" will naturally result in the development of immunological defects. In poultry, the virus of infectious bursal disease acts primarily on the lymphoid cells of the bursa of Fabricius to cause necrosis. This virus is not completely specific for the bursa, since it may also cause damage to the spleen and thymus. However, these tissues usually recover, whereas the bursa atrophies. The consequences of this infection, as might be predicted, are most evident in young birds infected immediately after hatching. These animals have a significantly reduced capacity for antibody production. If infection with the bursal disease virus is delayed for several weeks after hatching, then, again predictably, antibody production tends to be unaffected.

Some viruses are capable of infecting and destroying secondary lymphoid organs. For example, canine distemper (CD) virus, although it can multiply in a wide variety of cells, has a predilection for cells of lymphatic tissues as well as for epithelia and nervous tissue. In experimentally infected dogs, the CD virus is found first in tonsils and bronchial lymph nodes, from which it spreads to the spleen, lymph nodes and bone marrow, where the virus replicates causing lymphoid destruction. The shedding of infected cells from these tissues enables the virus to reach epithelial tissues and the brain. The destruction of lymphoid tissues and epithelium in this disease and the consequent immunosuppression account, in large part, for the clinical disease. If germ-free dogs are infected by virulent distemper virus, they suffer from a relatively mild disease, presumably because secondary infection cannot occur.

As well as in CD, depletion of lymphoid tissues is seen in feline panleukopenia (FPL), feline leukemia (FeLV) and African swine fever, where the virus tends to localize in germinal centers. Bovine virus diarrhea (BVD) can cause destruction of lymphocytes in the lymph nodes, spleen, thymus and Peyer's patches. The destruction of the Peyer's patches causes local ulceration and permits secondary bacterial invasion. BVD also exerts a generalized immunosuppressive effect through stimulation of interferon production, and it is capable of depressing some neutrophil functions such as degranulation and antibody-dependent cellular cytotoxicity (ADCC).

The results of virus-induced lymphoid tissue destruction are readily seen as a lymphopenia or a depression in the capacity of circulating lymphocytes to respond to mitogenic stimuli. For example, the response of peripheral blood lymphocytes to the plant lectin phytohemagglutinin is depressed in influenza, canine distemper, Marek's disease, Newcastle disease, bovine virus diarrhea and lymphocytic choriomeningitis. The immunosuppression observed in Newcastle disease infection is possibly due to the action of viral neuraminidase on lymphocyte membranes, which modifies their circulation within the lymphoid organs. Destruction of lymphoid tissue may also be reflected in hypogammaglobulinemia or a depressed ability to respond to antigen either with humoral antibodies or by graft rejection.

The effect of some viruses on the immune system may be relatively complex or anomalous. In canine distemper, for instance, lymphocyte reactivity to phytohemagglutinin is depressed but graft rejection is normal. In visna, a neurologic disease of sheep caused by a retrovirus, cell-mediated immune reactions such as graft rejection are suppressed while B-cell responses are enhanced. Some leukemia viruses can exert selective depressive effects, so that depression of the 7S antibody response is greater than that of the 19S antibody response. In equine infectious anemia, the IgG(T) response is variably depressed whereas synthesis of the other immunoglobulin subclasses remains unaffected. It has been claimed that, although chickens infected with Marek's disease show enhanced graft-versus-host reactivity (Chapter 16), they exhibit depressed graft rejection.

MECHANISMS OF ANTIVIRAL RESISTANCE

Nonimmunological Defense Mechanisms.   Just as nonimmunological factors influence susceptibility to bacterial disease, they modify and control the outcome of many viral infections. Lysozyme, for example, is capable of destroying several viruses, as are many of the intestinal enzymes. Bile is a powerful neutralizer of some viruses, so much so that Koch first successfully vaccinated cattle against rinderpest with the bile of animals dying from that disease.

INTERFERENCE AND INTERFERONS.   Probably the most important of the nonimmunological antiviral defense mechanisms is interference. Interference is the name given to the inhibition of viral replication by the presence of other viruses. One cause of this inhibition is the production of interferons. Interferons are released from virus-infected cells within a few hours after viral invasion, and high concentrations of interferon may be achieved within a few days *in vivo*, at a time when the primary immune response is still relatively ineffectual (Fig. 14–2). For example, in cattle that receive infectious bovine rhinotracheitis (IBR) virus intravenously, peak interferon levels in serum may be reached one to two days later and then decline, but they are still detectable by seven days. In contrast, antibody production is usually not apparent until five to six days after virus administration.

Interferons make up a class of glycoproteins with molecular weights that vary according to the method used to induce them but that generally lie between 20,000 and 34,000 daltons. Three major classes are recognized in humans and mice (Table 14–2): interferon α (IFN-α), a family of at least five different molecules derived from virus-infected leukocytes; interferon β (IFN-β) derived from virus-infected fibroblasts; and interferon γ (IFN-γ), a lymphokine derived from antigen-stimulated T cells. IFN-α and IFN-β are stable at pH2, whereas IFN-γ is labile at low pH. All are heat stable

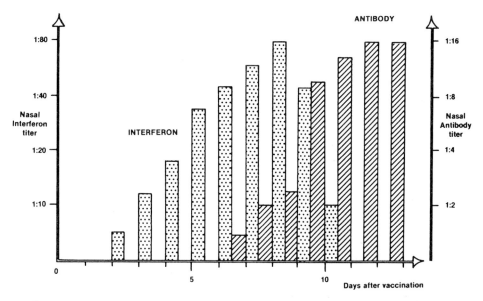

Figure 14–2 The sequential production of interferon and antibody following intranasal vaccination of calves with infectious bovine rhinotracheitis vaccine. (From data kindly provided by Dr. M. Savan.)

and only weakly antigenic. Production of IFN-α and IFN-β is brought about by the association between viral genetic material and host cell ribosomes, resulting in derepression of target cell DNA coding for interferon production. Interferons act on uninfected cells by derepressing their DNA so that they produce a protein known as translation-inhibitory-protein (TIP). TIP in turn can block the takeover of cell ribosomes by viral RNA (Fig. 14–3) and hence inhibit virus replication.

Virus-induced interferons are relatively species-specific; for example, bovine interferon appears to be most effective when acting on bovine cells. They are not, however, virus-specific, and interferon induced by one virus may be equally effective when acting against other, unrelated viruses. The capacity of cells to produce interferon varies. T cells appear to represent the major source of interferon in many virus diseases (Chapter 7), whereas other cells such as those from the kidney are relatively poor interferon producers, and neutrophils produce no interferon.

Although live or inactivated viruses are normally considered to be the most important stimulators of interferon production, interferons may also be produced under circumstances other than virus infection. For example, bacterial endotoxins appear to be able to stimulate the release of interferon from target cells within a few minutes of exposure. This interferon differs both in size and in heat stability from that produced by virus-infected cells and is probably released from stores within cells. Other substances that can induce interferon production include some plant extracts such as

Table 14–2 THE CLASSIFICATION OF INTERFERONS

SOURCE	NAME	TARGET	EFFECT
Leukocytes	IFN-α ⎫	Virus-infected cells	Blocking of viral replication
Fibroblasts	IFN-β ⎬	Suppressor cells	Immunosuppression
T, B or NK cells	IFN-γ ⎭	T and NK cells	Enhanced cytotoxicity

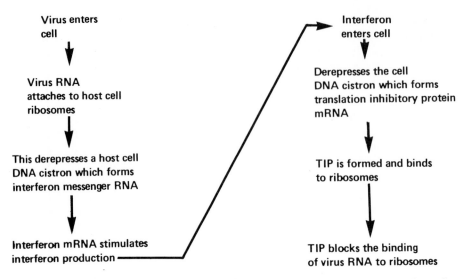

Figure 14–3 The mechanism by which interferon prevents viral replication within cells.

phytohemagglutinin and synthetic polymers, which act by mimicking the action of viral RNA. One of the most potent of these synthetic polymers (Poly I:C) consists of inosinic and cytidilic acids. Poly I:C may increase survival in experimental virus infections.

A second and probably much more important role for the interferons is the regulation of immune reactivity (Chapter 7). Interferons can enhance both suppressor and cytotoxic cell activity (see Fig. 7–5). The result of stimulating cytotoxic cells, especially NK cells, is enhancement of antitumor and anti–virus-infected-cell immunity.

Table 14–3 MECHANISMS OF ANTIVIRAL IMMUNITY

COMPONENTS EMPLOYED	TARGET ANTIGEN	RESULT
Antibodies	Virus surface antigen	Blocking of viral adsorption or penetration; phagocytosis
Complement	Virus surface antigen	Virolysis by the alternate pathway
Antibodies and complement	Virus surface antigen	Virolysis, phagocytosis, blocking of viral adsorption or penetration
	Cell-bound viral antigen	Cytolysis of infected cells, blocking of viral shedding
Antibodies, complement and cytotoxic cells	Cell-bound viral antigen	Cytolysis of infected cells, blocking of viral shedding
Cell-mediated immunity: activated macrophages	Cell-bound viral antigen	Macrophage-mediated phagocytosis or cytolysis
Cell-mediated immunity: cytotoxic lymphocytes	Cell-bound viral antigen	Cytolysis of infected cells
Cell-mediated immunity: NK cells	Cell-bound viral antigen	Cytolysis of infected cells

Destruction of Viruses and Virus-Infected Cells by Antibody (Table 14–3). Being protein, the capsid of viruses is antigenic, and it is against this component and the envelope that antiviral immune responses are largely mounted. Antibodies may destroy viruses or prevent infection of cells in many ways. The combination of antibody and virus need not be viricidal in itself, since the splitting of virus-antibody complexes may lead to the release of infectious virus. Antibody can act, however, to prevent cell infection by blocking the adsorption of coated virus to its target cell, by stimulating phagocytosis of viruses by macrophages, by initiating complement-mediated virolysis or by causing clumping of viruses, thus reducing the number of infectious units available for cell invasion. Circulating antibody is, therefore, considered to be well capable of virus neutralization. Of course, this neutralizing capacity of serum antibody is limited to areas reached by antibody, so that, for example, although chicks hatched from Newcastle disease–immune hens are resistant to systemic virus disease, they remain susceptible to local respiratory tract infection because they possess no local immunity.

Not only are antibodies active against the protein coat of free virions, they are also active against infected cells carrying viral antigens on their surface, so that these cells are also susceptible to destruction. Virus infections in which antibody-mediated cytolysis of infected cells occurs include Newcastle disease, rabies, bovine virus diarrhea, infectious bronchitis of birds and feline leukemia. Antibody may cause destruction of these modified cells not only through complement-mediated cytolysis but also through the activities of cytotoxic cells (e.g., ADCC). (These cytotoxic cells include lymphocytes, macrophages and neutrophils that possess an Fc receptor, through which they can bind to antibody-coated target cells (Chapter 6)).

The immunoglobulins involved in virus neutralization include both IgG and IgM in serum and IgA in secretions. It is possible that IgE also plays a protective role, since humans with a selective IgE deficiency appear to have an enhanced susceptibility to respiratory infections. As in antibacterial immunity, IgG is quantitatively the most significant immunoglobulin, whereas IgM is qualitatively best at virus neutralization.

Destruction of Viruses and Virus-Infected Cells by Cell-Mediated Immune Mechanisms. Although serum antibodies are capable of neutralizing viruses, it is probable that cell-mediated immune mechanisms constitute the most important pathway for the control of viral diseases in general. This can be readily seen in humans who have a defect in their capacity to mount an antibody-mediated response (Bruton-type agammaglobulinemia). These individuals suffer severely from recurrent bacterial infections but tend to respond normally to smallpox vaccination and to recover from mumps, measles, chickenpox, poliomyelitis and influenza. In contrast, humans who have a congenital deficiency in their cell-mediated immune response (thymic aplasia) are commonly resistant to bacterial infection but highly susceptible to virus diseases, and they may die from generalized vaccinia if vaccinated against smallpox. In spite of this, it is probable that both antibodies and the cell-mediated immune response work together in most cases, so that antibodies eliminate circulating virus while the cell-mediated immune system acts to eliminate infected cells. An example of this is seen in rabbit fibroma infections, in which antibody eliminates circulating virus while the cell-mediated immune response causes tumor regression.

New antigens develop on cell surfaces because viral genes code for new cell-surface determinants. These new antigens are found not only on cells from which virus particles bud, but also on virus-induced tumor cells, where viruses may code for tumor-specific antigens and tumor-specific transplantation antigens on the cell surface. Virus-infected cells may therefore be recognized by the body as foreign and eliminated in a manner analogous to graft rejection. Although antibody and complement or antibody with cytotoxic cells can play a role in this process, cytotoxic T cells are considered to be the major mechanism through which this destruction is achieved, and it is probable that these T cells recognize modified histocompatibility antigens. Evidence for this concept has been provided by studies showing that cytotoxic T cells will destroy canine distemper–infected cells only if both the cytotoxic cell and the virus-infected target cell have identical histocompatibility antigens. From this it has been postulated that the capacity of the body to recognize foreign or modified histocompatibility antigens has evolved, at least in part, as a mechanism for the recognition and elimination of virus-infected cells.

A second mechanism by which virus-infected cells are destroyed involves the activities of NK cells. These are a poorly defined population of lymphocytes found in normal, nonimmunized animals (Chapter 16). Activated by the presence of interferon, they have the ability to recognize and destroy abnormal cells.

Acquired cell-mediated immunity, mediated by macrophages that have been activated by T cell–derived interferon (Chapter 6), is also a feature of some virus diseases. For example, macrophages derived from birds immunized against fowlpox show an enhanced antiviral effect against Newcastle disease and will prevent the intracellular multiplication of *Salmonella gallinarum*, a feature that is not a property of normal macrophages. The rickettsia *Coxiella burnetii* (the causal agent of Q fever) is capable of replicating within normal macrophages, where it is insusceptible to the destructive effects of antibody. However, macrophages activated by T cell products acquire the capacity to destroy *C. burnetii*, and it is therefore probable that acquired cell-mediated immunity is of consequence in the development of resistance of animals to Q fever.

ADVERSE CONSEQUENCES OF THE IMMUNE RESPONSES AGAINST VIRUSES

Like the immune response to bacterial infections, the response to viruses can on occasion be disadvantageous. The destruction of virus-infected cells by antibody is classified as a type II hypersensitivity reaction (Chapter 18) and although normally beneficial may exacerbate the disease. For example, passive administration of antibodies to animals suffering from Aleutian disease of mink may intensify the severity of the lesions. The demyelinating encephalitis commonly seen in canine distemper may be a form of type II hypersensitivity, since most animals suffering from this syndrome possess antibodies to myelin proteins, and the level of these antibodies is related to the severity of the lesions. The active participation of these antibodies in the demyelinating syndrome may be demonstrated *in vitro*, since some sera from affected dogs can cause demyelination in cultures of canine cerebellum. Old dog encephalitis, a disease of middle-aged dogs, is perhaps a variant of this postdistemper lesion. Since the production of antimyelin antibodies has also been reported to occur in man following a wide variety of destructive lesions within the central nervous system, it is probable that this is a nonspecific sequel to any process that involves myelin destruction.

Type III (immune complex) lesions (Chapter 19) are very commonly associated with viral diseases, particularly those in which viremia is prolonged. For example, membranoproliferative glomerulopathies resulting from the deposition of immune complexes in glomeruli are not uncommon complications of equine infectious anemia, Aleutian disease of mink, feline leukemia, chronic hog cholera, bovine virus diarrhea–mucosal disease, canine adenovirus infections and feline infectious peritonitis. A generalized vasculitis due to deposition of immune complexes through the vascular system is seen in equine infectious anemia, Aleutian disease of mink, malignant catarrhal fever and, possibly, equine viral arteritis.

If immune complexes are deposited in the pulmonary vascular bed, damage may occur as a result of cellular infiltration and subsequent lysosomal enzyme release. A severe pneumonitis of this type is occasionally seen when children previously vaccinated with inactivated measles vaccine are exposed to virulent measles virus. This pneumonitis is due to the vaccine having stimulated a systemic IgG response but no local IgA response in the respiratory tract. Measles virus entering by the respiratory tract will therefore not be neutralized but can replicate. When this virus encounters serum antibody, extensive immune complex formation may occur in the alveolar walls, resulting in severe lung damage.

In feline infectious peritonitis, the virus appears to multiply within blood vessels of the peritoneal serosa. As a result of the cat's immune response, large quantities of antibodies are produced and immune complexes are deposited within these serosal vessels (Fig. 14–4). The resulting hypersensitivity reaction causes the severe peritonitis that is characteristic of this infection.

In dogs infected with canine adenovirus 1 (infectious canine hepatitis), two other forms of immune complex–derived lesions have been reported in addition to a focal

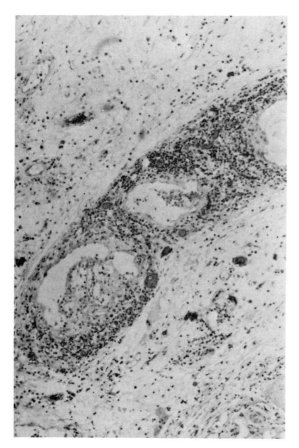

Figure 14–4 Granulomatous vasculitis of serosal blood vessels in an 8-year-old Siamese cat with feline infectious peritonitis. Note the marked mononuclear cell infiltration in the vessel adventitia and media. This may be due to chronic immune complex deposition in vessel walls. × 200. (From Weiss R. 1978. Modern Veterinary Practice. *59* 832. Used with permission.)

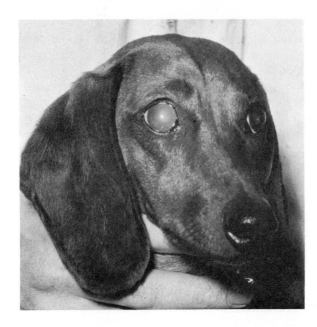

Figure 14—5 Blue-eye, a type III hypersensitivity reaction to canine adenovirus 1 (ICH) occurring in the cornea. (Courtesy of Dr. H. Reed.)

glomerulonephritis. One of these is the condition known as "blue-eye," a transient uveitis seen both in infected dogs and in dogs vaccinated with live attenuated vaccine (Figs. 14–5 and 14–6). This condition results from the release of virus into the anterior chamber of the eye with immune complex formation, complement fixation and consequent neutrophil accumulation. The neutrophils release enzymes that damage the corneal epithelial cells. As a result of this damage, corneal edema and opacity occurs. The condition resolves spontaneously in about 90 per cent of affected dogs. In addition, it has been shown experimentally that dogs rendered partially immune to CAV by immunization and subsequently infected with virulent CAV may suffer from a chronic fibrosing hepatitis despite the rapid disappearance of the second dose of virus. It is possible that this hepatitis is also due to a type III hypersensitivity reaction.

Finally, many virus diseases are associated with the occurrence of rashes. The pathology of these is complex but may reflect type II, type III or even type IV hypersensitivity reactions occurring as the host responds to the presence of viral antigen in the skin.

Feline Leukemia Virus (FeLV). The response of cats to feline leukemia virus demonstrates some of the immunological problems encountered in response to virus infections. FeLV is a retrovirus that can cause a number of different diseases in cats, including leukemia and other tumors, thymic atrophy, anemia, panleukopenia, abortions and profound immunosuppression. The leukemia caused by this virus is usually a T-cell neoplasm, although the FeLV grows in cells of many types and is not restricted to lymphoid tissues. Some FeLV alimentary lymphomas may be of B-cell origin.

Cats infected with FeLV may either become viremic within a few weeks or develop neutralizing antibodies and eliminate the infection. The presence of viremia may be readily detected either by a direct immunofluorescent test on a buffy coat smear using antibodies to group-specific antigen (Fig. 14–7) or by an enzyme-linked immunosorbent assay (ELISA) on a whole-blood sample. The latter test detects soluble viral antigen and may therefore detect infection prior to the development of viremia, since virus antigens are shed into the bloodstream. Of those cats that fail to make

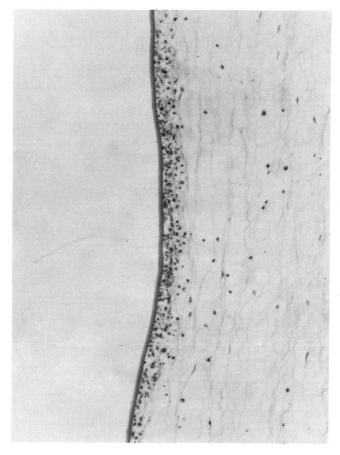

Figure 14–6 Histological section from the cornea of a dog suffering from blue-eye. The lesion consists of a polymorphonuclear cell infiltration of the posterior surface of the cornea as a result of virus-antibody complex deposition in this region. (From Carmichael LE. 1964. Pathol Vet. 1:73–95. Used with permission.)

neutralizing antibodies to FeLV and hence remain viremic, about 80 per cent develop antitumor activity by making antibodies against feline oncornavirus cell membrane antigen (FOCMA) (Fig. 14–8). FOCMA is not a component of the virus but is coded for by viral nucleic acid and is found on the surface of virus-induced tumor cells but not on normal cat cells. Thus, a cat that makes antibodies to FOCMA can usually destroy virus-induced tumor cells. Unfortunately, the possession of antibodies to FOCMA does not confer protection against the other FeLV disease syndromes, and viremic cats who fail to produce anti-FOCMA antibodies are fully susceptible to all the FeLV syndromes, including lymphosarcoma.

Because infected cats remain persistently viremic, those that make antiviral antibodies may suffer from type III (immune complex–mediated) hypersensitivity. Many of these animals develop a severe glomerulonephritis as the immune complexes are deposited in the kidney. As might be expected, viremic cats are also hypocomplementemic, since the immune complexes bind complement. If viral antigen binds to feline erythrocytes, the immune response can cause a severe antiglobulin-positive hemolytic anemia.

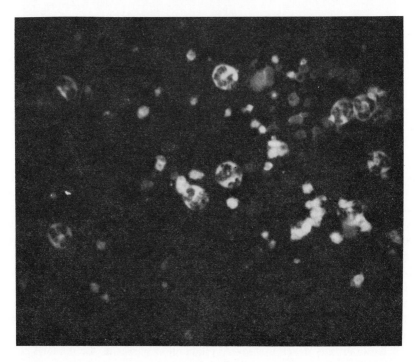

Figure 14–7   Fluorescent antibody tests for FeLV in cats. *Top,* Leukocytes in a peripheral blood smear from a FeLV-negative, normal cat. *Bottom,* Cytoplasmic FeLV virion (internal) antigen in granulocytes, lymphocytes and platelets from a cat with naturally occurring lymphosarcoma. (From Hardy WD. 1974. Vet Clin N Am *4(1)* 141. Used with permission. Courtesy of Dr. Hardy.)

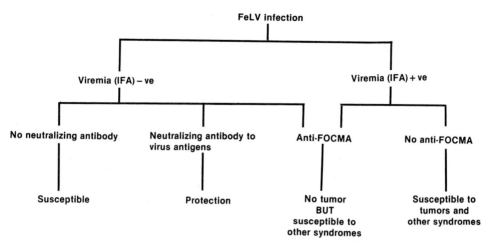

Figure 14–8   The alternative consequences of FeLV infection in cats.

FeLV-infected cats are usually severely immunosuppressed. Virus capsid antigens can directly suppress the T cells of such cats so that FeLV-infected cats may carry foreign skin grafts for about twice as long as normal cats (24 days as compared to 12). This immunosuppression predisposes viremic cats to secondary diseases such as feline infectious peritonitis, hemobartonellosis, toxoplasmosis, septicemia and fungal infections.

Attempts to produce a vaccine against FeLV must aim to provoke both neutralizing antibodies and anti-FOCMA. Two approaches to this problem are currently being investigated. One method uses an attenuated live virus vaccine that generates antigenic FOCMA by infecting cells in vaccinated animals. An alternative approach, which might be much safer, involves the use of a vaccine containing both inactivated virus, in order to induce neutralizing antibodies, and purified FOCMA, in order to induce antitumor immunity.

Aleutian Disease of Mink (ADV).   Although immune complex–mediated lesions are usually only of passing interest in many infectious diseases, they generate some of the major pathological lesions in Aleutian disease of mink.

Aleutian disease is a persistent virus infection first recognized in mink with the "Aleutian" coat color. Although all strains of mink are susceptible to this virus, Aleutian mink appear to be genetically predisposed to the development of severe lesions. (Aleutian mink are also affected by the Chediak-Higashi syndrome (Chapter 22)). Infected mink develop a marked plasmacytosis, which has been compared to a myeloma-like neoplasm, since it results in a marked polyclonal or monoclonal gammopathy (see Fig. 22–9). They also develop lesions of systemic type III hypersensitivity (Chapter 19), including glomerulonephritis and arteritis, and they show signs of autoimmunity by possessing autoantibodies to their own immunoglobulins (rheumatoid factors) and to DNA (antinuclear antibodies).

The immune complex–derived lesions are associated with the development of an arteritis in which IgG, C3 and viral antigen may be detected within vessel walls, and a glomerulonephritis in which "lumpy-bumpy" deposits of immune complexes containing virus and antibody may be identified. In addition, infected mink are anemic. Their erythrocytes can be shown to be coated with antibody, which, when eluted, can be demonstrated to be directed against the Aleutian disease agent. It is likely, therefore, that the erythrocytes of infected animals adsorb virus-antibody complexes from plasma. These coated erythrocytes are then rapidly removed from the circulation by mononuclear-phagocytic cells.

As might be predicted, the use of immunosuppressive agents such as cyclophosphamide or azathioprine in infected mink prevents the development of many of these lesions and so prolongs survival, whereas experimental vaccination with inactivated ADV increases the severity of infections.

Equine Infectious Anemia (EIA). EIA is a persistent virus infection of horses, many of the lesions of which are attributable to the development of hypersensitivity reactions. The most obvious lesion is a hemolytic anemia in which the erythrocytes of infected horses appear to adsorb circulating virus-antibody-complement complexes onto their surfaces, as a consequence of which the erythrocytes are cleared from the circulation rather more rapidly than normal. In addition to the anemia, infected horses may also develop a glomerulonephritis as a result of immune complex deposition on basement membranes and in mesangial areas. If infected horses are treated with immunosuppressive drugs, the glomerulonephritis does not occur. The presence of circulating immune complexes also appears to be immunosuppressive, so that infected horses possess unusually low levels of IgG(T), although their circulating lymphocytes appear to be unaffected and respond normally to mitogens such as phytohemagglutinin.

EVASION OF THE IMMUNE RESPONSE BY VIRUSES

As discussed at the beginning of this chapter, the relationship between host and virus must be established on the basis of mutual accommodation so that its long-term continuation is ensured. Failure to do this results in elimination of either host or virus. One aspect of this adaptation involves the avoidance by the virus of the attentions of the immune system.

This evasion may be accomplished by several techniques, one of the simplest of which is antigenic variation. The most significant example of this is seen among the influenza viruses. The influenza viruses possess a number of different surface antigens, of which the hemagglutinins and neuraminidases are most important. There are 13 different hemagglutinins and nine neuraminidases among the type A influenza viruses,

Table 14–4   EXAMPLES OF INFLUENZA A VIRUSES AND THEIR ANTIGENIC STRUCTURES

SPECIES	VIRUS STRAIN	ANTIGENIC STRUCTURE*
Human	A/Brazil/11/78**	H1N1
	A/Bangkok/1/79	H3N2
	A/New Jersey/76 (Swine Flu)	H1N1
Equine	A/Equine/Prague/1/56	H7N7
	A/Equine/Miami/1/63	H3N8
Swine	A/Swine/Iowa/15/30	H1N1
Avian	A/Fowl Plague/Dutch/27	H7N7
	A/Duck/England/56	H11N7
	A/Turkey/Ontario/6118/68	H8N4

*There are many other antigens known among the human and avian influenza viruses.
**The first number is the isolate number; the second is the year of isolation.

and they are identified according to a nomenclature system recommended by the World Health Organization (Table 14–4). Thus, the hemagglutinin of the swine influenza virus is classifed as H1 and its neuraminidase as N1. The two equine influenza viruses are A/equine/Prague/56, which is H7N7, and A/equine/Miami/63, which is classified as H3N8. Influenza viruses in a human population show an antigenic drift as mutation and selection gradually change the hemagglutinins and neuraminidases in a seemingly random fashion, as a result of which there is great antigenic variation within each subtype. This drift permits the virus to persist in a population for many years. In addition, influenza viruses sporadically exhibit a major antigenic shift in which a new strain develops whose hemagglutinins show no apparent relationships to the hemagglutinins of previously known strains. Such a major change cannot be produced by mutation and is probably due to recombination between two virus strains. It is the development of these influenza viruses with a completely new antigenic structure that accounts for the periodic pandemics of this disease in humans. In horses and pigs, in contrast, the rapid turnover of the population ensures the persistence of influenza without the necessity for antigenic drift. As a result, the antigenic structure of equine and swine influenza viruses has remained relatively stable since they were first described.

A second form of virus adaptation is seen in equine infectious anemia (EIA), Aleutian disease (AD) of mink and African swine fever. Although infected animals mount an immune response, the antibodies formed are incapable of virus neutralization. Thus, virus-antibody complexes from AD-infected mink or EIA-infected horses are fully infectious. The precise reason for the inability of antibody to neutralize these viruses is not clear, although it is assumed that antibody must bind to a "noncritical" site on the virus. It has also been suggested that some form of antigenic variation may occur.

An alternative evasive process has been observed in measles-infected cells in humans. Antibody against measles virus will normally kill measles-infected cells. If, however, there is insufficient antibody present to be immediately lethal, then an infected cell may respond by removing the measles antigens from its surface. Once these antigens are lost, the infected cells are refractory to cytolysis, although presumably the virus is itself unable to spread. Removal of the measles antibody permits reexpression of measles antigen.

In contrast to the immune response against bacteria, antiviral immunity is, in many cases, very long lasting. The reasons for this are not completely clear, but they appear to be related to virus persistence within cells, perhaps in a slowly replicating or a nonreplicating form as typified by the herpesviruses. The persistent virus may periodically boost the immune response of the infected animal and in this way generate long-lasting immunity to superinfection. This type of infection, exemplified by feline rhinotracheitis virus (a herpesvirus) can only be countered by an immune response directed against the target cell, and even this may be ineffective if the virus does not influence the antigenic structures on the cell surface. The immune responses in these cases, although not capable of eliminating virus, may serve to prevent the development of clinical disease and therefore serve a protective role. Immunosuppression of animals persistently infected in this way may permit disease to occur. The association between stress and the development of some virus diseases is well recognized, and it is likely that the increased levels of steroid production occurring in stressful situations may be sufficiently immunosuppressive to permit activation of latent viruses or infection by exogenous ones.

SOME COMMENTS ON VIRAL VACCINES AND
SPECIFIC VIRUS DISEASES

Because of the lack of chemotherapeutic antiviral agents, vaccination has become the major method of control of virus diseases in the domestic animals. As a result, the development of viral vaccines is, in some ways, more advanced than that of their bacterial counterparts. In particular, it has proved relatively easy to attenuate many viruses so that effective vaccines containing modified live virus (MLV) derived from tissue culture are readily available

As discussed in Chapter 12, MLV vaccines are usually good immunogens, but their use may involve certain risks. The most important problem encountered in the use of MLV vaccines is residual virulence. One serious example of this is the development of clinical rabies in some dogs following administration of low-egg-passage Flury-strain rabies vaccine and in cats following the use of SAD(ERA)-strain MLV rabies vaccine. Some strains of infectious bovine rhinotracheitis and equine herpesvirus vaccine may cause abortion when given to pregnant cows or mares, respectively, and MLV bluetongue vaccines may cause disease in fetal lambs if given to pregnant ewes (Chapter 11). More commonly, the residual virulence causes a relatively mild disease. Thus, intraocular/intranasal feline rhinotracheitis/calicivirus vaccine may cause a transient conjunctivitis or rhinitis, whereas some MLV canine distemper vaccines can cause transient thrombocytopenia. MLV infectious bursal disease vaccines can cause a mild immunosuppression, and older strains of BVD vaccine caused mild mucosal disease.

Transient side effects like these, which may otherwise be regarded as inconsequential, can be of major significance in the broiler chicken industry, where even a minor slowing in growth can have major economic consequences. Thus, two strains of infectious bronchitis vaccine are available. The Massachusetts strain is mildly pathogenic but a good immunogen, whereas the Connecticut strain is nonpathogenic but a poor immunogen. It is common, in order to minimize complications, to use the Connecticut strain for primary vaccination and, if boosters are required, to use the Massachusetts strain subsequently. Similarly, of the two major vaccine strains of Newcastle disease, the LaSota strain is a good immunogen but may provoke mild adverse reactions. In contrast, the B1 strain is considerably milder but is less immunogenic, especially if given in drinking water.

Because of problems of this nature, persistent attempts have been made to minimize residual virulence in vaccines. One successful method involves the use of temperature sensitive (ts) mutants. Ts strains of IBR virus that are now available will grow only at temperatures a few degrees lower than normal body temperature. As a result, when this organism is administered intranasally, it is able to colonize the relatively cool nasal mucosa but is unable to invade the rest of the body. Thus, the vaccine can stimulate a local immune response without incurring the risk of systemic invasion.

Some strains of IBR vaccine may persist in vaccinated animals and give rise to a prolonged carrier state. Although this is probably a unique problem, concerns have been expressed that the widespread use of MLV vaccines may serve to seed viruses into animal populations and that untoward consequences may develop in the future. This is a threat not to be taken lightly; indeed, it has been suggested that the sudden and widespread appearance of canine parvovirus in 1978 may have been facilitated by the use of MLV feline panleukopenia vaccines.

An alternative approach to overcoming the problems caused by MLV vaccines involves the increasing use of inactivated and subunit vaccines. Excellent inactivated vaccines are available against diseases such as foot-and-mouth disease, equine rhino-pneumonitis, pseudorabies, feline panleukopenia, feline herpes (rhinotracheitis) and rabies. At their best, these vaccines confer immunity comparable in strength and duration to that induced by MLV vaccines, with the assurance that they are free of residual virulence. A general trend toward the use of more inactivated virus vaccines in the future is anticipated.

ADDITIONAL SOURCES OF INFORMATION

Allison AC, Beveridge WIB, Cockburn WC, *et al*. 1972. Virus-associated immunopathology: animal models and implications for human disease. Bull WHO *47* 257–274.

Gresser I. 1977. On the varied biological effects of interferon. Cell Immunol *34* 406–415.

Hardy WD. 1979. Current status of FeLV diseases. Friskies Research Digest *15:2* 1–3; *15:3* 1–3.

Horzinek MC, and Osterhaus ADME. 1978. Feline infectious peritonitis: a coronavirus disease of cats. J Small Anim Pract *19* 623–630.

Humphrey GL, Bayer EV, and Constantine DG. 1978. Canine rabies vaccine virus infection. Review of the probable risk of such infections in vaccinated dogs in California during the 4-year period 1974–1977. Calif Vet *32:7* 13–17.

Johnson AW. 1976. Equine infectious anemia: the literature 1966–1975. Vet Bull *46* 559–574.

Krakowa S, Higgins RJ, and Koestner A. 1980. Canine distemper virus: review of structural and functional modulations in lymphoid tissues. Am J Vet Res *41* 284–292.

Lutz H, Petersen NC, Harris CW, *et al*. 1980. Detection of feline leukemia virus infections. Feline Pract 1980 *10* 13–23.

Mathes LG, Olsen RG, Hebebrand LC, *et al*. 1978. Abrogation of lymphocyte blastogenesis by a feline leukemia virus protein. Nature *274* 687–689.

Notkins AL. 1975. Viral Immunology and Immunopathology. Academic Press, New York.

Pastoret PP, Babiuk LA, Misra V, and Griebel P. 1980. Reactivation of temperature-sensitive and non–temperature sensitive infectious bovine rhinotracheitis vaccine virus with dexamethasone. Infect Immun *129* 483–488.

Rouse BT, and Babiuk LA. 1979. Mechanisms of viral immunopathology. Adv Vet Sci Comp Med *23* 103–136.

Wright NG. 1976. Canine adenovirus: its role in renal and ocular disease. A review. J Small Anim Pract *17* 25–33.

15

Immunity to Protozoa and Helminths

The essence of successful parasitism is accommodation and survival; that is, the success of any parasite is measured not by the disturbances it imposes on a host but on its ability to adapt and integrate itself within a host's internal environment. From an immunological point of view, a parasite can be considered a success if it succeeds in integrating itself into a host in such a way that it is not regarded as foreign.

These considerations apply not only to the protozoa and helminths that we conventionally consider parasites but also to other infectious agents, including bacteria and viruses. On this basis we may regard the intracellular bacteria and algae that serve as mitochondria and chloroplasts within animal and plant cells as the epitome of successful parasitism.

IMMUNITY TO PROTOZOA

Parasitic protozoa may be classified according to their degree of adaptation to a specific host. Some organisms such as the free-living amebae of the genus *Naegleria* are, apparently, totally unadapted to life in animal tissues. Because of this, their inadvertent invasion of the human nasal mucosa, which occurs as a consequence of swimming in contaminated water, leads to the development of hyperacute meningitis that is almost invariably fatal. Another example of an organism that is poorly adapted to its host is *Trypanosoma rhodesiense*. Although human trypanosomiasis caused by *Trypanosoma gambiense* has been known for hundreds of years and gives rise to a chronic disease usually lasting several years, disease due to *T. rhodesiense* is relatively recent, having been first recorded in 1908. It is not surprising, therefore, that the disease caused by this organism is rapidly progressive, with death occurring in some infected individuals within a few weeks. At the other extreme, *Toxoplasma gondii*, the causal agent of toxoplasmosis, is an organism that almost completely lacks species specificity in its tachyzoite stage, being capable of infecting any species of mammal and many species of birds. Not surprisingly, *T. gondii*, being so adaptable, causes clinical disease in only a very small proportion of infected animals, and most carry the parasite throughout their lives without showing any ill effects.

MECHANISMS OF RESISTANCE TO PROTOZOA

Nonimmunological Defense Mechanisms. Although the nonimmunological mechanisms of resistance to protozoa have not been fully clarified, they appear, in general, to be qualitatively similar to those that operate in bacterial and viral diseases. Species influences are perhaps of most significance; for example, *Trypanosoma lewisi* is found only in the rat and *Trypanosoma musculi* in the mouse, where neither cause disease. *Trypanosoma brucei*, *Trypanosoma congolense* and *Trypanosoma vivax* appear not to cause disease in the wild ungulates of East Africa but are highly virulent for domestic cattle, presumably as a result of lack of mutual adaptation. Similarly, the coccidia are extremely host specific; they include *T. gondii*, which in its tachyzoite stages can infect any species of mammal but in its coccidian stages will affect only felids (cats, tigers, etc.).

Presumably, these species' differences are but a development of somewhat more subtle genetic influences. Thus, some strains of African cattle, most notably N'Dama, show an increased resistance to the pathogenic trypanosomes, which is probably based on a continuing selection of the most resistant animals over many years. Perhaps the best analyzed case of genetically determined resistance to protozoan disease is sickle cell anemia in humans. Individuals who inherit the sickle cell trait possess hemoglobin S (HbS) in which a residue of valine has replaced a residue of glutamic acid present in normal hemoglobin. The changes in the shape of the hemoglobin molecule induced by this substitution cause deoxygenated hemoglobin molecules to aggregate, thus distorting the shape of the erythrocytes and resulting in increased erythrocyte fragility and clearance. Individuals who are homozygous for the sickle cell gene die when young from the results of severe anemia. Heterozygous individuals are also anemic, but in west central Africa the fact that red cells containing hemoglobin S are not parasitized by *Plasmodium falciparum* ensures that affected individuals are resistant to malaria. As a consequence of this, more of these individuals tend to survive to reproductive age than normal persons. The mutation is therefore maintained in the human population at a relatively high level.

Immunological Defense Mechanisms. The obvious inadequacies of the immune responses to many parasites led early investigators to conclude that successful parasites were, in general, poorly immunogenic. This is not the case; most parasites are fully antigenic, but in their adaptation to a parasitic existence they have developed mechanisms through which they may survive in the presence of an immune response. Therefore, like other antigenic particles, protozoa can stimulate both humoral and cell-mediated immune responses. In general, antibodies serve to control the level of parasites that exist free in the blood stream and tissue fluids, whereas cell-mediated immune responses are directed largely against intracellular parasites.

Serum antibodies directed against protozoan surface antigens may opsonize, agglutinate or immobilize them. Antibodies together with complement and cytotoxic cells may kill them, and some antibodies (called ablastins) may act to inhibit protozoan enzymes in such a way that their replication is prevented. In infections of the genital tract due to *Tritrichomonas fetus* and *Trichmonas vaginalis*, a local antibody response is stimulated in which, at least in humans, IgE production is prominent. Not only does the local type I hypersensitivity reaction that ensues provoke intense discomfort, but also, by increasing vascular permeability, it permits IgG antibodies to reach the site of infection and immobilize and eliminate the organisms.

The major immune response to the parasite *T. gondii* is cell-mediated. *T. gondii* is an obligate intracellular parasite whose tachyzoite stages replicate within cells (Fig. 15–1). When the number of intracellular organisms becomes excessive, the infected cell ruptures and the organisms released invade other cells. They penetrate these cells by a poorly understood mechanism that resembles phagocytosis. When toxoplasma tachyzoites invade normal macrophages, however, they are not destroyed. In the normal process of phagocytosis, once a particle has been enclosed in a phagosome, it is usual for lysosomes to move through the cytoplasm and to empty their hydrolytic enzymes into the space around the particle. This does not happen in cells that have phagocytosed toxoplasma. The lysosomes may move toward the phagosome but they do not fuse with it. The toxoplasma tachyzoites therefore remain free to replicate within the cell in an environment devoid of antibodies or lysosomal enzymes.

Normally, both antibody production and a cell-mediated immune response occur in response to toxoplasma infection. The antibodies acting in conjunction with complement can eliminate organisms found free in body fluids and thus reduce the spread of the organism between cells, but they will naturally have little or no influence on the intracellular forms of the parasite. These intracellular organisms are destroyed through a cell-mediated immune response similar to that described for *Listeria monocytogenes* and the mycobacteria (Fig. 15–2) (Chapter 6). Sensitized T lymphocytes release lymphokines in response to toxoplasmal ribonucleoproteins. These lymphokines can act on macrophages, first to make them resistant to the lethal effects of toxoplasma and second to assist them in killing the intracellular organism, presumably through

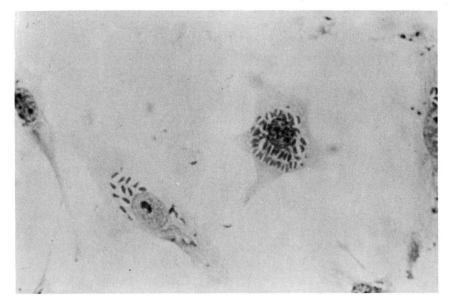

Figure 15–1 Mouse macrophages growing in tissue culture and infected with tachyzoites of *Toxoplasma gondii*. (Courtesy of Dr. C. H. Lai.)

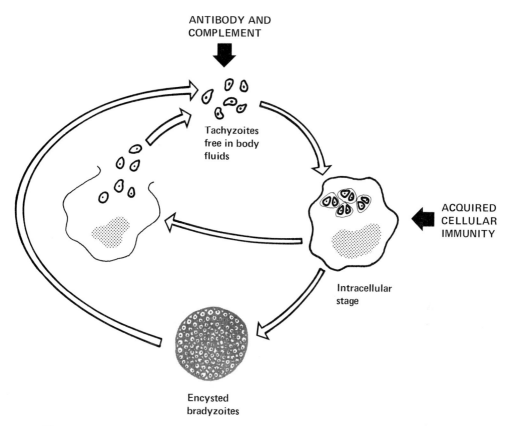

ANTIBODY AND
COMPLEMENT

Tachyzoites
free in body
fluids

ACQUIRED
CELLULAR
IMMUNITY

Intracellular
stage

Encysted
bradyzoites

Figure 15–2   The points in the life cycle of *Toxoplasma gondii* at which the immune response can exert a controlling influence.

removal of the block preventing lysosome-phagosome fusion. In addition, cytotoxic T cells can also destroy toxoplasma tachyzoites and toxoplasma-infected cells. Interferon is active against toxoplasma because of its ability to activate macrophages and stimulate cytotoxic T cells. In these ways, antibody-mediated and cell-mediated immune responses act together to ensure the elimination of the tachyzoite stage of this organism. However, *T. gondii* can exist in a cystic form. The cysts develop within cells during the course of infection. They appear to be nonimmunogenic and nonpathogenic, since on histological examination no host response, as shown by the presence of inflammatory cells, can be seen. It is possible that this cyst stage is not recognized as foreign.

The evidence for a significant role for cell-mediated immune responses in other protozoan diseases of animals is less complete, although it is a very prominent feature of *Trypanosoma cruzi* and *Leishmania tropica* infections in humans. In *Theileria parva* infection (East Coast fever) of cattle, animals that have recovered from the disease are solidly immune. Antibody alone is not protective, but cytotoxic T cells can destroy parasitized cells. Similarly, in histomoniasis of turkeys, recovered birds show a short-lived resistance to reinfection that is not transferable by serum.

In some protozoan diseases, notably those due to coccidia, the mechanisms of protective immunity are unclear. For example, infection of chickens with some strains of the intestinal parasite *Eimeria maxima* leads to the development of a form of immunity that is capable of preventing reinfection. This immune response acts by inhibiting the growth of the trophozoite, the earliest invasive stage, within intestinal epithelial cells. This growth inhibition is reversible, since arrested stages may be transferred to normal animals and complete their development uneventfully. The mechanism of this resistance is unclear. Antibodies to *E. maxima* can be readily detected in the serum of immune chickens, and the phagocytic cells of these birds show an increased ability to ingest coccidian sporocysts. The results of attempts to detect a local immune response have been equivocal, although a slight measure of resistance can be provided by oral administration of IgA. In spite of all this, neither neonatal bursectomy, thymectomy nor the use of antilymphocyte serum significantly modifies the course of experimental disease.

Immunity to intestinal coccidia is also observed in mammals. Infections by coccidia in lambs and by the coccidian stage of *T. gondii* in cats both effectively stimulate an immune response that is capable of inhibiting reinfection. In cats the shedding of toxoplasma oocysts, which ceases abruptly about three weeks after infection, coincides with the appearance of serum antibodies. It is not entirely clear, however, whether it is these antibodies that effectively inhibit oocyst production. Bovine transfer factor produced from sensitized calf lymphocytes can transfer delayed hypersensitivity reactions to *Eimeria bovis* as well as confer partial protection to recipient cattle. This imples that cell-mediated immunity must be of significance in this infection.

For many years it was thought that a common feature of protozoan infection was premunition. Premunition is the term used to describe resistance that is only effective if the parasite persists in the host and wanes rapidly when all parasites are eliminated. It was believed, for example, that only cattle actually infected with babesia were resistant to clinical disease. If all organisms were removed from an animal, then resistance was considered to wane immediately. Further studies have shown that this is not in fact true. For example, cattle cured of babesia infection by chemotherapy have been shown to be resistant to challenge with the homologous strain of that organism for up to 2½ years afterward. Nevertheless, the presence of infection does appear to be mandatory for protection against heterologous strains. Babesiosis is also of interest since splenectomy of animals carrying the organisms will cause recrudescence of clinical disease. Not only does the spleen serve as a source of antibodies in this disease, but it also removes infected erythrocytes. Cessation of these functions through splenectomy is apparently sufficient to allow the clinical disease to reappear.

EVASION OF THE IMMUNE RESPONSE BY PROTOZOA

Most important protozoan parasites have evolved mechanisms for evading the consequences of their hosts' immune responses. In general, these mechanisms resemble those evolved by other types of organism. For example, many protozoa are immunosuppressive. Thus, *Theileria parva* invades and destroys T cells specifically. Other protozoa such as the trypanosomes are also potently immunosuppressive, but their mode of action is unclear. It has been suggested that trypanosomes may promote the development of suppressor cells. Other evidence suggests that they stimulate the B-cell system to exhaustion, while other investigators believe that they release immunosuppressive factors.

Parasite-induced immunosuppression may be of great assistance to the parasite. For example, *Babesia bovis* is immunosuppressive for cattle. As a result, its host vector, the tick *Boophilus microplus*, is more able to survive on an infected animal. Consequently, infected cattle have more ticks than noninfected animals and the efficiency of transmission of *B. bovis* is greatly enhanced. It must also be pointed out, however, that parasite-induced immunosuppression commonly leads to the death of host animals as a result of secondary infection, so it is not necessarily always beneficial to the parasite.

In addition to immunosuppression, protozoa have evolved two other extremely effective immunoevasive techniques. One involves becoming either hypo- or nonantigenic, and the other involves acquiring a capacity for the rapid and repeated alteration of surface antigens. An example of a hypoantigenic organism is the cyst stage of *T. gondii*, which, as mentioned previously, appears not to stimulate a host response. As an alternative to the evolution of nonimmunogenic stages, some protozoa can become functionally nonantigenic by masking themselves with host antigens. Examples of these include *Trypanosoma theileri* in cattle and *Trypanosoma lewisi* in rats. These are both nonpathogenic trypanosomes, which can survive in the bloodstream of infected animals because they become covered with a layer of host serum proteins and so are not regarded as foreign. There is also some evidence to suggest that *T. brucei*, a pathogenic trypanosome of cattle, may adsorb either host serum proteins or red cell antigens and so become functionally nonantigenic.

Although the absence of antigenicity may be considered the ultimate stage in the evasive process, many protozoa, especially the trypanosomes, have evolved the technique of antigenic variation to a high degree of sophistication. If cattle are infected with the pathogenic trypanosomes *T. vivax*, *T. congolense* or *T. brucei* and the parasitemia is checked at regular intervals, it is found that the numbers of circulating organisms fluctuate greatly, with periods of high parasitemia alternating regularly with periods of low or undetectable parasitemia (Fig. 15–3). Serum taken from infected animals will react with trypanosomes isolated prior to the time of bleeding but not with those taken subsequently. Each peak period of high parasitemia corresponds to problems is carefully analyzed. Under the more rigorous economic conditions of

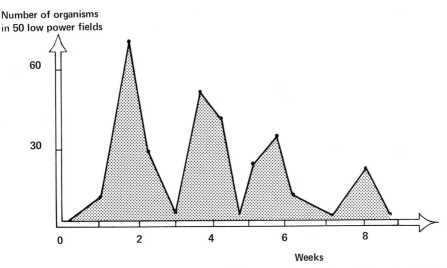

Figure 15–3 The course of *Trypanosoma congolense* parasitemia in an infected calf. Each parasitemic peak represents the development of a new antigenically original population of organisms.

the development of a population of trypanosomes of a new antigenic type. The elimination of a population of one antigenic type leads to a fall in blood parasite levels. From the survivors, however, a proportion of parasites develop new surface antigens and a fresh population arises to produce yet another period of high parasitemia (Fig. 15–4). This cyclical fluctuation in parasite levels with each peak reflecting the appearance of a new antigenic variant population can continue for a long time.

The sequence of antigens produced appears to be entirely random and is not provoked by antibody. Trypanosomes grown in tissue culture also show spontaneous antigenic variation. By means of electron microscopy, it can be shown that the variant antigen forms a thick coat over the surface of the trypanosome. When antigenic change occurs, the proteins in the old coat are shed and replaced by an antigenically different protein. Analysis of the genetics of this process indicates that the trypanosomes possess a large number of genes for coat protein and that antigenic variation occurs as a result of random gene rearrangement and selection.

Trypanosomiasis is not the only protozoan infection in which antigenic variation is seen. Minor antigenic variations have been recorded in babesiosis in which relapse strains appear to be antigenically different from the original strains. Antigenic variation is also seen in malaria, although the range of antigens and the differences between them are relatively small.

Since parasitic protozoa seek to evade the immune responses, it is not surprising that they also invade immunosuppressed individuals. Organisms that are normally maintained in a relatively quiescent state by the immune response, such as the cyst forms of *T. gondii*, are capable of changing to a more active form and producing severe disease in immunosuppressed animals. For this reason, acute toxoplasmosis is not uncommonly seen in patients immunosuppressed for transplantation purposes or for cancer therapy.

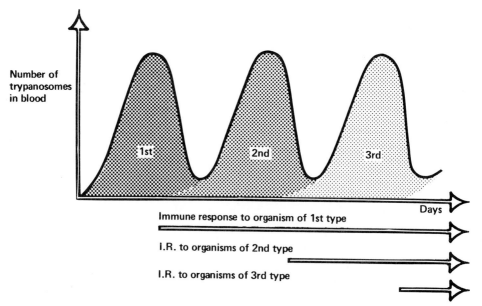

Figure 15–4 Schematic diagram depicting how antigenic variation may account for the cyclical parasitemia observed in trypanosomiasis. Each peak represents the growth of a new antigenic variant.

ADVERSE CONSEQUENCES OF THE IMMUNE RESPONSE TO PROTOZOA

As with the groups of organisms described earlier, the immune response against protozoa can give rise to each of the hypersensitivity types described in Chapter 8, and these may, under some circumstances, contribute significantly to the pathogenesis of the disease process.

Type I hypersensitivity, as has been mentioned, is a feature of trichomoniasis and results in local irritation and inflammation in the genital tract. Type II cytotoxic reactions, which contribute to the development of anemia, are of significance in babesiosis and trypanosomiasis. In babesiosis, parasitized erythrocytes carry parasite-derived antigens on their surfaces and are thus recognized as foreign and eliminated by immune cytolysis and phagocytosis. In trypanosomiasis, either fragments of effete organisms or possibly preformed immune complexes bind to erythrocytes and provoke their immune elimination, thus contributing to the development of anemia. Immune complex formation on circulating erythrocytes is not the only problem of this type in trypanosomiasis. In many cases, systemic immune complex formation can also lead to the development of vasculitis and glomerulonephritis (type III hypersensitivity; Chapter 19). The actual cause, or causes, of death in animal trypanosomiasis is not clear, but it is likely that systemic immune complex deposition may contribute to the demise of infected animals.

It is probable that a type IV hypersensitivity reaction contributes to the inflammatory reaction that occurs when toxoplasma cysts break down and release fresh tachyzoites. Extracts of *T. gondii* (toxoplasmin), if administered intradermally to infected animals, will result in the development of a delayed hypersensitivity response (see Fig. 20–1), and this phenomenon has been used on occasion as a diagnostic test for this infection. Finally, it has been observed by several workers that an association appears to exist between the occurrence of lymphosarcoma and *T. theileri* infection in cattle. Nevertheless, although it is known that *T. theileri*–infected cattle have a lymphocytosis and that *T. theileri* can act as a lymphocyte mitogen, it has never been proved that this organism either causes or promotes bovine lymphosarcoma.

VACCINATION AGAINST PROTOZOAN INFECTIONS

Successful vaccination against protozoan infections of domestic animals is currently limited to babesiosis. The Babesia species constitute a heterogeneous group of organisms transmitted by ixodid ticks, which parasitize erythrocytes and so cause anemia. A number of factors contribute to the resistance of animals against babesiosis, including genetic factors (humped cattle are more resistant to disease than European cattle) and age (cattle show a significant resistance to babesiosis in the first six months of life). Animals that recover from acute babesiosis are immune, and this immunity has been considered to be a form of premunity (see page 230). It is possible to infect young calves deliberately so that they will acquire infection while they are still relatively insusceptible to disease, and thereafter be resistant to reinfection. The organisms employed for this procedure are first attenuated by repeated passage through splenectomized calves and then administered to recipient animals in whole blood. As might be anticipated, the side effects of this type of controlled infection may be relatively severe and chemotherapy is commonly required to control them. The transfer of blood from one calf to another may also lead to sensitization and the production of isoantibodies against red cells. These antibodies complicate any attempts at blood transfusion in later life and may provoke hemolytic disease of the newborn in calves born from sensitized cows (Chapter 18).

Many attempts have been made to immunize poultry against coccidia, but it is clear that only infection with viable organisms can induce protective immunity. Thus, repeated dosing with small numbers of oocysts can provide some protection. Unfortunately, this technique may provoke severe reactions that require treatment with coccidiostats. Alternatively, oocysts may be attenuated by ionizing radiation. The results obtained by this method suggest that any protection obtained is due to patent infection by coccidia whose life cycles have not been interrupted by the radiation.

In the case of a well-adapted organism such as *T. gondii*, not only does infection rarely lead to disease, but it also results in the development of strong lifelong immunity to reinfection. Because of this, it would be difficult to produce a vaccine against this organism that would improve significantly on the natural infection. It may, however, be desirable to develop a vaccine for cats, which could inhibit oocyst production and thus break that segment of the transmission cycle.

IMMUNITY TO HELMINTHS

The immune system has not been conspicuously successful in producing absolute resistance to helminth infections in mammals. In a sense it has been detrimental, since the IgE-mediated immune reactions appear to have evolved largely for the control of these parasites. In Western society where parasites are largely controlled by hygienic measures, the problem of allergies is probably of much greater social significance than parasitism. On a worldwide basis, however, and in relation to domestic animals, helminth parasites remain of major significance.

It is not surprising that the immune system is relatively inefficient in controlling helminth parasites. After all, these organisms have adapted to an obligatory parasitic existence, and presumably this adaptation has involved dealing with the immune system and either overcoming or evading it. Helminths are, therefore, not maladapted pathogenic organisms but fully adapted obligate parasites whose very survival depends on reaching some form of accommodation with the host. Consequently, if an organism of this type causes disease, it is likely to be expressed either very mildly or subclinically. Only when helminth parasites invade a host to which they are not fully adapted or in unusually large numbers does acute disease occur.

MECHANISMS OF RESISTANCE TO HELMINTHS

Nonimmunological Defense Mechanisms. The factors that influence the course of helminth infections are many and complex. They include not only the influences of host-derived factors but also of factors derived from other helminths within the same host. For example, both intraspecies and interspecies competition are known to occur. In the former case, it is evident, particularly with respect to cestode infections, that the presence of adult worms in the intestine delays the further development of larval stages in the tissues. Consequently, for example, calves infected with *Cysticercus bovis* appear to be resistant to further infection by this organism. Similarly, lambs acquire resistance to *Echinococcus granulosus* to the extent that multiple dosing with ova does not result in the development of massive worm burdens. It is hypothesized that the original dose of eggs may stimulate "rejection" of subsequent doses. In interspecies competition, competition between helminths for mutual habitats and nutrients serves to control the numbers and composition of an animal's helminth population.

The factors of host origin that influence helminth burdens include the age, breed and sex of the host. The influence of sex and age on helminth burdens appears to be largely hormonal. In animals whose sexual cycle is seasonal, parasites tend to synchronize their reproductive cycle with that of the host. For instance, ewes show a "spring rise" in fecal nematode ova, which coincides with lambing and the onset of lactation. Similarly, the development of helminth larvae ingested by cattle in autumn tends to be inhibited until spring. Perhaps the most evolved organisms in this respect are the nematodes of the genus *Toxocara*, the larvae of which may migrate from an infected bitch to the liver of the fetal puppy, resulting in a congenital infection. Once born, the infected pups can reinfect their mother by the more conventional fecal-oral route.

A good example of genetically mediated resistance to helminths is the superior resistance of sheep with hemoglobin AA to infestations with *Haemonchus contortus* and *Ostertagia circumcincta*, as compared to sheep with hemoglobin BB. The reasons for this are unclear, but AA sheep mount a better immune response to many other antigens as well.

Immunological Defense Mechanisms

HUMORAL MECHANISMS. Helminths, in general, can be found in two situations in the body: in tissues as larval forms or within the gastrointestinal or respiratory tracts as adults. Obviously, the form of the immune response that is most effective against these stages differs considerably.

Although conventional antibodies of the IgM, IgG and IgA classes are produced in response to helminth antigens, an increasing body of evidence suggests that the most significant immunoglobulin class involved in resistance to helminths is IgE. For example, IgE levels are usually extremely elevated in parasitized individuals; many helminth infestations are associated with the characteristic signs of type I hypersensitivity, including eosinophilia, edema, asthma and urticarial dermatitis; and many helminth infections such as oesophagostomiasis, ancylostomiasis, strongyloidiasis, taeniasis and fascioliasis are accompanied by a positive passive cutaneous anaphylaxis (PCA) reaction to worm antigens (Chapter 17).

Many helminth antigens preferentially stimulate IgE production, so investigators who handle helminths regularly may become sensitized to worm antigens. These indiviuals then suffer from asthmatic attacks or cutaneous wheal-and-flare reactions (urticaria) on exposure to worms. In addition to being potent stimulators of IgE production against themselves, helminth antigens are also capable of acting as adjuvants, specific for IgE production against other, nonhelminth antigens.

Although IgE production and the allergies that result from it are considered by some to be only a nuisance, they appear to be of considerable benefit in controlling worm burdens. One of the best examples of this is the "self-cure" reaction seen in sheep infected with gastrointestinal nematodes, particularly *H. contortus*. These worms, which are embedded in the intestinal and abomasal mucosa, secrete antigens during their third ecdysis that act as allergens. As a result, the development of a worm burden provokes a local acute type I hypersensitivity reaction in the parasitized regions of the intestine. The combination of helminth antigens with mast cell–bound IgE leads

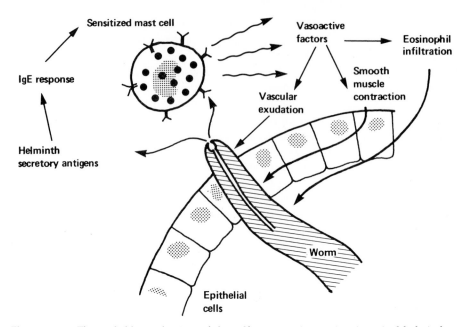

Figure 15-5 The probable mechanism of the self-cure reaction against intestinal helminths.

to mast cell degranulation and the release of vasoactive amines. These compounds stimulate smooth muscle contraction and increase vascular permeability. Thus, in the self-cure reaction, violent contractions of the intestinal musculature and an increase in the permeability of intestinal capillaries occur allowing an efflux of fluid into the intestinal lumen. This combination results in dislodgment and expulsion of the major portion of the animal's gastrointestinal worm burden (Fig. 15-5). In sheep that have just undergone self-cure, their PCA antibody titer is high (Chapter 17) and experimental administration of helminth antigens will result in acute anaphylaxis, confirming the role of type I hypersensitivity in this phenomenon. A similar reaction is seen in fascioliasis in calves in which peak PCA titers coincide with expulsion of the parasite.

IgE has other roles to play in the reduction of helminth burdens in animals. For example, macrophages may bind to helminth larvae through an IgE-mediated pathway to cause their destruction. Also, by mediating mast cell degranulation, IgE stimulates release of ECF-A (eosinophil chemotactic factor of anaphylaxis). This material, in turn, will mobilize the body's eosinophil pool, which results in the release of large numbers of eosinophils into the circulation. It is for this reason that eosinophilia is so characteristic of helminth infections. The eosinophils appear to serve in at least two roles. First, they contain enzymes capable of neutralizing the vasoactive agents released from mast cells (Chapter 17). Second, in conjunction with antibodies and complement, eosinophils are capable of killing some helminth larvae and hence also serve a protective function. Eosinophils attach to helminths by means of IgG. They then degranulate, releasing their granule contents onto the helminth cuticle (Fig. 15-6). The major basic protein of the granules can cause direct damage to the cuticle and also promote the adherence of additional eosinophils. The cytotoxic effects of major basic protein are enhanced by mast cell-derived factors such as histamine as well as by complement.

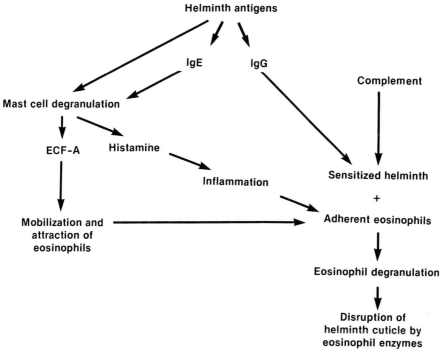

Figure 15−6 The mechanism by which mast cells, IgE, IgG and eosinophils interact to destroy helminths. Recent evidence suggests that Eosinophils may also attach to helminths through IgE.

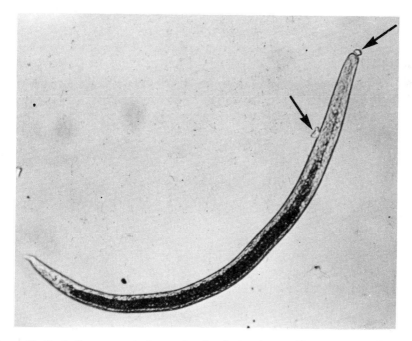

Figure 15−7 A *Toxocara canis* larva after incubation in specific antiserum. The immune precipitates at the oral and exretory pores are indicated by arrows. (Courtesy of Dr. D. H. De Savigny.)

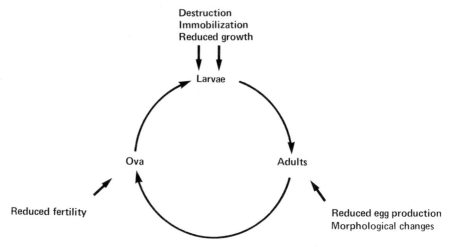

Figure 15–8   The effects of the immune responses on various stages of helminth development.

While the IgE-eosinophil–mediated antihelminth response is perhaps the most significant mechanism of resistance to helminths, antibodies of the other immunoglobulin classes also play a protective role. The mechanisms involved include antibody-mediated neutralization of the proteolytic enzymes used by larvae to penetrate tissues, blocking of the anal and oral pores of these larvae by immune complexes as antibodies combine with their excretory and secretory products (Fig. 15–7) and prevention of ecdysis and inhibition of larval development by antibodies directed against exsheathing antigens. Other enzyme pathways may be blocked by antibodies acting against adult worms, causing possible arrest of egg production or even interference in the development of anatomical structures (Fig. 15–8). Thus, female *Ostertagia ostertagi* worms fail to develop vulvar flaps when grown in immune calves. Similarly, spicule morphology may be altered in *Cooperia* males derived from immune hosts. Larvae also tend to cause tissue destruction and inflammation, attracting large numbers of neutrophils (Fig. 15–9).

CELL-MEDIATED IMMUNITY.   Many helminths, particularly those that undergo tissue migration, may be considered as functional xenografts. It is somewhat remarkable, therefore, that they are not precipitously rejected by the cell-mediated immune system. Their survival is a reflection of the success of their adaptation to existence within mammalian tissues. Nevertheless, there is evidence to suggest that sensitized T lymphocytes may successfully attack helminths that are either deeply embedded in the intestinal mucosa or undergoing prolonged tissue stages. For example, cell-mediated immune reactions have been shown to occur in *Trichinella spiralis* and *Trichostrongylus colubriformis* infections. In the former, immunity can be transferred to normal animals by lymphoid cells, and infected animals show delayed hypersensitivity reactions to intradermally inoculated worm antigens. *In vitro* tests for cell-mediated immunity such as MIF production and lymphocyte proliferation are also positive in these infections. (Trichinosis is also characterized by the occurrence of a massive eosinophilia. This appears to be associated with the presence of T cells and may be due to the activity of an eosinophil-stimulating lymphokine.) In the case of *T. colubriformis*, immunity can be transfered to normal animals from immune ones by both cells and serum, and the site of worm attachment is subjected to a massive lymphocyte infiltration.

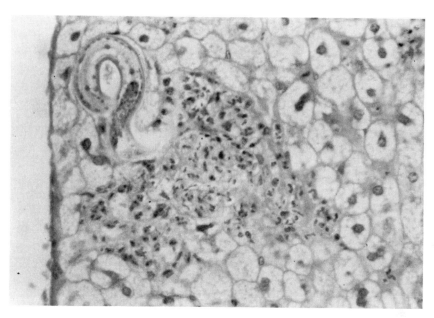

Figure 15−9 The cellular response to a helminth larva. This is a *T. canis* larva in the liver of a rabbit, 48 hours after oral administration of infective eggs. Most of the cells present are neutrophils. (Courtesy of Dr. J. P. Lautenslager.)

The cell-mediated immune responses participate in resistance against a number of other helminth infections. Thus, lymphocytes from sheep infected with *H. contortus* will release MIF and undergo blastogenesis in response to worm antigen, and it has been claimed that immunity to this organism can be transfered by allogeneic mesenteric lymph node cells or transfer factor from immune to normal animals.

Sensitized T lymphocytes depress the activities of helminths by two mechanisms. First, the development of an inflammatory response of the delayed hypersensitivity type tends to attract mononuclear cells to the site of larval invasion and renders the local environment unsuitable for growth or migration. Second, cytotoxic lymphocytes may be capable of causing larval destruction. In connection with this it has been shown that the treatment of experimental animals with BCG vaccine, a treatment that stimulates the T cell system (Chapter 6), inhibits the metastases of hydatid cysts (*E. granulosus*) and in these treated animals the space that surrounds the cysts may be filled with large lymphocytes. It is also not uncommon to observe large lymphocytes adhering firmly to migrating nematode larvae *in vivo*.

EVASION OF THE IMMUNE RESPONSE BY HELMINTHS

Although the preceding discussion has noted a number of mechanisms whereby animals resist helminth infection, it is obvious, even to a casual observer, that these responses are not fully effective. The success of this adaptation is seen at its most marked extent in cestode infections where cysticerci, in particular, appear to be able to survive indefinitely in the presence of a host response. Several mechanisms may be considered to play a ·role in this adaptation. They include mimicry of host antigens, absorption of host antigens, antigenic variation, blocking of antibodies and tolerance.

The first of these mechanisms introduces the concept that helminths may synthesize histocompatibility or blood group antigens to match those of their host. It is clear that a helminth cannot synthesize all antigens it could possibly require, since this would demand the existence of a genetic system similar in complexity to the antibody-producing system. Nevertheless, partial mimicry of host antigens is indeed possible, so that, for example, sheep respond to fewer antigens of *H. contortus* than do rabbits. This suggests that *H. contortus* possesses a closer antigenic similarity to sheep, its natural host, than to rabbits, which it does not normally infect. It has also been shown that many trematodes and cestodes are capable of synthesizing blood group antigens, which, if they happen to be identical to those of the host, also serve to reduce the effective antigenicity of the worm.

Second, there is a considerable amount of evidence that suggests that tissue helminths may be protected from the consequences of their hosts' immune response by the adsorption of host antigens onto their surface. An example of this is the adult *Schistosoma mansoni*, a trematode that lives in the mesenteric blood vessels of humans and which is capable of adsorbing host erythrocyte and histocompatibility antigens to its surface. Cysticerci can also adsorb histocompatibility antigens in this way.

A third mechanism of evasion of the immune response involves antigenic variation. Although helminths have not evolved a system as efficient as that seen in trypanosomiasis, gradual antigenic variation is recognized. Thus, the cuticular antigens of *T. spiralis* larvae show extensive changes following each moult. Even during their growth phase they show quantitative changes in the expression of surface protein antigens.

Another response that may contribute to the survival of parasitic helminths is immunosuppression. For example, sheep infected with *H. contortus* become specifically suppressed so that they are unreactive to *H. contortus* even though they remain responsive to unrelated antigens. The mechanisms involved in this response are unknown. They may involve induction of specific suppressor cells, as has been demonstrated in filariasis or, alternatively, they may result from the production of blocking antibody in a manner analogous to that seen in pregnancy and in some neoplastic conditions (Chapter 16). In other helminth infections, such as trichinosis, infected animals are nonspecifically immunosuppressed. This immunosuppression is reflected in a lowered resistance to other infections, a poor response to vaccination and a prolongation of skin graft survival.

It is theoretically possible that tolerance could occur in young animals that receive a high dose of parasite antigen either *in utero* as in toxocariasis, or very soon after birth.

VACCINATION AGAINST HELMINTHS

It is not surprising, considering the ineffectiveness of the host response to helminths, that vaccines are not widely available. Since vaccines consisting of dead organisms or extracts of organisms have been uniformly unsuccessful in conferring protection, studies have tended to concentrate on the use of irradiated material. Experimentally it has been shown, for instance, that irradiated metacercariae can reduce a *Fasciola hepatica* burden in calves, while irradiated ova of *Ascaridia galli* protect chickens against challenge by this helminth. However, only very few of these preparations have been commercially produced with any success. Perhaps the most important of those that have is the vaccine that is used to protect calves against verminous pneumonia caused by the lungworm *Dictyocaulus viviparus*. In this vaccine, second-stage larvae hatched from ova in culture are exposed to 40,000 R x-irradiation, and two doses of these larvae are then fed to calves. The larvae succeed in penetrating the calf's intestine, but, since they are unable to develop to the third stage, they never reach the lung and for this reason are nonpathogenic. During their exsheating process, however, they stimulate the development of antibodies that are then capable of blocking reinfection. The efficiency of this vaccine, like other vaccines, depends very much on the challenge dose, since vaccinated calves may show mild pneumonic signs if placed on grossly infected pastures.

A similar type of vaccine has been used to protect puppies against the hookworm *Ancylostoma caninum*. In this case irradiated larvae are administered three days after birth in order to provide immunity. Interestingly, passive immunity from the bitch does not appear to interfere with the development of resistance in the puppy.

ADDITIONAL SOURCES OF INFORMATION

Bloom BR. 1979. Games parasites play: how parasites evade immune surveillance. Nature *279* 21–26.

Butterworth AE, and David JR. 1981. Current concepts: eosinophil function. New Engl J Med *304* 154–156.

Callow LL, and Stewart NP. 1978. Immunosuppression by *Babesia bovis* against its tick vector *Boophilus microplus*. Nature *272* 818–819.

Capron A, Dessaint JP, and Capron M. 1979. Immunoregulation of parasite infections. J Allergy Clin Immunol *66* 91–96.

Ciba Foundation. 1974. Parasites in the immunized host: mechanisms of survival. Ciba Foundation Symposium 25 (new series). Excerpta Medica Foundation, New York.

Cohen S, and Sadun E (eds). 1976. Immunology of Parasitic Infections. Blackwell Scientific Publications, Oxford.

Jarrett EEE. 1973. Reaginic antibodies and helminth infections. Vet Rec *93* 480–483.

Miller TA. 1978. Immunology in intestinal parasitism. Vet Clin North Am (Small Animal Practice) *8* 707–720.

Mitchell GF. 1979. Effector cells, molecules and mechanisms in host-protective immunity to parasites. Immunology *38* 209–223.

Urquhart GM. 1980. Application of immunity in the control of parasitic disease. Vet Parasitol *6* 217–239.

16

Surveillance and Elimination of Foreign and Abnormal Cells

Although the immune responses first attracted the attention of scientists by virtue of the body's capacity to recognize and eliminate invading microorganisms, the observation that animals also possess the capacity to reject foreign skin grafts has led to the development of a much broader view of the function of the system as a whole.

In a complex multicellular organism, mechanisms for interaction between cells must exist. These interactions are generally mediated by means of surface structures or receptors through which "signals" are transmitted (see Fig. 7–1). If, for some reason, a cell becomes abnormal and, as a consequence, its surface structure becomes modified, then it is possible for this change to be recognized by other cells. The cell-mediated immune system appears to be designed so that cells with modified surfaces may be identified and then promptly eliminated. The cell surface structures that function as "recognition units" in this way are the class I and II histocompatibility antigens. These antigens are characteristic of an individual animal rather than of particular organs or cell types, although their distribution is not uniform throughout the body. The cells that are capable of recognizing and responding to these altered histocompatibility antigens include the T lymphocytes and an ill-defined population of natural killer (NK) cells.

HISTOCOMPATIBILITY ANTIGENS AND GRAFT REJECTION

The survival of an allograft is directly related to the histocompatibility differences between graft and recipient. Differences at the major histocompatibility locus lead to rapid, irreversible graft rejection. Differences at minor histocompatibility loci provoke slow, easily reversed rejection. The major antigens against which the rejection process is directed are those of the class I and class II histocompatibility antigens (Chapter 7).

Class I antigens of the major histocompatibility complex are identifiable by the use of specific antisera and are described as serologically defined (SD) antigens. It is possible to obtain specific antisera against each SD antigen and to determine which of these antisera will kill an animal's leukocytes in the presence of complement. By using a set of these antisera it is possible to identify, or "type," each of the antigens on the cells of both the recipient and the potential donors and so select the closest "match." About 15 different SD antigens (alleles) have been described in the dog; they are located at three loci (DLA-A, DLA-B, DLA-C.) (Fig. 16–1).

Probably of more importance in influencing graft rejection are the class II antigens found on lymphocytes, macrophages, epidermal cells and sperm. These antigens are detectable by measuring their ability to stimulate allogeneic lymphocytes to divide and are called lymphocyte-defined (LD) antigens. LD antigens may be detected by mixing lymphocytes from donor and recipient *in vitro*. If incompatible, both cell populations are stimulated to divide by the presence of foreign histocompatibility antigens; this division may be quantitated by measuring the rate of uptake of tritium(^{3}H)-labeled thymidine. (Thymidine is used only by dividing cells that are

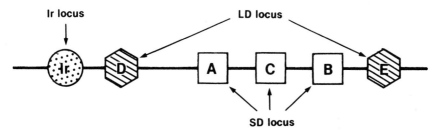

Figure 16–1 The structure of the major histocompatibility complex in the dog (DLA). A, B and C are serologically defined; D and E are lymphocyte defined. Ir is an immune response locus.

actively synthesizing DNA.) This technique is known as the mixed lymphocyte reaction (MLR). If one of the cell populations is prevented from reacting by pretreatment with an immunosuppressive drug (see page 251), then the inactivated cells act as "targets" and it is possible to "type" the LD antigens on the inactivated cells. In dogs, at least 11 LD antigens have been identified at two loci (DLA-D and DLA-E) (Fig. 16–1).

When dogs are given kidney grafts from donors incompatible at both the SD and the LD loci, they survive for about 10 days (Table 16–1). If, on the other hand, they are compatible at all these loci, graft survival is prolonged to about 40 days. A more impressive result is obtained with canine liver grafts, which survive for about 8 days in unrelated animals and for 200 to 300 days in DLA-identical recipients. The failure of DLA-compatible grafts to survive indefinitely is due to the cumulative effects of a large number of minor histocompatibility differences.

A simple and rapid test for histocompatibility is to take lymphocytes from a potential graft recipient and inject them into the skin of a potential donor. If the injected cells are not compatible with the recipient, then both injected lymphocytes and the recipient's lymphocytes will attack and destroy the nearest foreign tissue and provoke an inflammatory skin reaction. This reaction is known as the "normal lymphocyte transfer test." It measures primarily compatibility at the LD loci, the intensity of the inflammatory response providing an indication of the degree of incompatibility between donor and recipient.

THE ALLOGRAFT REACTION

If a kidney allograft is transplanted between unrelated mongrel dogs, it will survive for about a week (Table 16–1). The rejection process is associated with disruption of the renal vasculature, oliguria and finally anuria. If a second graft from the same donor dog is made, it will be rejected by the recipient within one to two days without ever becoming functional. This accelerated reaction to a second graft is known as a "second-set" reaction and is a form of secondary immune response. The second-set reaction is specific for a graft from the original donor or from a donor syngeneic with the first. It is not restricted to any particular site or to any specific organ, since histocompatibility antigens are present on most nucleated cells.

Histology of Allograft Rejection.   The events that take place during graft rejec-

Table 16–1   MEAN SURVIVAL TIMES OF CANINE TISSUES TRANSPLANTED BETWEEN DLA-INCOMPATIBLE MONGREL DOGS*

ORGANS	SURVIVAL TIME (DAYS)
Skin	12.0
Kidney	7.0
Liver	7.7
Pancreas	10.5
Lung	5.8
Small intestine	8.1
Heart	8.4
Tracheal cartilage	250.0
Parathyroids	< 14.0

*Survival times are usually significantly longer in grafts between DLA-incompatible beagles.

tion vary among different types of grafts. For example, if a skin graft is placed on an animal, it takes some time for vascular and lymphatic connections to be established between the graft and the host. Only when these connections are made can host cells penetrate the graft and commence the rejection process. The first indication of this process is a transient neutrophil accumulation around the blood vessels at the base of the graft, and this is followed by an infiltration of mononuclear cells (lymphocytes and macrophages) that eventually extends throughout the grafted skin. The first signs of tissue damage are observed in the capillaries of the graft, whose endothelium becomes destroyed, and as a result thrombosis, vascular stasis and infarction follow rapidly. In renal grafts, the blood supply to the transplanted kidney is established at the time of transplantation. As a result, the whole organ gradually becomes infiltrated with mononuclear cells (Fig. 16–2), which cause damage to the endothelium of small intertubular blood vessels. This vascular damage is progressive, and tubular destruction, infarction, hemorrhage and death of the grafted kidney follow thrombosis of these vessels.

In a second-set reaction, vascularization of skin grafts usually does not have time to occur, since an extensive and destructive mononuclear cell and neutrophil infiltration occurs in the graft bed. Similarly, the blood vessels of second kidney grafts become rapidly thrombosed as a result of the action of serum antibodies and complement on the vascular endothelium. Xenografts are usually rejected extremely promptly. For example, porcine renal xenografts transplanted to dogs are hyperacutely rejected in 10 to 20 minutes because of the presence of natural antibodies to pig antigens in dog serum.

Mechanism of Allograft Reactions (Fig. 16–3).   As described above, the rejection of grafts are of two general types. In first-set reactions, grafts are rejected in a matter of days. In second-set reactions or xenografts, rejection is a hyperacute process. Both processes occur as a result of damage to vascular endothelium. The first-set reaction may be divided into two stages. First, information about the antigenic structure of the graft must reach antigen-sensitive cells, usually located in the draining

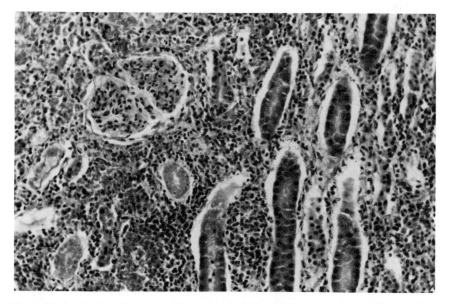

Figure 16–2   Section of a canine kidney that had been rejected after 14 days by an allogeneic canine recipient. × 360. (From a specimen kindly provided by Dr. R. G. Thomson.)

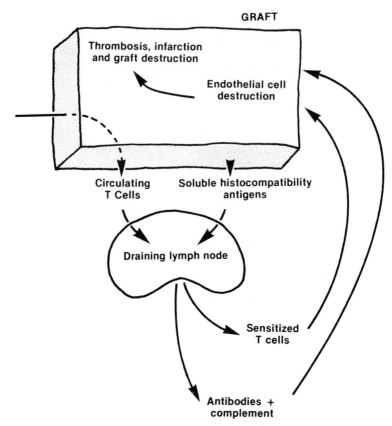

Figure 16–3 The mechanism of graft rejection.

lymph node. Second, effector cells from this lymph node must invade the graft and mediate its destruction.

SENSITIZATION OF THE RECIPIENT. Information on graft antigens may reach the antigen-sensitive cells of the recipient by two routes. Either graft cells may release their histocompatibility antigens in soluble form, or, more importantly, circulating T cells may, on passing through the blood vessels of the graft, recognize foreign histocompatibility antigens. These cells may then pass from the graft in either the lymphatics or the blood vessels and eventually lodge in the draining lymph node as a consequence of local triggering of the lymphocyte "trap" (Chapter 5). It is probable, at least in skin grafts, that the lymphatic route is of most importance, since if a graft is prevented from developing lymphatic connections with the host, then rejection is considerably delayed.

The cells that first recognize the graft as foreign are capable of recruiting, in some way, specific effector T cells within the draining lymph node. The thymus-dependent paracortical regions of lymph nodes draining a graft contain increased numbers of cells, among which are clusters of large pyroninophilic cells. The numbers of these cells are greatest about six days after grafting and decline rapidly once the graft has been rejected. In addition to these signs of an active T cell–mediated immune response, it is also usual to observe some germinal center formation in the cortex and plasma cell accumulation in the medulla, suggesting that a humoral immune response also occurs.

DESTRUCTION OF THE GRAFT. As a result of the events that occur in the draining lymph node, effector T lymphocytes, recruited by the cells that recognize the graft as foreign, leave the node in the efferent lymph and reach the graft through the vascular system. When these cells enter the grafted tissue, they attach to and destroy the vascular endothelium by direct cytotoxicity. As a result of this microvascular damage, hemorrhage, platelet aggregation, thrombosis and infarction occur, and because of this failure in its blood supply, the grafted tissue dies. There is evidence to suggest that the intensity of the graft rejection process may be related to the number of allogeneic lymphocytes in the grafted tissue, and it has been suggested that a form of graft-versus-host response may contribute to the rejection process.

Although sensitized T cells are the most important destroyers of foreign grafted tissues, it is clear that antibodies also play a significant role in graft destruction (Table 16–2). This antibody-mediated destruction is brought about by antibodies, complement and neutrophils or through antibody-dependent cytotoxic cell activity (Chapter 6) and is particularly important in second-set and xenograft reactions.

REJECTION OF CARDIAC ALLOGRAFTS. In humans and dogs that have received heart transplants, the pathology of the rejection process is uniquely different. The major lesion observed in these grafts is extensive endothelial cell proliferation in the walls of cardiac blood vessels (Fig. 16–4). The resulting obliteration of the blood vessel lumen eventually results in cardiac failure and death. A similar lesion is sometimes seen in renal allografts undergoing chronic rejection.

Graft-versus-Host (GVH) Reaction. In a previous section the normal lymphocyte transfer reaction, in which lymphocytes from a potential graft recipient are injected into a potential donor animal, was discussed. These transferred lymphocytes recognize that their new host is foreign and therefore attack nearby cells, as a consequence of which a local inflammatory response occurs. In other words, the graft attacks the host! In a normal lymphocyte transfer reaction, the results of this graft-versus-host reaction are not usually serious, since the host is capable of destroying the

Table 16–2 SOME MECHANISMS OF CYTOTOXICITY IMPORTANT IN THE DESTRUCTION OF GRAFTS

MECHANISM	*CELLS INVOLVED*	*PATHWAY*	*RELATIVE IMPORTANCE IN GRAFT REJECTION*
Cell-mediated cytotoxic reactions	T cells	Direct contact	$+ + + +$
	T cells	Through lymphotoxin	$+$
	Macrophages	Through SMAF*	$+$
	Macrophages	Nonspecifically activated	$+$
Antibodies and cells	Null-lymphocytes Macrophages Neutrophils	Through Fc receptors and antibody	$+ +$
Antibodies and complement	—	Complement-mediated cytolysis	$+ + +$

*SMAF = specific macrophage arming factor.

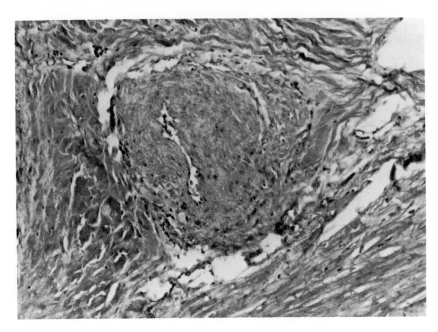

Figure 16–4 A section of coronary artery from a canine cardiac allograft, showing severe narrowing of the lumen. × 100. (From Penn OC, et al. 1976. Transplantation 22 313. © The Williams & Wilkins Co., Baltimore. Used with permission.)

foreign lymphocytes and thus terminating the attack. If, however, the host animal cannot for some reason reject the grafted lymphocytes, then these cells may cause uncontrolled destruction of the host's tissues, which will eventually lead to death. This type of GVH reaction can occur if the recipient of the lymphoid cells has been immunosuppressed or is immunodeficient. It has been observed in foals or puppies that receive normal lymphoid tissue transplants in an attempt to cure congenital immunodeficiencies (Chapter 22). Animals suffering from a GVH reaction develop lymphocytic infiltration of the intestine, skin and liver, which results in mucosal destruction and diarrhea, ulcerative dermatitis and stomatitis, hepatic necrosis and jaundice. The eventual result is cessation of growth (runting) and death.

Grafts That Are Not Rejected

PRIVILEGED SITES.   Certain areas of the body, such as the anterior chamber of the eye, the cornea and the brain, lack effective lymphatic drainage. As a consequence, although antigen derived from grafts made in these sites will reach lymphoid tissue, cytotoxic effector cells cannot reach the graft and these grafts survive relatively well. It is for this reason that corneal allografting is a successful procedure in human and canine surgery.

PREGNANCY.   Because the fetus and its placenta possess paternal antigens, they may be considered an allograft within the mother. Nevertheless, the fetus is consistently successful in establishing and maintaining itself through pregnancy, in spite of great histocompatibility differences. The reasons for this acceptance of the fetus and its placenta are not completely understood. It is known, however, that the uterus is not a privileged site, since grafts of other tissues, such as skin, made into the uterine wall are readily rejected. In fact, under some circumstances the mother may make antibodies against fetal blood group antigens, and these can destroy fetal red cells either *in*

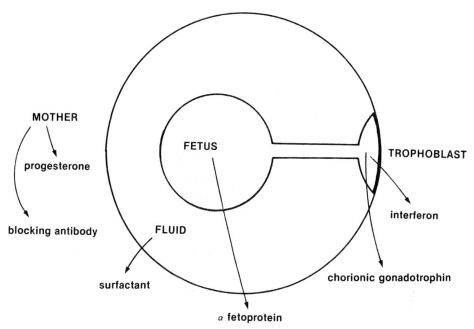

Figure 16–5 Some of the immunosuppressive factors that act to protect the fetus from immunological rejection.

utero, as in humans, or in newborn animals following ingestion of colostrum (Chapter 18).

The immunological destruction of the fetus is prevented by the combined activities of several different specific and nonspecific immunosuppressive mechanisms (Fig. 16–5). First, the fetus is protected from the mother's immune system by the trophoblast, which is that part of the placenta in closest contact with maternal tissue. Trophoblast cells have very low concentrations of histocompatibility antigens on their surface and are also covered by a layer of nonimmunogenic sulfated mucoprotein.

Second, the fetus is a source of immunosuppressive factors. These include the hormones estradiol and progesterone and possibly also chorionic gonadotrophin. α-Fetoprotein, the major protein in fetal serum, is immunosuppressive as a result of its ability to stimulate suppressor cell function. In addition, a number of pregnancy-associated glycoproteins, including α_2-macroglobulin, and placental interferon have immunosuppressive properties, and amniotic fluid is rich in immunosuppressive phospholipids.

Third, both "blocking antibody" and suppressor cells are produced in response to fetal antigens. These interfere with the maternal anti-fetal immune response. The blocking antibody coats placental cells, thus preventing their destruction by maternal T cells. This antibody can be eluted from the placenta and shown to be capable of suppressing other cell-mediated immune reactions against paternal antigens, such as graft rejection. Absence of this blocking material has been shown to account for some cases of recurrent abortion in women.

It must not be assumed from the foregoing list of immunosuppressive factors that the pregnant female is grossly immunosuppressed. In fact, the immunosuppression generated by the fetus is very local in nature. Pregnant animals have only minor deficiencies in cell-mediated immune reactivity to nonfetal antigens, showing, for example, a slight delay in the rejection of skin grafts, or transient unreactivity to the tuberculin skin test (Chapter 20).

CULTURED OR STORED ORGANS. If an organ or tissue is grown in tissue culture or stored frozen, its potential for successful transplantation is greatly enhanced. This is probably because any lymphocytes living within the tissue are destroyed. Thus, thyroid cells and islet cells have been successfully transplanted to allogeneic hosts after prolonged tissue culture. Freeze-dried pig dermis is very useful in covering extensive wounds in horses and dogs, and there have been reports of successful bone and aortic allografts in domestic animals after storage of the grafts in liquid nitrogen.

IMMUNOLOGICALLY FAVORED ORGANS. On some occasions, pigs and dogs that have received a whole liver graft do not appear to mount an allograft response against it, whereas in others, a response may be mounted that is relatively weak and easily suppressed. The liver grafts may, by their presence, be capable of protecting another graft, such as a kidney allograft from the same donor, resulting in the prolonged survival of the kidney graft. It is likely that these effects occur in response to the release from the liver of immunosuppressive factors such as hepatic glycoferroprotein and bilirubin (Chapter 7).

In some circumstances, such as in dogs that have maintained functioning renal allografts for a long period of time (several years), immunosuppressive therapy may be gradually reduced and eventually totally discontinued as graft acceptance becomes complete. It is probable that this phenomenon is an example of high dose tolerance—that is, tolerance that results when the amount of antigen is in excess of the capacity of the antigen-sensitive cells to respond to it (Chapter 7). In the case of graft acceptance following immunosuppression, antigen-sensitive cells are gradually eliminated by the immunosuppressive agents. Once their numbers are sufficiently low, the relatively large mass of grafted tissue may be sufficient to establish and maintain tolerance.

SUPPRESSION OF THE ALLOGRAFT RESPONSE

The many techniques available for inhibiting the allograft response may be classified into three general groups. First, the most widely employed techniques involve drugs or radiation that, by inhibiting cell division, serve to reduce the multiplication of antigen-sensitive cells upon encountering antigen. This approach is crude and dangerous, since other rapidly proliferating cell populations such as intestinal epithelium and bone marrow cells of the myeloid and erythroid series also may be severely depleted, with potentially disastrous consequences. Second, it is possible to employ techniques that serve to selectively eliminate T cells. This can be done by means of specific anti-T cell serum, by selective drugs or by thoracic duct drainage. Third, the normal immune responses are well controlled by the body, and although not widely employed at present, these natural control mechanisms are likely to provide potentially useful techniques for the control of the allograft response in the future.

Nonspecific Immunosuppression

RADIATION. X-radiation exerts its effect on cells by several different mechanisms. The simplest of these is through ionizing rays hitting an essential, unique molecule within the cell. The most important of these molecules are the nucleic acids, particularly DNA. A loss of even one nucleotide entails a permanent mutation of a gene, with potentially lethal effects on the progeny of the affected cell. Another technique involves radiation of aqueous solutions, which results in ionization and the formation of highly reactive free hydrogen and hydroxyl radicals. These free radicals can react with dissolved oxygen to form peroxides that may have toxic effects on many cell processes. Although x-radiation is of some use in prolonging graft survival in many experimental animals, the amount of radiation required for effective prolongation of graft survival in the dog is usually lethal.

CORTICOSTEROIDS. Corticosteroids are immunosuppressive for several reasons. First, they are "toxic" for some lymphoid cells, particularly those in the thymus. Second, steroids are capable of "stabilizing" lysosomal membranes, thus inhibiting the release of lysosomal enzymes and impairing antigen processing. Third, it has been suggested that steroids may render macrophages unresponsive to lymphokines. Steroids are also potent anti-inflammatory agents, since they reduce the release of hydrolytic enzymes from neutrophils and macrophages. Thus, when applied directly to skin grafts, steroids may inhibit rejection without causing systemic immunosuppression.

CYTOTOXIC DRUGS. The major immunosuppressive drugs, having been designed to inhibit cell division, act largely on various stages of nucleic acid synthesis and activity. Thus, many of these drugs are analogues that interfere with nucleic acid synthesis through competitive blocking of substrate binding sites on enzymes. For example, azaserine blocks glutamine synthesis; azathioprine, 6-mercaptopurine, and 6-thioguanine block purine synthesis; 5-fluorouracil blocks pyrimidine synthesis; and methotrexate blocks folic acid synthesis (Fig. 16–6).

The other major group of immunosuppressive drugs comprises the alkylating agents, which act by cross-linking DNA helices, preventing their separation and thus inhibiting template formation. The alkylating agents include cyclophosphamide, chlorambucil and the antibiotics actinomycin and mitomycin C. The final group of commonly employed cytotoxic drugs are those that inhibit cell division by disrupting microtubule formation. They include drugs such as colchicine and the vinca alkaloids, vincristine and vinblastine.

All these cytotoxic drugs are immunosuppressive by virtue of their ability to prevent the replication of antigen-sensitive cells in response to antigen. The relative sensitivity of T cells and B cells to these drugs may vary. Thus, azathioprine, a very commonly used drug in human renal transplantation, tends to inhibit the cell-mediated rejection process in doses that leave the humoral immune response unimpaired, whereas cyclophosphamide tends to selectively prevent B cell responses.

Specific Methods of Immunosuppression

DEPLETION OF LYMPHOCYTES. Because of the many adverse side effects of the nonspecific immunosuppressive agents (not the least important of which is an increased predisposition to infection) there has been considerable effort made to establish more specific alternative immunosuppressive procedures. One relatively simple technique that largely depletes T cells is cannulation of the thoracic duct. The recirculating lymphocytes that pass through the duct are mainly T cells, and interference with their recirculation in this way can precipitate a dramatic drop in the number of T lymphocytes. Obviously, this procedure does not lend itself readily to routine use, and an alternative procedure is to administer an antiserum specific for T lymphocytes. Antilymphocytic serum (ALS) can be made by inoculating a recipient of a different species with a purified lymphocyte suspension. The antiserum produced must be refined to ensure that it is specific for lymphocytes. Thus, it is usual to attempt to remove antibodies for the other blood elements by repeated absorption. ALS suppresses the cell-mediated immune response and leaves the humoral immune response relatively intact. Theoretically, it is, therefore, a great improvement on other immunosuppressive

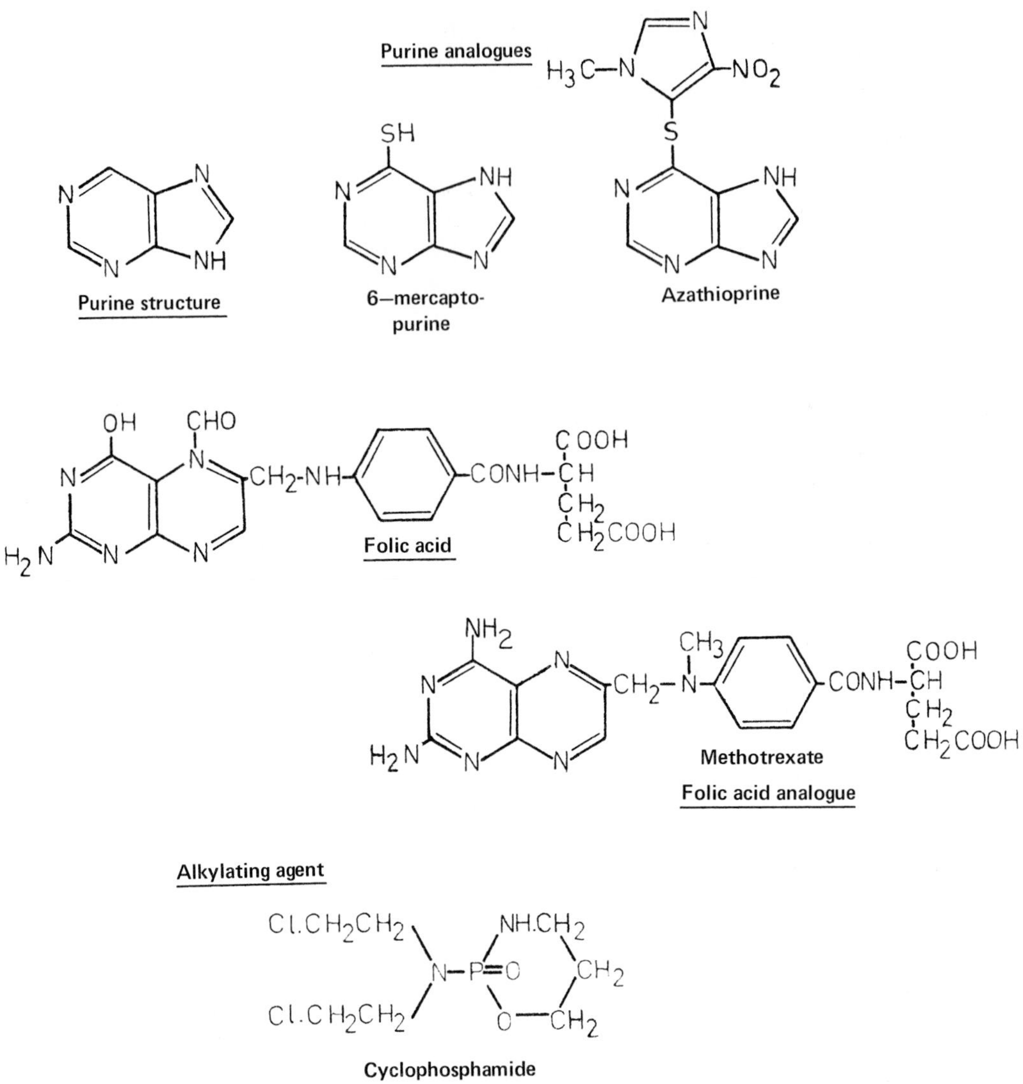

Purine analogues

Purine structure

6—mercapto-
purine

Azathioprine

Folic acid

Methotrexate

Folic acid analogue

Alkylating agent

Cyclophosphamide

Figure 16–6 The structure of some commonly employed immunosuppressive drugs and the normal compounds with which they compete. Cyclophosphamide is an alkylating agent that cross-links DNA chains and hence prevents their separation.

techniques. In practice, however, ALS has proved to be of variable efficiency. In experiments in mice, ALS-treated animals have been shown to accept rat xenografts, whereas clinical use of ALS in humans has not been universally accepted as being useful. Being a foreign antigen, ALS induces an immune response against itself, a feature that prevents prolonged therapy and increases the risks of anaphylaxis and serum sickness. Finally, since ALS is a suppressor of all cell-mediated immune functions, it may render treated animals susceptible to virus infections, permitting, for instance, the development of distemper and hepatitis in vaccinated dogs.

CYCLOSPORIN A. Cyclosporin A is a cyclic polypeptide derived from certain fungi. It acts a specific suppressor of the T cell response by blocking the response of T cells to interleukin-1 so that they fail to produce interleukin-2 (Chapter 6). It also blocks the response of effector T cells to interleukin-2. The net effect of the action of cyclosporin A is, therefore, blocking of the T cell response without affecting nonresponding lymphocytes. Unfortunately, some patients receiving cyclosporin A have developed B cell lymphomas. If it were not for this problem, cyclosporin A would be an almost perfect immunosuppressive agent.

UTILIZATION OF NATURAL CONTROL MECHANISMS. For many years, the administration of blood transfusions to potential renal allograft recipients prior to transplantation was discouraged on the grounds that they might sensitize the recipient and so hasten graft rejection. Experience has shown, however, that multiple transfusions given prior to transplantation greatly enhance graft survival not only in humans but also in pigs and dogs. The mechanisms are unclear, but the response may be due to stimulation of blocking antibodies similar to those found in pregnant animals.

TUMORS AS ALLOGRAFTS

When organ transplantation became a common and widespread procedure in humans as a result of the development of potent immunosuppressive agents, it was observed that patients with prolonged graft survival and immunosuppressive therapy were 80 to 100 times more likely to develop neoplasia than were nonimmunosuppressed individuals. It was therefore suggested that the immunocompetent cells suppressed by the therapy were also responsible for the prevention of neoplasia. It was from this suggestion that the concept of a surveillance function for the immune system was developed, providing a stimulus for a growing interest in the role of the immune responses in neoplastic diseases.

Experimental evidence has shown that this simple view of the T cell system as a device used to identify and destroy tumor cells is no longer tenable. For example, nude mice, which have no T cells, are not more susceptible to tumors, either natural or induced, than are normal mice. The resistance of these animals to tumors does not lie in the T cell system but is due to natural killer (NK) cells. It is probable therefore, that if a surveillance system does exist, then it is mediated by NK cells rather than by the conventional immune system. The increase in cancer seen in immunosuppressed individuals is probably due to destruction of NK cells. Although the original surveillance hypothesis has had to be greatly modified, there is good evidence to show that some tumor cells may be antigenic and that immunological techniques may be used to treat cancer. It should be pointed out, however, that there is a great difference between the massive immune response triggered by allogeneic grafts and the host's responses to the very weak antigens associated with tumor cells.

Tumor Antigens. Tumor cells that are functionally different from their normal precursors may also be antigenically different, in that they may gain or lose antigens. For example, they may lose histocompatibility or blood group antigens, and some tumors of the intestine, such as colon carcinomas, may lose the ability to produce mucus. More commonly, tumor cells gain antigens, and some naturally occurring tumors of adult humans are characterized by the production of antigenic proteins normally found only in the fetus. For example, tumors of the gastrointestinal tract may produce a glycoprotein known as carcinoembryonic antigen (CEA), which is usually found only in the fetal intestine. The appearance of CEA in serum may indicate the presence of a colon or rectal adenocarcinoma. Other examples of the generation of a fetal antigen by tumor cells include production of α-fetoprotein by hepatoma cells (α-fetoprotein is normally found only in the fetal liver), and squamous cell carcinoma cells of horn may possess antigens also found in normal bovine fetal liver and skin.

Tumors induced by oncogenic viruses tend to gain new antigens characteristic of the inducing virus. These antigens, although coded for by the viral genome, are not part of the virus particle. Examples of this type of antigen include the FOCMA antigens found on the lymphoid cells of cats infected with feline leukemia virus (Chapter 14) and MATSA (Marek's tumor-specific antigens) found on Marek's disease–infected cells.

Chemically induced tumors are different from the virus-induced variety in that they carry surface antigens unique to the tumor and not to the inducing chemical. Tumors induced by a single chemical in different animals of the same species may be antigenically quite unrelated, and even within a single chemically induced tumor mass it is possible to demonstrate the existence of antigenically distinct subpopulations of cells.

Immune Responses to Tumor Antigens.   In general, if tumor cells are antigenically sufficiently different from normal, they will be regarded as foreign and attacked. The major mechanisms of tumor cell destruction involve NK cells and cytotoxic T cells, although activated macrophages may also participate in this process.

NK CELLS AND INTERFERON.   Natural killer cells are large granular lymphocytes derived from bone marrow. Although they possess some T cell characteristics, they are part of the null cell population in peripheral blood. NK cells are not phagocytic, but they effectively destroy tumors and virus-infected cells by direct cytotoxicity in the absence of prior antigenic stimulation. They possess Fc receptors and may therefore also participate in antibody-dependent cellular cytotoxicity (ADCC). NK cells produce interferon upon encountering target cells. The interferon then acts to enhance NK activity by promoting the rapid differentiation of pre-NK cells. (Interferon also enhances T cell- and macrophage-mediated cytotoxicity (Chapter 6)).

The NK cell-interferon system probably plays a critical role in resistance to tumors, and it may be shown that mice or humans deficient in NK cells (Chédiak-Higashi syndrome, Chapter 22) have a greatly increased susceptibility to cancer. Neutralization of interferon by means of specific antisera enhances tumor growth in mice, presumably by depressing NK cell activity. Finally, preliminary studies suggest that interferon treatment may be useful in human cancer therapy.

SPECIFIC IMMUNITY.   It is occasionally possible to detect a cell-mediated response to tumor antigens either by skin testing or by an *in vitro* test such as macrophage migration inhibition. It is also possible to show that lymphocytes from some tumor-bearing animals may exert a cytotoxic effect on tumor cells cultured *in vitro*. Antibodies to tumor cells are commonly found in many tumor-bearing animals; for instance, about 50 per cent of sera from dogs with lymphosarcomas contain precipitating antitumor antibodies. These antibodies may be of some protective significance, since in conjunction with complement, antibodies may be capable of lysing tumors of dispersed cells. Antibodies do not appear to be effective in lysing solid tumors.

Failure of the Immune Responses to Tumor Cells.   The fact that neoplasisms are so readily induced in experimental animals and are so relatively common in domestic animals and in humans testifies to the inadequacies of the immunological protective mechanisms. Studies of tumor-bearing animals have indicated the existence of a number of mechanisms by which immune systems fail to reject tumors.

IMMUNOSUPPRESSION.   It is commonly observed that tumor-bearing animals are severely immunosuppressed. This suppression is most clearly seen in animals bearing lymphoid tumors; in these animals, tumors of B cells appear to suppress antibody formation whereas tumors of T cell origin generally suppress the cell-mediated immune responses (see Table 22–1). The suppression observed in leukemia virus infections is possibly a reflection of generalized disturbances in the lymphoid cell system brought about by these viruses. In contrast, immunosuppression observed in animals bearing chemically induced tumors appears to be due, at least in some cases, to the release of immunosuppressive factors such as prostaglandins from the tumor cells. Finally, it should be pointed out that the presence of actively growing tumor cells represents an extremely severe protein drain on an animal. This protein loss may be reflected in an impaired immune response.

INHIBITORS OF THE CELL-MEDIATED IMMUNE RESPONSE. Although tumor cells are antigenic and may stimulate a protective cell-mediated immune response, the humoral immune response commonly has an opposite effect. Thus, the serum of a tumor-bearing animal when given to a second tumor-bearing animal may cause the tumor of the second animal to grow even faster — a phenomenon known as enhancement. Serum of this type may also effectively inhibit the *in vitro* cytotoxicity of T cells for tumor cells. The nature of the blocking material that causes tumor enhancement is not clear, but it may be either antigen or an immune complex consisting of antibody complexed to tumor cell antigen. Certainly many tumors release large quantities of cell surface antigen, and this may bind to cytotoxic T cells, saturating their antigen receptors and so blocking their capacity to bind to target cells. Of more importance is the production of blocking antibodies — non–complement-fixing antitumor antibodies that effectively mask tumor antigens and thus protect the tumor cells from attack by cytotoxic T cells. In general, the presence or absence of these blocking factors correlates well with the state of progression or regression of a tumor.

TUMOR CELL SELECTION. There are two possible mechanisms by which the biological activity of tumor cells might influence their survival. One is "sneaking through," the process by which a tumor may not provide sufficient stimulus to induce an immune response until it has reached a size at which it cannot be controlled by the host. Second, tumor cells that are very different from the host cells will be rapidly identified and eliminated without leading to disease. Those tumors that do develop must, therefore, be selected for minimal antigenicity and for their inability to stimulate the host's immune system.

TRANSMISSIBLE VENEREAL SARCOMA. Transmissible venereal sarcoma of dogs is a tumor transmitted between animals by transplantation. In order to successfully colonize a new host, it must be able to establish itself in the face of gross histoincompatibility. It is not always successful, and after an initial growth phase the tumor often regresses. Nevertheless, lethal metastases do occasionally occur. Exposed dogs, whether or not they develop progressive tumors, develop antibodies to tumor cells, although the serum of dogs with regressive tumors is more effective in inhibiting tumor growth. If recipient dogs are immunosuppressed, the tendency to malignant growth is enhanced.

TUMOR IMMUNOTHERAPY (Table 16–3)

Two general approaches have been used in attempts to cure or modify tumor growth through immunotherapy. The simplest is to nonspecifically stimulate the immune system. Obviously, any improvement in an animal's immune capabilities will tend to enhance its resistance to tumors, although a cure may be expected only if the tumor mass is small or is surgically excised. The most widely used immune stimulant

Table 16–3 SOME APPROACHES TO TUMOR IMMUNOTHERAPY

1. Nonspecific stimulation of the immune systems
   e.g., BCG, *Propionibacterium acnes*
2. Specific immunization
   a.   Attempted immunization with chemically modified cells
        e.g., neuraminidase-, or glutaraldehyde-treated cells
   b.   Antiviral vaccination
        e.g., Marek's disease, warts
   c.   Attempted transfer of cell-mediated immunity
        e.g., transfer factor therapy

is the attenuated strain of *Mycobacterium bovis,* bacille Calmette-Guérin (BCG). This organism has a nonspecific effect on cell-mediated immune reactivity. It may be given systemically, or, more effectively, it may be inoculated directly into the tumor mass. Techniques such as this have been employed with success in the treatment of equine sarcoid and ocular squamous cell carcinoma in cattle.

Other immunostimulants that have been employed, although generally with less success than BCG, include *Corynebacterium parvum*, thymus hormones, levamisole (Chapter 3) and various mixed bacterial vaccines. A related technique that has been used to treat human skin tumors is to paint them with the contact allergen dinitro-chlorobenzene. The local hypersensitivity reaction provoked by this compound appears to preferentially damage the tumor cells and cause tumor regression.

Specific immunotherapy, the second major approach, has also been attempted by many investigators. This may be achieved by active immunization — that is, vaccinating the animal with tumor cells or antigens. One such technique is to take tumor cells, emulsify them in Freund's complete adjuvant and reinoculate the mixture into the host. This method has achieved some success in the treatment of canine lymphosarcoma. Lyophilized phenol-saline extracts of bovine ocular squamous cell carcinomas have produced encouraging remissions in cattle.

Because so many tumors can evade the immune response, it is usual to treat the tumor cells in an attempt to enhance their antigenicity. Thus, x-irradiated cells and neuraminidase- or glutaraldehyde-treated cells have been used in tumor vaccines with limited success.

Adoptive transfer of immune lymphocytes is, at least in theory, a logical method of conferring immunity against a tumor in an animal. In practice, however, this technique is not feasible, although some success has been achieved with transfer factor extracted from these cells. Since transfer factor functions across species barriers, it is possible that it may be harvested from domestic animals and used therapeutically in humans.

Passive immunization using serum from immune animals is generally considered undesirable because of the risk of tumor enhancement through transfer of blocking antibody. Nevertheless, as described above, serum from immune donors accelerates the regression of canine venereal sarcoma. Normal cat serum causes rapid regression of FeLV-induced tumors for unknown reasons.

In contrast to the techniques described above, most of which have met with only partial success, there do exist a number of successful techniques for vaccination against tumor viruses. The most important of these is the vaccine against Marek's disease, a T cell tumor of chickens caused by a herpesvirus. The immune response evoked by this vaccine has two components. First, humoral and cell-mediated responses act directly on the virus to reduce the quantity available to infect cells. Second, an immune response against antigens generated by the virus on the surface of tumor cells is provoked. These antigens, known as MATSA (Marek's tumor-specific antigens), provoke successful antitumor immunity. Both the antiviral and antitumor immune responses act synergistically to protect the birds. Success has also been achieved with formolized wart vaccines in cattle. In view of this, it is perhaps possible to predict that future successes are more likely to be due to the development of vaccines against oncogenic viruses such as these rather than to more esoteric immunological approaches directed toward the destruction of the tumor cells.

ADDITIONAL SOURCES OF INFORMATION

Allison AC, and Ferluga J. 1976. How lymphocytes kill tumor cells. N Engl J Med 295 165–167.

Beer AE, and Billingham RE. 1978. Immunoregulatory aspects of pregnancy. Fed Proc 37 2374–2378.

Barker CF, and Billingham RE. 1977. Immunologically privileged sites. Adv Immunol 25 1–54.

Broder S, and Waldmann TA. 1978. The suppressor-cell network in cancer. N Engl J Med 299 1281–1284, 1335–1341.

Carpenter CB, d'Apice AJF, and Abbas AK. 1976. The role of antibodies in the rejection and enhancement of organ allografts. Adv Immunol 22 1–65.

Chism SE, Burton RC, and Warner NL. 1978. Immunogenicity of oncofetal antigens: a review. Clin Immunol Immunopathol 11 346–373.

Essex M, and Grant CK. 1979. Tumor immunology in domestic animals. Adv Vet Sci Comp Med 23 183–228.

Freedman SO, and Gold P. (eds). 1977. Immunology as it relates to reproductive biology. Clin Obstet Gynecol 20 665–772.

Grebe SC, and Streilen JW. 1976. Graft-versus-host reactions: a review. Adv Immunol 221 119–221.

Kelly GE. 1977. Current prospects for renal transplantation in veterinary practice. Aust Vet J 53 53–60.

Kolb M, Sale GE, Lerner KG, et al. 1979. Pathology of acute graft-versus-host disease in the dog. Am J Pathol 96 581–594.

Marx JL. 1980. Natural killer cells help defend the body. Science 210 624–626.

Oettgen HF. 1977. Immunotherapy of cancer. N Engl J Med 297 484–491.

Perryman LE, and Liu IKM. 1980. Graft-versus-host reactions in foals with combined immunodeficiency. Am J Vet Res 41 187–192.

Rowlands DT, Hill GS, and Zmijewski CM. 1976. The pathology of renal homograft rejection: a review. Am J Pathol 85 774–812.

Russell PS, and Cosimi AB. 1979. Transplantation. N Engl J Med 301 470–479.

17

Type I Hypersensitivity:
Allergies and Anaphylaxis

Type I hypersensitivities are inflammatory reactions mediated by certain classes of immunoglobulins, especially IgE, bound to mast cells and basophils; the reactions result from the release of pharmacologically active factors (Fig. 17–1).

Of all the adverse consequences of the immune response, the most dramatic are those of type I hypersensitivity. These reactions are variously termed immediate hypersensitivity, allergies or anaphylaxis. Because they cause so much discomfort and distress, any possible beneficial effects are not immediately obvious; nevertheless, certain features of this type of hypersensitivity do give us indications of a beneficial positive biological function. First, it is probable that the localized acute inflammatory response that occurs in this condition plays a significant role in antigen elimination. Second, this type of hypersensitivity is commonly associated with helminth antigens and appears to play a role in resistance to these parasites (Chapter 15). Third, statistical evidence suggests that individuals who suffer from allergies are less likely than unaffected people to die from cancer. The mechanism and significance of this phenomenon are unknown.

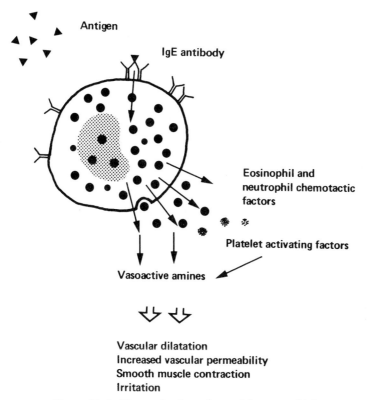

Figure 17–1 The mechanism of type I hypersensitivity.

TERMINOLOGY

Before the antibodies that mediate type I hypersensitivity were characterized as IgE, they were known as *reagins* or *reaginic antibodies*. Because they bind to cells, they are also *cytotropic* or *cytophilic*. If they can bind only to cells of their own species, they are said to be *homocytotropic*. IgE is not, strictly speaking, homocytotropic, since it may bind to cells of several species of animals. The type of reaction that IgE mediates is an *immediate hypersensitivity*, so called because of its prompt occurrence following exposure to antigen. This type of hypersensitivity reaction is also known as *allergy*. Antigens that stimulate allergies may be termed *allergens*. However, many clinicians and laymen use the term allergy to describe any unpleasant reaction of immunological or quasi-immunological origin. If an immediate hypersensitivity reaction is systemic and severe, it is termed *anaphylaxis*. In this chapter, the term type I hypersensitivity is employed as much as possible, since it has an etiologic connotation that many of the other terms now lack.

INDUCTION OF TYPE I HYPERSENSITIVITY

Type I hypersensitivity is mediated by antibodies of the IgE class. The conditions under which IgE rather than IgG antibodies are produced are not entirely clear. The antigens that induce IgE antibodies have no discernible unique biochemical features. Certain antigens are, however, uniquely potent stimulators of this type of response. These include proteins of pollen grains, some helminth antigens and some proteins in insect venoms. Freund's complete adjuvant or killed *Bordetella pertussis* organisms may act to preferentially stimulate IgE production in some animals.

In many species, including dogs and humans, the capacity to respond to antigen by production of IgE antibodies is largely inherited, and some individuals therefore have a higher than normal tendency to mount an IgE response. These individuals are said to be atopic, and about 1 to 2 per cent of the dog population in North America is affected in this way. If both parents are atopic, then most of their progeny will be atopic also and will suffer from type I hypersensitivities. If only one parent is atopic, then the percentage of atopic offspring varies. There also appears to be a breed disposition to atopy, so that atopic dermatitis, for instance, is most commonly observed in terriers (Cairn, West Highland white, Scottish), Dalmatians and Irish setters. It is rarely seen in cocker spaniels.

IMMUNOGLOBULIN E

IgE is a heat-labile immunoglobulin of conventional four-chain structure. Because of the addition of an extra constant homology region near the hinge, its heavy chain contains four C_H regions and one V_H region, and IgE thus has a molecular weight of 196,000 daltons, which is somewhat greater than that of IgG. IgE is produced by plasma cells, most of which are located near epithelial surfaces. It is found in serum in exquisitely small quantities (9 to 700 μg/ml in dogs). Much is normally bound through its C_H3 and C_H4 regions to mast cells and basophils. The precise level in serum appears to be related to the parasite burden of the animal.

Some IgG subclasses may also bind to mast cells and participate in type I hypersensitivity reactions. However, the affinity of these IgG subclasses for mast cell receptors is considerably lower than that of IgE, and they may be considered to be of much less practical importance.

MAST CELLS AND BASOPHILS

Mast cells are large, round cells (15 to 20 μm diameter) distributed throughout the body in connective tissue (Figs. 17–2 and 17–3). Their most characteristic feature is cytoplasm packed with large granules that stain metachromatically with dyes such as toluidine blue. The granules usually mask the relatively large, bean-shaped nucleus.

Mast cells, at least in rodents and humans, fall into two populations differentiated on the bases of their origins and functions. Ordinary connective-tissue mast cells arise from precursors in fetal liver and bone marrow. Their numbers increase slowly in tissues, although irritation may cause local proliferation. In contrast, the mast cells found in the epithelial mucosa are apparently derived from a thymus-cell precursor. They differ from connective tissue mast cells in several respects. For example, they tend to have fewer granules and these granules stain differently. It has been suggested that these submucosal mast cells respond specifically to nematode antigens. Mast cells carry receptors for the Fc region of IgE and hence are able to bind free IgE molecules.

No visible change occurs in the structure of mast cells as a result of their combination with IgE. However, when cell-bound IgE combines with an antigen that

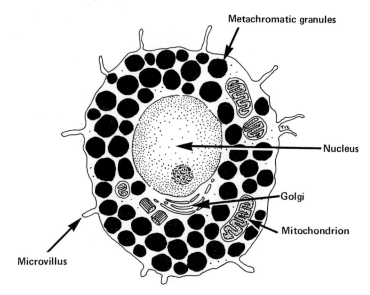

Figure 17–2 A schematic diagram showing the structure of a mast cell.

cross-links two IgE molecules, the mast cell responds dramatically by abruptly exposing its granules to extracellular fluid. One mechanism by which this occurs is by the
expulsion of granules from the interior of the cell into the extracellular environment.
Alternatively, channels may open in the cell cytoplasm, permitting the extracellular
fluid to penetrate to the granules. These mast cell responses are extremely rapid,
occurring only a few seconds after immune complex formation on the cell surface
(Fig. 17–4). Degranulated mast cells do not die, but they are difficult to identify

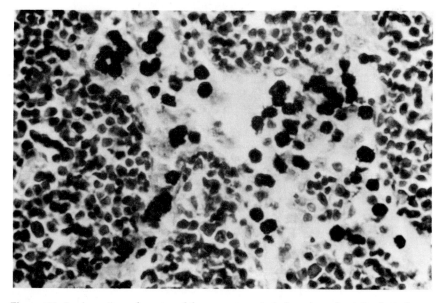

Figure 17–3 A section of a normal human mesenteric lymph node stained to show mast
cells. The mast cells stain intensely because of the presence of their cytoplasmic granules.

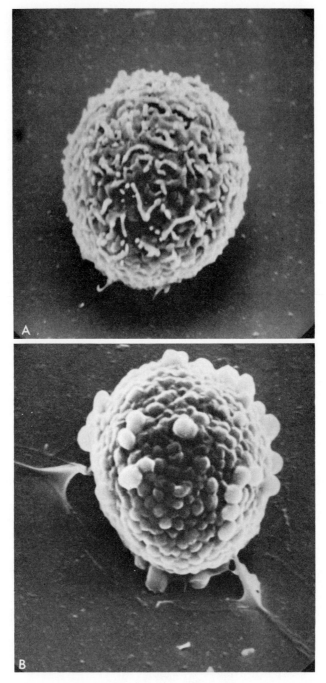

Figure 17–4 Scanning electron micrographs of a normal rat mast cell (*A*) and a sensitized mast cell fixed five seconds after exposure to antigen (*B*).

because of an absence of characteristic morphological features. It is thought that some are identical to the so-called globule leukocytes seen in the intestinal wall of animals after elimination of helminth infections as a result of the process of "self-cure" (Chapter 15).

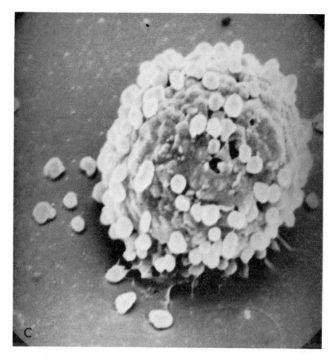

Figure 17−4 *Continued*   A sensitized mast cell fixed 60 seconds after exposure to antigen (C). × 3000. (From Tizard IR, and Holmes WL. 1974. Int Arch Allergy Appl Immunol *46* 867–879. Used with permission from the publisher, S. Karger, Basel.)

Strictly speaking, peripheral blood basophils should not be considered simply circulating mast cells. They may, however, be passively sensitized with IgE, and they will respond to antigen in a manner apparently similar to that of mast cells.

Agents that initiate mast cell degranulation by nonimmunological mechanisms include drugs such as the antibiotic polymyxin B, morphine, and tubocurarine and the basic polypeptides C3a and C5a released in the complement cascade. These peptides are known as anaphylatoxins.

BIOLOGICALLY ACTIVE AGENTS RELEASED IN TYPE I HYPERSENSITIVITY

On exposure to extracellular fluid, mast cell granules release their content of vasoactive agents into the surrounding tissue fluid. In addition, the combination of IgE with antigen on the surface of these cells provokes the formation of other vasoactive substances. It is these agents, both those released preformed from granules and those newly synthesized, that generate the characteristic lesions of type I hypersensitivity (Table 17–1).

Histamine.   Histamine is an amine formed by the decarboxylation of histidine and stored, preformed, within the mast cell granules. Once these granules are exposed to the extracellular fluid, histamine is released through exchange with sodium ions. Histamine possesses a number of biological activities that particularly affect blood vessels and smooth muscle. For example, it dilates most micro blood vessels (e.g., capillaries and venules) but contracts certain specific vessels, including the pulmonary

Table 17–1 MAJOR MEDIATORS INVOLVED IN TYPE I HYPERSENSITIVITY

MEDIATOR	*MAJOR ACTIONS*
PREFORMED MEDIATORS	
Histamine	Smooth muscle contraction, increased vascular permeability, pruritis, increased exocrine secretion
Serotonin	Vasospasm and smooth muscle contraction
ECF-A	Eosinophil chemotaxis
Platelet activating factor	Platelet aggregation and secretion
NCF-A	Neutrophil chemotaxis
MEDIATORS GENERATED DE NOVO	
Prostaglandins	Very complex; influence vascular and smooth muscle tone, platelet aggregation and immune reactivity
Leukotrienes C and D	Characteristic smooth muscle contraction and increased vascular permeability
Leukotriene B	Neutrophil and eosinophil chemotaxis
Bradykinin	Smooth muscle contraction and increased vascular permeability
Serotonin	Smooth muscle contraction and vasospasm

vessels of herbivores and the hepatic veins of dogs. It also causes increased permeability of microvessels so that intradermal inoculation of histamine gives a "wheal and flare" reaction. Histamine causes smooth muscle contraction, particularly of the bronchi, gastrointestinal tract, uterus and bladder. Finally, it is a potent stimulator of exocrine secretions, stimulating bronchial mucus secretion, lacrimation and salivation. The importance of this latter function is seen in dogs with mast cell tumors. These animals occasionally present with gastric ulcers due to the histamine-mediated stimulation of gastric secretion.

In small quantities, histamine is chemotactic for eosinophils, which, possessing large quantities of histaminases, can readily break it down. Other tissue enzymes that can inactivate histamine include diamine oxidase (histaminase); coenzyme A, which can acetylate histamine; and imidazole N-methyl transferase, which can methylate it.

Serotonin (5-Hydroxytryptamine). Serotonin, a derivative of the amino acid tryptophan, is released from the mast cells of some species of rodents and the large domestic herbivores. It also exists preformed in platelets, in central nervous tissue and in the argentophil cells of the intestine. It is released from platelets through the activity of a number of factors including the platelet activating factors (see page 265). Serotonin stimulates the heart and causes vasoconstriction that results in a rise in blood pressure (a fall in cattle). It appears to have little effect on vascular permeability, except in rats and in mice in which serotonin readily induces wheal and flare reactions.

Factors Derived from Arachidonic Acid. Arachidonic acid, an unsaturated long-chain fatty acid, is metabolized by two alternative pathways. Under the influence of enzymes known as lipoxygenases, it yields leukotrienes. Under the influence of enzymes known as cyclooxygenases, it yields prostaglandins and thromboxanes.

LEUKOTRIENES. Four major groups of leukotrienes are synthesized by mast cells upon stimulation by antigen. Leukotriene B acts to stimulate neutrophil and eosinophil chemotaxis; indeed, it is the most potent chemotactic factor known. It also stimulates random motility of these cells and enhances their expression of C3b receptors. The other major leukotrienes, leukotrienes C, D and E collectively, may represent what was formerly known as slow-reacting substance of anaphylaxis (SRS-A) — that is, they provoke a slow contraction of smooth muscle. Leukotrienes C and D are up to 20,000 times more potent than histamine in contracting the smooth muscle of bronchioles in certain species. They also increase vascular permeability.

PROSTAGLANDINS.   Prostaglandins are a family of complex lipids with a wide range of activities. Some prostaglandins such as $PGF_{2\alpha}$ and thromboxane (TxA_2) cause smooth muscle to contract and provoke vasoconstriction. Other prostaglandins such as PGE_1, PGE_2 and prostacyclin (PGI_2) cause smooth muscle relaxation and vasodilation. PGI_2, PGE_1, and $PGF_2\alpha$ inhibit platelet aggregation, and PGE_2 and TxA_2 promote platelet aggregation and the release of platelet mediators such as serotonin. $PGF_{2\alpha}$ promotes mast cell–mediator release. As pointed out earlier, the E prostaglandins are potently immunosuppressive.

Since each target tissue may be able to synthesize many different prostaglandins, the ultimate response to prostaglandins represents the sum of a large number of interactions.

Eosinophil Chemotactic Factor of Anaphylaxis (ECF-A).   There are at least two ECF-As, both acidic tetrapeptides with molecular weights of less than 1000 daltons which exist preformed within mast cells. When released they act as powerful chemotactic agents for eosinophils. Not only do they attract eosinophils to the site of mast cell degranulation; they subsequently desensitize them so that the eosinophils can move away. These factors account, at least in part, for the eosinophilia so characteristic of type I hypersensitivity reactions, including helminth infestations.

Platelet Activating Factor.   A phospholipid closely related to lecithin, platelet activating factor makes platelets aggregate and release their contents, especially serotonin, and also promotes platelet prostaglandin synthesis. Platelet activating factor is inactivated by the enzyme phospholipase D found in eosinophils.

Other Biologically Active Factors.   Mast cell granules appear to be modified lysosomes. Upon phagocytosis of particles by mast cells, the granules form phagolysosomes. It is, therefore, not surprising that they contain hydrolytic enzymes such as kallikreins and enzymes of the respiratory burst such as superoxide dismutase. Other factors found in the granules include a neutrophil chemotactic factor (NCF-A) and a neutrophil immobilization factor. The latter factor, as its name suggests, stops the movement of neutrophils after they have been attracted to the area by the chemotactic factor. It does not interfere with the phagocytic activities of the cells.

Heparin is found in mast cell granules and probably is largely responsible for their metachromatic staining properties. It is released from the granules independently of histamine. Because of the anticoagulant properties of heparin, blood from animals suffering from anaphylaxis and from dogs with mast cell tumors may fail to coagulate.

Kinins are basic polypeptides, the most important of which is bradykinin. They are derived from kininogens (α-globulins) by the activity of the proteolytic enzymes called kallikreins (kininogenases). Kallikreins may be produced directly from mast cells and basophils or indirectly from activated platelets. They may also be produced in plasma by the action of Hageman factor (factor XII) on an inert prekallikrein (kallikreinogen). Kinins increase vascular permeability and stimulate smooth muscle contraction.

CONTROL OF TYPE I HYPERSENSITIVITY

Regulation of the IgE Response. It is well recognized, at least in humans, that not all individuals are equally able to mount an IgE response. The reasons for this are primarily genetic. The ability to mount an IgE response is probably regulated by several different immune response genes. From studies of the immune system of atopic individuals, it is clear that some individuals have a deficiency of suppressor cells, as a result of which their IgE-producing B cells can function at a higher rate than normal. It has proved possible to remedy this deficiency of suppressor cells by the use of "desensitizing" injections of antigen. The original rationale for administering antigen to atopic individuals was to stimulate the production of IgG antibodies. It was anticipated that these would compete with IgE for antigen and hence prevent the antigen from reaching the mast cells. However, it is now believed that desensitizing injections may promote suppressor cell activity and in some way directly reduce the sensitivity of mast cells to antigen.

In desensitization therapy, antigen is administered in a form designed to stimulate the immune response while reducing, as far as possible, the risks of anaphylactic shock. Thus, antigen may be administered in a suspension with alum or in a water-in-oil emulsion to form a depot. It is also possible to use allergoids, which are formaldehyde-treated allergens. The first injections contain only a very small quantity of allergen. Over a number of weeks, the dosage is gradually increased. If an animal's allergy is of the seasonal type, the course of injections should be timed to reach completion just prior to the anticipated antigen exposure.

A newer approach to the selective stimulation of suppressor cells in atopic individuals is to modify the allergen by attaching it to a nonimmunogenic polymer such as polyethylene glycol. This molecule can, when bound to an allergen, promote specific suppression of the IgE response.

Regulation of Mast Cell Degranulation. The release of vasoactive agents from mast cells is modulated by intracellular cyclic nucleotides. Elevation of cyclic AMP or depression of cyclic GMP inhibits mast cell degranulation, whereas depression of cyclic AMP or elevation of cyclic GMP enhances degranulation. The precise relationship between these two compounds is complex, and the final response may depend on the cyclic AMP–to–cyclic GMP ratio.

On the surface of mast cells there are two types of receptor for adrenergic agents (adrenoceptors), named α and β. Compounds that stimulate the α receptor enhance mast cell degranulation because they depress intracellular cyclic AMP (Table 17–2). Compounds that stimulate the β receptor have the reverse effect and thus depress mast cell degranulation. Drugs that either stimulate the α receptor, such as norepinephrine and phenylephrine (propranolol), or block the β receptor therefore enhance mast cell degranulation. Drugs that stimulate the β receptor, thus raising cyclic AMP levels and inhibiting mast cell degranulation, include isoproterenol, epinephrine and salbutamol. Recently, it has become clear that β-receptor impairment can also contribute to the atopic state. The effects of β-receptor activation can be inhibited by certain respiratory tract pathogens such as *B. pertussis* or *Hemophilus influenzae* or by autoantibodies directed against the β receptor. Because of this impairment, affected individuals are more susceptible to hypersensitivity conditions such as chronic asthma.

Regulation of the Response to Mast Cell–Derived Mediators. The α and β adrenoceptors are found not only on mast cells but also on secretory and smooth muscle cells throughout the body. Stimulators of α adrenoceptors mediate vaso-

Table 17–2   EFFECTS OF STIMULATING α AND β ADRENOCEPTORS

SYSTEM	STIMULATION OF α ADRENOCEPTOR	STIMULATION OF β ADRENOCEPTOR
Cyclic nucleotides	Lowers cAMP Raises cGMP	Raises cAMP Lowers cGMP
Mast cell degranulation	Enhances	Depresses
Smooth muscle	Contracts	Relaxes
Blood vessels	Constricts	Dilates

constriction (Table 17–2). Consequently, α adrenergic agents may be of use in the treatment of anaphylaxis, reducing edema and raising blood pressure. Stimulators of β adrenoceptors mediate smooth muscle relaxation and may therefore be useful in modulating the severity of smooth muscle contraction.

Pure α and β stimulants are of only limited use in the treatment of anaphylaxis because each alone is insufficient to counteract all the effects of mast cell–derived factors. Epinephrine, on the other hand, has both α and β adrenergic activity and therefore, in addition to causing vasoconstriction in skin and viscera, its β effects cause smooth muscle to relax. This combination of effects is well suited to combat the

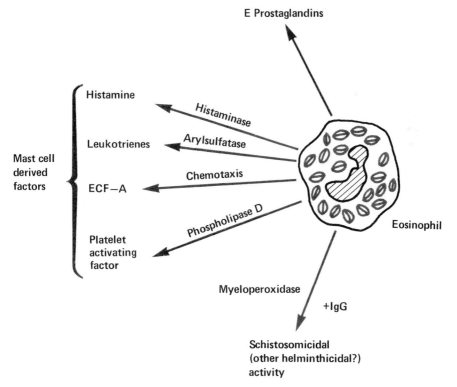

Figure 17–5   The functions of eosinophils. These cells are attracted to the sites of mast cell degranulation by ECF-A. Their enzymes neutralize many of the factors released by mast cells while the E prostaglandins further inhibit mast cell degranulation through stimulation of adenyl cyclase and elevation of cyclic AMP.

vasodilation and smooth muscle contraction produced by histamine. Ideally, epinephrine (1:1000) solution should be available whenever potential allergens are administered to animals.

The Destruction of Released Mediators.   Eosinophils are attracted to the site of mast cell degranulation by ECF-A, leukotriene B and histamine and its breakdown products. Once they have arrived, most if not all of the various factors released by mast cells are destroyed by eosinophil enzymes (Fig. 17–5). Eosinophils contain histaminases, which break down histamine; arylsulfatase B, which destroys the leukotrienes; and phospholipase D, which breaks down platelet activating factor. In addition, eosinophils promote the production of prostaglandin E_1, which raises the mast cell cyclic AMP levels, thus inhibiting degranulation.

It is clear, therefore, that one function of eosinophils is to modulate the inflammatory effects of mast cell degranulation by destroying the vasoactive factors released by these cells.

MEASUREMENT OF TYPE I HYPERSENSITIVITY

The term hypersensitivity is used to denote a severe reaction that occurs in response to normally harmless material. For example, normal animals do not react to antigens injected intradermally. If, however, IgE antibodies are produced to the injected antigen and if these antibodies bind to skin mast cells, then intradermal inoculation of antigen, even in very dilute solution, will provoke a local hypersensitivity reaction. Because of the nature of the mast cell response, vasoactive agents are released within minutes to produce erythema as a result of capillary dilatation, and circumscribed edema (a wheal) due to increased vascular permeability. The reaction may also involve an erythematous flare due to arteriolar dilatation brought about by a local nerve reflex. This type of response to antigen reaches maximal intensity within 30 minutes and tends to fade and disappear within a few hours.

Two other skin testing techniques may be used to detect reaginic antibodies to specific antigens. One, named the Prausnitz-Küstner or P-K test, is a skin test in which serum from a test animal is injected intradermally into a normal animal. After a period of 24 to 48 hours, which allows antibodies to fix to skin mast cells, the antigen is injected at the same site. In a positive reaction, a wheal and flare reaction occurs within one to two minutes. Alternatively, several separate injections of serum at different dilutions may be used and the antigen solution then administered intravenously. If positive, each injection site will show an immediate inflammatory response. This test is known as the passive cutaneous anaphylaxis (PCA) test. In the PCA test it is sometimes difficult to detect very mild skin reactions. One way to render them more visible is to inject the test animal intravenously with a dye such as Evans blue. This normally binds to serum albumin and will not, therefore, leave the blood stream. In areas of the skin where vascular permeability is increased, such as in an acute inflammatory reaction, the dye-labeled albumin may enter tissue spaces and form a striking blue patch. The size of this patch may be used as a measure of the intensity of the inflammatory reaction (Fig. 17–6).

An *in vitro* experimental test of immediate hypersensitivity is the Schultz-Dale technique. In this test, a strip of smooth muscle such as intestine is removed from a sensitized animal, washed and suspended in physiological saline. If this tissue is then exposed to specific antigen, degranulation of the mast cells within it will cause it to

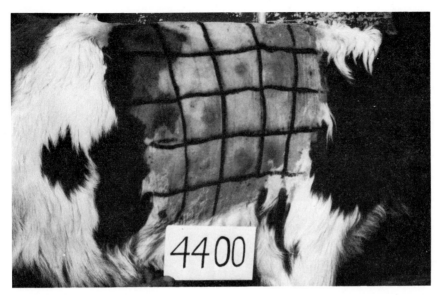

Figure 17−6   Passive cutaneous anaphylaxis (PCA) reactions in a calf. A number of different sera were tested for PCA activity in the flank of a normal calf. (Courtesy of Dr. P. Eyre.)

contract violently. This test may be modified by preincubating the smooth muscle from a normal animal in serum derived from a sensitized one. This passively sensitized muscle may then also contract in response to exposure to specific antigen. Other smooth muscle–containing tissues, such as the uterus, bronchus or trachea and certain blood vessels, may also be employed to demonstrate Schultz-Dale reactions.

CLINICAL MANIFESTATIONS OF TYPE I HYPERSENSITIVITY

All the clinical signs of type I hypersensitivity relate to the release of vasoactive substances from mast cells and basophils. The severity and location of the conditions depend on the number and location of the mast cells stimulated, and this, in turn, is dependent on the amount of antigen and its route of administration. In its most extreme form, antigen administered rapidly and intravenously will cause generalized mast cell degranulation. If the rate of release of vasoactive agents in this situation is in excess of the body's capacity to respond to the rapid changes in its vascular system, the animal will suffer from anaphylactic shock and may die. If, on the other hand, antigen is administered either locally in small quantities or slowly, then the clinical signs of hypersensitivity will be very much less severe, since the animal will have had an opportunity to compensate for the vascular changes provoked by the mast cell–derived factors.

Acute Systemic Anaphylaxis (Table 17–3).   In cattle, acute anaphylaxis is characterized by profound systemic hypotension and pulmonary hypertension. The major organ involved in the reaction is the lung. The pulmonary hypertension occurs as a result of constriction of the pulmonary vein and results in severe dyspnea with pulmonary edema. Other events that take place include contraction of the smooth muscle of the bladder and intestine, resulting in urination, defecation and bloating. It

Table 17−3 COMPARISON OF ANAPHYLAXIS IN VARIOUS SPECIES*

SPECIES	MAIN SHOCK ORGAN	SYMPTOMS	PATHOLOGY	MAJOR PHARMA-COLOGICAL MEDIATORS
Cattle and sheep	Respiratory tract	Cough, dyspnea, collapse	Lung edema, emphysema, hemorrage	Leukotrienes, kinins, histamine
Horse	Respiratory tract, intestine	Cough, dyspnea, diarrhea	Emphysema, intestinal hemmorrhage	Histamine, serotonin, kinins
Swine	Respiratory tract, intestine	Cyanosis, itch, staggering, collapse	Systemic hypotension	Histamine (uncertain)
Cat	Respiratory tract, intestine	Itch, vomiting, dyspnea, diarrhea	Lung edema, intestinal edema	Histamine, leukotrienes
Dog	Hepatic veins	Vomiting, diarrhea, dyspnea, collapse	Hepatic engorgement, visceral hemorrhage	Histamine, leukotrienes
Chicken	Respiratory tract	Dyspnea, convulsions, collapse	Lung edema	Histamine, serotonin, leukotrienes
Man	Respiratory tract	Urticaria, dyspnea	Lung edema, emphysema	Histamine, leukotrienes

*Modified from Eyre P. 1972. The biochemical pharmacology of allergic reactions in domestic animals. Vet Rev 23 3–16. Used with permission.

seems likely that the main mediators of anaphylaxis in the bovine are serotonin, kinins and SRS-A (leukotrienes?). Histamine is of much lesser importance. Dopamine also functions in bovine anaphylaxis by enhancing histamine and SRS-A release from the lung, thus exerting a form of positive feedback. Cattle are also of interest since, in contrast to the other species, drugs that stimulate the β adrenoceptor, such as isoproterenol, potentiate histamine release from leukocytes, whereas drugs that stimulate the α receptor, such as norepinephrine, inhibit histamine release. In addition, epinephrine potentiates histamine release in the bovine. The significance of these anomalous effects is unclear.

In sheep, too, pulmonary signs predominate in acute anaphylaxis as a result of constriction of the bronchi and pulmonary vessels. Smooth muscle contraction also occurs in the bladder and intestine with predictable results. The major mediators of type I hypersensitivity in sheep are histamine, serotonin, leukotrienes and kinins.

The major shock organs of horses are the lungs and the intestine. Bronchial and bronchiolar constriction in anaphylaxis leads to coughing, dyspnea and eventually apnea. On necropsy, severe pulmonary emphysema and peribronchiolar edema are commonly seen. In addition to the lung lesions, edematous hemorrhagic enterocolitis may occur, resulting in severe diarrhea. Pathologically, the intestinal lesion resembles that of colitis X, a disease probably due to salmonellosis. It is tempting to suggest that an anaphylactic reaction may play a role in colitis X. The major mediators in horses are probably histamine and serotonin.

In pigs, acute systemic anaphylaxis is largely the result of systemic and pulmonary hypertension leading to dyspnea and death. In some pigs the intestine shows signs of involvement, whereas in others no gross lesions are observed. The most significant mediator so far identified in this species is histamine.

Dogs differ from the other domestic animals in that the major organ involved in acute anaphylaxis is not the lung but the liver, specifically the hepatic veins. Clinically, acute anaphylaxis in the dog is less spectacular, the animal showing initial excitement followed by vomiting, defecation and urination. As the reaction progresses, the dog collapses with muscular weakness and depressed respiration, becomes comatose, convulses and dies within an hour. On necropsy, the liver and intestine are massively engorged, perhaps holding up to 60 per cent of the animal's total blood volume. All these signs are due to occlusion of the hepatic vein, which results in portal hypertension and visceral pooling. The mechanism of this is probably a combination of smooth muscle contraction in the vessel walls and of occlusion secondary to hepatic swelling.

In cats, the shock organ is the lung. Cats undergoing anaphylaxis will show vigorous scratching around the face and head as histamine is released into the skin, followed by dyspnea, salivation, vomiting, incoordination and collapse. On necropsy, there is bronchoconstriction, emphysema, pulmonary hemorrhage and edema. The relative importance of the major pharmacological mediators in this species is not known.

The signs of acute anaphylaxis in chickens are similar to those in mammals. They show increased salivation, defecation, ruffling of feathers, dyspnea, convulsions, cyanosis, collapse and death. The major target organ is probably the lung, and death is due to pulmonary arterial hypotension, right heart dilatation and cardiac arrest. The pharmacological agents involved include histamine, serotonin, the kinins and the leukotrienes.

Specific Allergic Conditions.   Although acute systemic anaphylaxis is the most dramatic of the type I hypersensitivity reactions, it is more common to observe local allergic reactions, the sites of which are referable to the route of administration of antigens. For example, inhaled antigens (allergens) provoke an initial response in the upper respiratory tract, trachea and bronchi, resulting in fluid exudation from the nasal mucosa (hay fever) and tracheobronchial constriction (asthma). Aerosolized antigen will also contact the eyes and provoke conjunctivitis and intense lacrimation. Ingested antigens may provoke diarrhea and colic as the intestinal smooth muscle contracts violently, and if sufficiently severe the resulting diarrhea may be hemorrhagic. Antigen reaching the skin will cause a local hypersensitivity reaction similar to that described following a skin test. The reaction is erythematous and edematous and is said to be of an urticarial type (*urtica* is Latin for "stinging nettle"). Urticarial lesions are extremely irritating because of the histamine released; consequently, the true nature of the lesion may be masked by self-inflicted trauma.

Milk Allergy.   Jersey cattle may become allergic to the α casein of their own milk. Normally, this material is synthesized in the udder, and, provided that the animals are milked regularly, nothing untoward occurs. If the milking is delayed, however, then the rising intramammary pressure forces milk proteins back into the blood stream. In allergic cattle, the result of this may vary from mild discomfort with urticarial skin lesions to acute systemic anaphylaxis and death. The condition can be readily treated by prompt milking, although some seriously affected animals may have to go for several lactations without drying off because of the severe reactions that occur on cessation of milking.

ALLERGIES TO FOODS.   It has been claimed that up to 30 per cent of cases of allergic dermatitis in dogs may be due to food allergies and that responses to ingested allergens may account for 1 per cent of cutaneous disease in dogs and cats. The clinical signs of food allergies are observed both in the digestive tract and on the skin.

The intestinal reaction may be mild, perhaps showing only as an irregularity in the consistency of the feces, or it may be severe, with vomiting, cramps, and violent, sometimes hemorrhagic diarrhea occurring soon after feeding. The skin reactions are usually urticarial and erythematous and may involve the feet, eyes, ears, axillae or perianal area. The lesion itself is commonly masked by self-inflicted trauma. In chronic cases the skin may be hyperpigmented, lichenified and secondarily infected. The foods involved vary but are usually protein-rich, e.g., cow's milk, wheat meal, fish, meat or eggs. In pigs, fishmeal and alfalfa have been incriminated, and in horses, wild oats, white clover and alfalfa have been recognized as allergens. Diagnosis of suspected food allergies is made by removing all potential allergens and then testing using a trial diet. Mutton and brown rice are said to be hypoallergenic for dogs, and a diet of this may be supplemented by various foods until the allergen is identified by a recurrence of clinical signs.

ALLERGIES TO INHALED ANTIGENS.   The most significant allergies of human beings are hay fever and asthma, which are caused by exposure to antigenic particles suspended in inhaled air. Hay fever is generally due to pollens, whereas asthma is etiologically complex, involving both pharmacological and psychological factors as well as allergy. It can be provoked by a number of allergens including fungal spores and mites present in house dust and may also occur as a result of food allergies.

In dogs and cats, inhalant allergy most commonly leads to an allergic dermatitis manifested primarily as pruritus. Many affected animals have a history of foot licking, face rubbing or axillary pruritus. The specific lesions vary greatly from acute erythema-edema to more chronic secondary changes including crusting, scaling hyperpigmentation and pyoderma. The major allergens implicated include molds; tree, weed and grass pollens; house dusts; animal danders; and fabrics such as kapok or wool. Most animals develop multiple sensitivities. Diagnosis is based primarily on history and identification of the offending antigens by direct skin testing.

Nasolacrimal urticaria (hay fever) is an uncommon manifestation of respiratory allergy in dogs and cats. Pollens usually provoke a rhinitis and conjunctivitis characterized by a profuse watery nasal discharge and excessive lacrimation. If the offending allergenic particles are sufficiently small, they may reach the bronchi or bronchioles (see Fig. 10–1), where the resulting local reaction can cause bronchoconstriction, wheezing and recurrent asthmalike paroxysmal dyspnea.

In Australia, a form of nasal granuloma occurs in cattle, which consists of numerous polypoid nodules, 1 to 4 mm in diameter, situated in the anterior nasal mucosa. The nodules contain large numbers of mast cells, eosinophils and plasma cells and probably arise as a result of repeated exposure to an unidentified antigen. These lesions are intensely pruritic and cause great distress to affected animals.

Chronic obstructive pulmonary disease (COPD) (as in asthma in humans or heaves in horses) may be due in part to bronchopulmonary hypersensitivity to atmospheric allergens. Horses suffering from COPD may show positive skin reactions to many fungal extracts (such as *Aspergillus* spp., *Alternaria* spp. and *Cladosporium* spp.) and always have large numbers of eosinophils and high titers of antibody to equine influenza in their bronchial secretions. The significance of the latter finding is not yet clear. There is no correlation between the severity of COPD and circulating levels of mast cell–derived mediators. Removal of clinically affected horses to air-conditioned stalls permits improvement of the disease, but this is reversed if the horses are returned to dusty stables.

ALLERGIES TO VACCINES AND DRUGS.   The induction of an IgE response is a potential hazard that may arise from the administration of any antigen, including vaccines, and this factor must be considered in undertaking any vaccination process. In practice, severe problems have been associated with the use of killed foot-and-mouth disease vaccines, rabies vaccines and contagious bovine pleuropneumonia vaccines in cattle.

It is not uncommon for an IgE response to occur following administration of drugs. Most drug molecules are too small to be antigenic, but many can bind to host proteins and then act in haptenic fashion. Penicillin allergy, for example, may be produced in animals either through therapeutic exposure or by ingestion of penicillin-contaminated milk. The penicillin molecule is degraded *in vivo* to a number of compounds, the most important of which contains a penicilloyl active determinant. This penicilloyl group can bind to proteins and stimulate the immune system (see Fig. 3–2). In animals sensitized in this way, parenteral administration of penicillin may lead to acute systemic anaphylaxis or milder forms of allergy, whereas feeding of penicillin-contaminated milk to these animals can lead to severe diarrhea.

Allergies to many other drugs and hormones have been reported in the domestic animals. Even substances contained in leather preservatives used in harnesses, in catgut sutures, or "vehicles" such as methyl cellulose or carboxymethylcellulose in vaccines may provoke local allergic responses.

ALLERGIES TO PARASITES.   The role of the IgE–mast cell–vasoactive amine system in immunity to helminths was first observed in the self-cure phenomenon (Chapter 15). In general, helminths appear to stimulate IgE responses preferentially, and helminth infestations are commonly associated with many of the signs of allergy and anaphylaxis; for example, animals with tapeworms may exhibit signs of respiratory distress or urticaria. Rupture of a hydatid cyst during surgery, or transfusion of blood from a dog infected with *Dirofilaria immitis* to a sensitized animal may provoke anaphylaxis.

Allergies are also commonly associated with the response of animals to arthropod parasites. Perhaps the most dramatic of these is the response of cattle infested with the warble fly (*Hypoderma bovis*). The pupae of this fly develop under the skin on the back of cattle after the larvae have migrated through the tissues from the site of egg deposition on the hind leg. Because the pupae are so obvious, it is tempting to remove them manually. Unfortunately, if they rupture during this process, the release of coelomic fluid into the sensitized animal may provoke an anaphylaxis-like response and even kill the animal. The precise role of anaphylaxis in this condition is unclear.

In horses and cattle, hypersensitivity to insect bites may cause an allergic dermatitis known as Queensland itch or "sweet itch." The flies involved include the midges (*Culicoides* spp.) and the black flies (*Simulium* spp.). If animals are allergic to substances in the saliva of these insects, biting results in the development of urticaria accompanied by intense itching. The itching may provoke severe self-mutilation with subsequent secondary infection that may mask the original allergic nature of the lesion.

In mange due to *Sarcoptes scabiei* in dogs and to *Octodectes cyanotis* in cats, a type I hypersensitivity may contribute to the development of the lesions. The infested dermis is infiltrated with mast cells, lymphocytes and plasma cells and an intradermal injection of mite antigen leads to an immediate wheal-and-flare response. Infested animals may also possess precipitins to mite antigens; it is therefore possible that immune complexes may also contribute to the development of the lesion.

IgE antibodies may be produced in some animals in response to bee, wasp and hornet stings so that a second sting in a sensitized animal may provoke acute systemic anaphylaxis. The response of animals to arthropod allergens is not inevitably of the immediate hypersensitivity type. Thus, the reactions to *Demodex* mites and to components of flea saliva are largely mediated by type IV hypersensitivity mechanisms (Chapter 20).

DISEASES OF POSSIBLE BUT AS YET UNPROVEN ALLERGIC ETIOLOGY.   Edema disease of pigs is a condition seen in rapidly growing weaned piglets. Many of these animals die suddenly, and on necropsy there is extensive edema of the intestinal tract and the subserous tissues, nervous tissue and the subcutis. The edema is associated with a sudden change in the dominant serotype of *E. coli* in the intestine. Although it is probable that this is primarily a toxemic disease, there is some evidence to suggest that an allergic component is also involved. It has been postulated that animals may be previously sensitized by exposure to small numbers of organisms of a given serotype. The hypothesis goes on to suggest that a sudden increase in the number of organisms of this serotype and the influx of antigens derived from these organisms into the body lead to an acute anaphylactic reaction that contributes to the development of edema and to the death of the piglets.

Laminitis is a syndrome seen in all the hoofed animals. It is etiologically complex and is associated with a wide variety of predisposing causes, but one of the factors that may play a role in some cases of laminitis is type I hypersensitivity. The condition occurs as a result of engorgement of the vascular bed of the laminae of the hoof. This engorgement, occurring in a tissue where there is no room for swelling to occur, leads to intense pain and discomfort. A condition resembling laminitis may be produced in some animals by intravenous histamine, and in affected calves blood histamine levels may be raised. However, the source of this histamine is not known. It may be derived directly from food or, alternatively, may represent a product of food allergy. In some cases, antihistamines may be of assistance in treatment.

PREVENTION AND TREATMENT OF TYPE I HYPERSENSITIVITY

In order to prevent type I hypersensitivity reactions, it is essential that the antigen be identified and removed. This may be extremely difficult and tedious. Intradermal skin testing using dilute solutions of a variety of potential antigens may be of assistance. Alternatively (or additionally) in food allergies a change of diet and the readdition of individual components on a test basis may enable the investigator to identify a specific antigen or, more commonly, a group of antigens.

When elimination of the offending allergen is not possible, as, for example, in allergies to pollens, desensitization therapy performed as described previously (see page 266) may prove effective.

Treatment of type I hypersensitivity reactions may be accomplished by means of a number of different drugs. One group comprises the sympathomimetic agents, which act as β adrenoceptor stimulants. These include epinephrine and isoprenaline. Salbutamol is a more selective β stimulant that causes bronchodilation. Sympathomimetics that act as α adrenoceptor inhibitors include methoxamine and phenylephrine. All have been used extensively in humans and are available for use in animals.

Another group of drugs widely employed in the treatment of type I hypersensitivity reactions are the specific pharmacological inhibitors. These drugs, by mimicking the structure of the active mediators, competitively block specific receptors. Thus, antihistamines such as pyrilamine, promethazine and diphenhydramine can effectively inhibit the activities of histamine. However, since histamine is but one of a large number of mast cell–derived mediators, antihistamines possess limited effectiveness in controlling hypersensitivity diseases. The tryptamine antagonist cyproheptadine can block receptors for both serotonin and histamine and may be of assistance in some situations.

Salicylates such as acetylsalicylic acid and phenylbutazone are antagonists of the leukotrienes and kinins and are widely used in veterinary medicine as anti-inflammatory agents. They may also be very useful in the treatment of acute hypersensitivities.

As an alternative to the specific pharmacological agents described above, considerable use is made of glucocorticosteroids as anti-inflammatory drugs. The corticosteroids can suppress all aspects of inflammation by stabilizing cell and lysosome membranes. Corticosteroids have a considerable palliative effect on chronic type I hypersensitivities, but it must be borne in mind that these drugs are immunosuppressive and increase an animal's susceptibility to infection.

Two other drugs that may be of assistance in the treatment of type I hypersensitivity are disodium cromoglycate, which interferes with the release of histamine and leukotrienes from mast cells, and diethylcarbamazine citrate, an anthelmintic with similar pharmacological properties.

ADDITIONAL SOURCES OF INFORMATION

Amos HE. 1976. Allergic drug reactions. *In* Turk JL (ed). Current Topics in Immunology. Edward Arnold, London.

Beaven MA. 1976. Histamine. N Engl J Med *294* 30–36, 320–325.

Black L. 1979. Hypersensitivity in cattle. Part I: Mechanisms of causation. Part II: Clinical reactions. Part III (with JF Burka) The mediators of anaphylaxis. Vet Bull *49* 1–9, 77–88, 303–307.

Chamberlain KW (ed). 1974. Symposium on Allergy in Small Animal Practice. Vet Clin North Am *4* 1–205.

Eyre P. 1980. Pharmacological aspects of hypersensitivity in domestic animals: a review. Vet Res Comm *4* 83–98.

Eyre P, and Burka JF. 1978. Hypersensitivity in cattle and sheep: a pharmacological review. J Vet Pharmacol Therapeut *1* 97–109.

Eyre P, and Lewis AJ. 1973. Acute systemic anaphylaxis in the horse. Br J Pharmacol *48* 426–437.

Jarrett EE, MacKenzie S, and Bennich H. 1980. Parasite-induced "nonspecific" IgE does not protect against allergic reactions. Nature *283* 302–303.

Katz DH. 1980. Recent studies on the regulation of IgE antibody synthesis in experimental animals and man. Immunology *41* 1–24.

Kay AB. 1979. The role of the eosinophil. J Allergy Clin Immunol *64* 90–104.

Kuehl FA, and Egan RW. 1980. Prostaglandins, arachidonic acid and inflammation. Science *210* 978–984.

Nesbitt GH. 1978. Canine allergic inhalant dermatitis: a review of 230 cases. JAVMA *172* 55–60.

Schatz M, Patterson R, and Fink J. 1979. Immunologic lung disease. N Engl J Med *300* 1310–1320.

Scott DW. 1978. Immunologic skin disorders in the dog and cat. Vet Clin North Am (Small Animal Practice) *8* 641–664.

Thoday KL. 1980. Canine pruritis: an approach to diagnosis. Stages III and IV: Allergy and idiopathy. J Small Anim Pract *21* 483–493.

18

Erythrocyte Antigens: The Immune Responses to Red Cells as an Example of Type II Reactions

Erythrocytes, like nucleated cells, possess characteristic cell-surface antigens. Unlike the histocompatibility antigens of nucleated cells, however, erythrocyte-surface antigens do not appear to be intimately linked with an animal's capacity to mount an immune response, although they do influence graft rejection. (Grafts incompatible in the major blood groups are rapidly rejected.)

Except in the case of the M-L antigens of sheep erythrocytes, which are associated with the membrane potassium pump, the exact functions of these antigens are unknown. Most erythrocyte-surface antigens are either carbohydrate or protein in nature and appear to be integral components of the cell membrane. Exceptions are those antigens that, although found on erythrocytes, are synthesized at other sites within the body. These antigens are found free in serum, saliva and other body fluids and are passively adsorbed onto erythrocyte surfaces. Examples of such antigens include the J antigens of cattle, the R antigens of sheep, the A and O antigens of pigs and the Tr antigens of dogs.

If normal erythrocytes are administered to an allogeneic recipient, their surface antigens will stimulate an immune response. This response results in the rapid elimination of the transfused erythrocytes through intravascular hemolysis mediated by antibody and complement and through extravascular destruction occurring as a result of opsonization and clearance by the cells of the mononuclear-phagocytic system. Cell destruction mediated by antibodies in this way is classified as a type II hypersensitivity reaction.

276

BLOOD GROUPS

The antigens found on the surface of erythrocytes are termed blood group antigens. There are many different blood group antigens on the surface of a red cell, and they vary in their antigenicity, some being of greater importance than others. The expression of blood group antigens is controlled by genes and inherited in conventional fashion. For each blood group system there exists a variable number of alternative alleles. (If alleles are invariably inherited together in groups of two or more, they are known as phenogroups.) The alleles or phenogroups control in turn a variable number of erythrocyte antigenic factors. Thus, the complexity of the erythrocyte blood group systems may vary greatly, ranging from simple ones like the L or N systems of cattle, which consist of two alleles controlling a single alloantigen system, to the highly complex B system. This system, also found in cattle, contains several hundred alleles or phenogroups that, together with the other cattle blood groups, may yield many billions of unique blood group combinations.

In addition to possessing blood group antigens on their cells, animals may also possess serum antibodies directed against foreign blood group factors. For example, J-negative cattle commonly carry antibodies to the J factor in their serum, while A-negative pigs can possess anti-A antibodies. These "natural isoantibodies" are thought to be derived not from prior contact with foreign red cells but as a consequence of exposure to similar or identical antigenic determinants (heterophile antigens) that commonly occur in nature. Many blood group antigens, for example, appear to be common structural components of a wide range of organisms including plants, bacteria, protozoa and helminths. The presence of these natural isoantibodies is not, however, a uniform phenomenon, and not all blood group factors are accompanied by the production of natural isoantibodies to their alternative alleles.

BLOOD TRANSFUSION AND CONSEQUENCES OF INCOMPATIBLE TRANSFUSIONS

Red cells can be readily transfused from one animal to another. If the donor erythrocytes carry antigens identical to those found on the recipient's erythrocytes, no immune response will result. If, however, the recipient possesses natural isoantibodies to antigens on donor erythrocytes, they will be subject to immediate attack. Natural isoantibodies are usually (but not always) of the IgM class. When these antibodies combine with foreign erythrocyte antigens, they may cause agglutination, immune hemolysis, opsonization and phagocytosis of the transfused cells. In the absence of naturally occurring antibodies, allogeneic erythrocytes stimulate an immune response in the recipient. The transfused cells then circulate for a period of time before antibody production takes place and immune elimination occurs. A second transfusion with identical allogeneic cells results in their immediate destruction.

Although the body is able to eliminate small numbers of effete red cells on a continuing basis, the rapid destruction of large numbers of foreign red cells can lead to the development of severe pathological reactions. The signs of this destructive process are, in general, referable to massive hemolysis. They include tremors, paresis and convulsions, disseminated intravascular coagulation, fever and hemoglobinuria. In some animals dyspnea, coughing and diarrhea may also be observed. Treatment of these transfusion reactions consists of stopping the transfusion and maintaining urine flow with a diuretic, since accumulation of hemoglobin within the kidney may result in renal tubular destruction. Recovery occurs following elimination of all the foreign erythrocytes.

The occurrence of transfusion reactions may be prevented by prior testing of the recipient for antibodies against donor red cells. The test for compatibility is known as cross-matching and is performed by mixing recipient serum with donor erythrocytes. It is usual to obtain serum and washed erythrocytes from both donor and recipient. Donor erythrocytes are mixed with recipient serum, and recipient erythrocytes are mixed with the donor serum and then incubated at 37° C for 30 minutes. If the donor's erythrocytes are lysed, or agglutinated by recipient serum, then no transfusion should be attempted with those cells. It is occasionally found that the donor's serum may be capable of reacting with the recipient's red cells. This is not of major clinical significance, since donor antibodies given intravenously are rapidly diluted within the recipient. Nevertheless, blood giving such a reaction is best avoided.

HEMOLYTIC DISEASE OF THE NEWBORN

Female animals may become sensitized to allogeneic red cells not only through incompatible blood transfusions given for clinical reasons but also through leakage of fetal erythrocytes into the maternal blood stream via the placenta. In animals sensitized by either of these routes, antibodies to the allogeneic erythrocytes are concentrated in colostrum. On ingestion by the newborn animal these colostral antibodies are absorbed through the intestinal wall and so reach the circulation. If the absorbed antibodies are directed against antigens present on the erythrocytes of the newborn animal, then the erythrocytes will be rapidly destroyed. The hemolytic disease arising from this massive erythrocyte destruction occurs in a number of the domestic animal species as well as in humans and is known as hemolytic disease of the newborn.

BLOOD GROUPS, BLOOD TRANSFUSION AND HEMOLYTIC DISEASE IN THE DOMESTIC ANIMALS (Table 18–1)

CATTLE.   Cattle possess at least 12 blood group systems, of which 2 (termed B and J) are of the greatest importance. J antigen, as mentioned earlier, is found free in body fluids and is passively adsorbed onto erythrocytes. It is absent from the erythrocytes of newborn calves but is acquired within the first six months of life. J-positive cattle are of two types. Some possess J antigen in high concentration, which may be detected both on their erythrocytes and in serum. Other J-positive animals possess low levels of this antigen, which is only with great difficulty detected on erythrocytes. J-negative cattle, lacking the J antigen completely, may possess natural anti-J antibodies, although the level of these antibodies shows a marked seasonal variation. Because of the presence of these antibodies, transfusion of J-positive erythrocytes into J-negative recipients may result in a transfusion reaction even in the absence of known prior sensitization.

The B blood group system of cattle is one of the most complex systems known, containing more than a thousand different alleles. Because of this complexity, it is generally impossible to obtain bovine blood from a donor animal that is absolutely identical to that of the recipient. Indeed, it has been suggested that the complexity of

Table 18-1 BLOOD GROUP SYSTEMS OF THE MAJOR DOMESTIC ANIMALS

	NUMBER OF SYSTEMS RECOGNIZED	*MOST IMPORTANT SYSTEMS*	*TECHNIQUES USED IN BLOOD TYPING*
Cattle	12	B, J	Hemolysis
Sheep	8	B, R	Hemolysis, agglutination
Swine	15	A, E	Hemolysis, agglutination, antiglobulin testing
Horses	8	Q, A, C	Hemolysis, agglutination
Dogs	11	A	Hemolysis, agglutination, antiglobulin testing

the B system is such that there exist sufficient different antigenic combinations to provide a unique identifying character for each bovine in the world. Naturally, such a system provides an ideal method for the accurate identification of individual animals, and many breed societies utilize blood grouping as a check on the identity of registered animals.

Hemolytic disease of newborn calves is rare but may occur as a result of vaccinating calves against anaplasmosis or babesiosis. These vaccines consist of blood derived from infected calves. In the case of anaplasma vaccines, the blood from a large number of donor animals is pooled, freeze-dried and then mixed with adjuvant before being administered to cattle. The vaccine against babesiosis consists of relatively fresh, infected calf blood. Both vaccines result in infection and, consequently, the development of premunity (Chapter 15) in the recipient animals. They also cause the production of antierythrocyte isoantibodies directed primarily against antigens of the A and F-V systems. Cows sensitized to erythrocyte antigens by these vaccines and then mated with bulls carrying the same blood groups can transmit colostral isoantibodies to their calves, which may then develop a hemolytic disease. The clinical signs of this condition vary with the amount of colostrum ingested. Calves are usually healthy at birth but commence to show symptoms from 12 hours to five days afterward. In acute cases, death may occur within 24 hours of birth, with the animals developing respiratory distress and hemoglobinuria. On necropsy they are found to have severe pulmonary edema, splenomegaly and dark kidneys. Less severely affected animals develop anemia and jaundice and may die during the first week of life. The erythrocytes of affected calves are antiglobulin-positive and may sometimes be lysed by the addition of hemolytic complement (fresh normal rabbit serum). Death is due to disseminated intravascular coagulation (DIC) as a result of the lysed erythrocytes activating the extrinsic clotting mechanism.

SHEEP. The blood groups of sheep resemble those of cattle. The ovine equivalent of bovine B is also termed B and, like the bovine system, is relatively complex, containing more than 50 different alleles. Sheep also possess an ovine equivalent of the bovine J system, which is known as R. R antigens are found free in serum and are passively adsorbed to erythrocytes. The recessive allele of R is termed r and it too may be found free in serum. Some sheep may possess neither R nor r as a result of being homozygous for a suppressor gene i. Erythrocytes from ii sheep may acquire R or r by incubation in appropriate serum. It is probable that the i gene prevents the production of both R and r substances, and animals homozygous for r will not produce

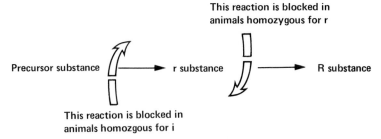

**This reaction is blocked in
animals homozygous for r**

Precursor substance ⟶ r substance ⟶ R substance

**This reaction is blocked in
animals homozgous for i**

Figure 18−1 The genes that regulate the development of R blood group antigens in sheep.

R substance (Fig. 18–1). This interaction between the i genes and the Rr system is known as an epistatic effect. A similar effect is seen in the A-O system of pigs (Example 1). Natural anti-R antibodies may be found in R-negative sheep.

Sheep erythrocytes are commonly used as a tool in immunological research, since they are a very economical source of antigen. Antibodies against these cells produced in species other than sheep tend to be directed mainly against sheep-specific antigens. Some of these species antigens are also heterophile, that is, they are found in a wide

---

Example 1. The inheritance of the A blood group system in pigs

In pigs, the expression of the A blood groups is under the control of two loci. One, the A locus, contains two alleles, A and O, of which A is dominant. The other, the S locus, also contains two alleles, S and its recessive allele s. The S locus controls the expression of the A system so that A or O blood group factors will only be expressed if the animal carries at least one S gene.

Possible genotypes are therefore

               AA   AO   OO   and SS, Ss and ss

These may be combined thus

    Animals that are   AASS ⎫
                       AASs ⎬ will all have A red cells
                       AOSS ⎪
                       AOSs ⎭
    Animals that are   OOSS ⎫ will all have O red cells
              or   OOSs ⎭
    Animals that are   AAss ⎫
                       AOss ⎬ will have neither A nor O red cells, i.e., − red cells
                       OOss ⎭

If we cross an animal of blood group O whose genotype is OOSs with an animal of blood group − whose genotype is AOss, then the offspring may be either

                    AOSs   with blood group A
                    OOSs   with blood group O
                    AOss ⎫
                    OOss ⎬ with blood group −

variety of different organisms, particularly bacteria. Consequently, "natural" anti-bodies to sheep erythrocytes are found in the serum of many normal animals. These heterophile antigens include the M antigen and the Forssman antigen. Antibodies against the M antigen are elevated in the virus infection of humans known as infectious mononucleosis. The Forssman antigen is a glycolipid common to the erythrocytes of many mammals, including horses, dogs, cats and mice, but is absent in humans, cattle, pigs, rabbits and rats.

SWINE. Of the 15 pig blood group systems that have been identified, the most important is the A–O system. A and O, like J in cattle and R in sheep, are soluble antigens found in serum and passively adsorbed onto red cells after birth. A suppressor gene (S) in the homozygous recessive state can prevent the production of the AO antigens. As a result, the amount of these antigens bound to red cells in these animals is reduced to an undetectable level (see Example 1). Natural anti-A antibodies may occur in A-negative pigs, and transfusion of A-positive blood into such an animal may cause transient collapse and hemoglobinuria.

Hemolytic disease of the newborn in piglets used to occur as a result of the use of hog cholera vaccine containing pig blood. This vaccine consisted of pooled blood from viremic pigs inactivated with the dye crystal-violet. Sensitization of sows by means of this vaccine led to the occasional occurrence of hemolytic disease of their offspring. There appeared to be a breed predisposition to this disease, which was most commonly seen in the offspring of Essex and Wessex sows. Affected piglets did not necessarily show clinical disease, although their red cells were shown to be sensitized by anti-body. Other piglets showed rapidly progressive weakness and pallor of mucous membranes preceding death, and those animals that survived longest showed hemo-globinuria and jaundice. The severity of the reaction did not appear to be directly related to the antierythrocyte antibody titer in the piglet serum. Since the withdrawal of all live hog cholera virus vaccines, the problems associated with their use have disappeared.

True isoimmunization of pregnancy has also been recorded in the pig. The isoantibodies responsible are usually directed against antigens of the E system. In addition to the development of hemolytic anemia in newborn piglets, the presence of antibodies to platelet antigens may result in the development of thrombocytopenia, reflected clinically as a neonatal purpura. Deprivation of colostrum in an attempt to prevent piglets from absorbing antierythrocyte antibodies may lead to difficulties as a result of the lack of resistance of the newborn colostrum-deprived animals to infection.

HORSES. Horses possess at least eight distinct blood group systems. Their major significance lies in the fact that hemolytic disease of the newborn foal is not uncom-mon. In mules, in which the antigenic differences between dam and sire are great, about 8 to 10 per cent of foals may be affected. In thoroughbreds the prevalence is considerably less, ranging from 0.05 to 1 per cent of foals. This is in spite of the fact that in up to 25 per cent of pregnancies the mare and the stallion are incompatible.

The mechanism of isoimmunization is unclear, but fetal erythrocytes are assumed to gain access to the maternal circulation throughout pregnancy (see Fig. 18–2). Mares have been shown to respond to fetal erythrocytes as early as day 56 post conception. The greatest leakage probably occurs during the last month of pregnancy and during parturition, as a result of breakdown of placental blood vessels. Necrotic foci are found in many equine placentas after birth.

The major sensitizing blood group antigen is Aa, followed (in decreasing order of importance) by Qa, R and S. Mares react to these antigens by making antibodies. The

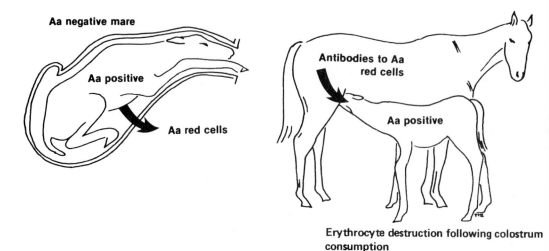

Figure 18–2 The mechanisms involved in the development of hemolytic disease in newborn foals. First, fetal erythrocytes leak into the circulation of the mother, where they provoke an immune response. Second, these antibodies are concentrated in colostrum. Third, the foal on suckling ingests and absorbs these antibodies. They then commence to destroy the foal's erythrocytes.

degree of maternal sensitization is usually relatively weak following a first pregnancy. If repeated pregnancies result in exposure to the same erythrocyte antigens, however, then her response will be stimulated considerably. Hemolytic disease is, therefore, only a problem in mares that have had several foals.

The antibodies produced by the mare do not cross the placenta; instead, they reach the foal via the colostrum. Affected foals are, therefore, born healthy but begin to sicken several hours after birth. The most potent antibodies formed are those directed against Aa, and disease due to these may develop within 12 hours. Anti-Qa produces a less severe disease of slower onset, whereas disease due to anti-R or anti-S is milder still. The earliest signs are those of weakness and depression. The mucous membranes of affected foals may be pale and may eventually show a distinct jaundice, and hemoglobinuria may be present. Some foals sicken and die so rapidly that they do not have time to develop jaundice.

Hemolytic disease is readily diagnosed by clinical signs alone. Hematological examination is of little diagnostic use but may be of assistance in assessing appropriate treatment. Definitive diagnosis requires that immunoglobulin be demonstrated on the surface of the red cells of the foal. In the case of anti-Aa or anti-Qa, addition of a source of complement (fresh normal rabbit serum) will cause rapid hemolysis. Since factors R and S are not as antigenic as Aa and Qa, antibodies to them can be detected *in vivo* only by means of a direct antiglobulin test involving an anti-equine globulin serum (Chapter 9). If hemolytic disease is anticipated, it is possible to test the serum of a pregnant mare for antibodies by means of an indirect antiglobulin test. By using erythrocytes from horses with the major sensitizing blood groups it is possible to show that the antibody titer may increase significantly in the month prior to parturition if sensitization is occurring. Testing of the foal's erythrocytes against the mare's colostrum is of limited usefulness because of the tendency of colostrum to induce marked rouleaux formation, which mimics agglutination.

The prognosis of hemolytic disease is good provided the condition is diagnosed sufficiently early and the appropriate treatment instituted rapidly. In acute cases, blood transfusion is necessary. Although exchange transfusion is efficient, it requires a donor capable of providing at least 5 liters of blood as well as a double intravenous catheter and an anesthetized foal. A much simpler technique is to transfuse washed cells from the mare. About 3 to 4 liters of blood are collected in sodium citrate and centrifuged, and the plasma is discarded. The red cells are washed once in saline and transfused slowly into the foal. The blood is usually given in divided doses about six hours apart. Milder cases of hemolytic disease may require only careful nursing.

If hemolytic disease is anticipated as a result of either a rising titer or the previous birth of a hemolytic foal, it may be prevented by stripping off the mare's colostrum and giving the foal colostrum from another mare. The foal should not be allowed to suckle its mare for 24 to 36 hours. Once suckling is permitted, the foal should only be allowed to take small quantities at first and should be observed carefully for any adverse side effects.

DOGS. In dogs, at least eleven blood group systems exist, but only one, the A system, is sufficiently strong to be of clinical significance. About 60 per cent of dogs are A-positive and the remainder are A-negative. Naturally occurring antibodies to A occur in about 10 per cent of A-negative dogs, but these are usually of low titer and not of clinical significance. Therefore, unmatched first transfusions in the dog are usually safe. If, however, an A-negative dog is sensitized by transfusion of A-positive blood, high titered anti-A may be produced. Subsequent transfusions of A-positive blood into such an animal could lead to a severe transfusion reaction. Similarly, if a bitch is sensitized in this manner, hemolytic disease may occur in her pups if she is mated to an A-positive dog. Natural hemolytic disease of the newborn in dogs is extremely rare.

CATS. In cats, only one major blood group system, with three alleles, has been reported. Hemolytic disease of the newborn can be produced artificially, but natural cases have not been recorded. It has been suggested that some cases of the fading kitten syndrome may be due to sensitization of the queen with cat tissue in panleukopenia vaccines, resulting in isoimmunization, disease and death in newborn kittens.

CHICKENS. Chickens are similar to mammals with respect to possessing blood group systems. They have at least twelve different blood group systems with multiple alleles. The erythrocyte B system is the major histocompatibility system in the chicken as well as in mammals. A hemolytic disease may be artificially produced in chicken embryos by vaccinating the hen with cock erythrocytes.

Hemolytic Disease of the Newborn in Man. In humans, hemolytic disease of the newborn is due almost entirely to isoimmunization against the antigens of the Rhesus (Rh) system. The condition is, or should be, of historical interest only, since a very simple but effective technique is available for its prevention. This is discussed here in anticipation of the development of a similar treatment for hemolytic disease in newborn animals.

The prevention of hemolytic disease in humans depends on preventing an Rh-negative mother from reacting to the Rh-positive fetal red cells that escape from the placenta into her circulation at parturition. Strong human anti-Rh globulin is obtained from male volunteers and given to mothers at risk soon after birth. It acts, just as other systems of passive immunization do, by specifically inhibiting the immune response to that antigen. Routine use of this material will therefore prevent maternal sensitization, antibody production and hemolytic disease.

DETECTION OF FREEMARTINS

In about 90 per cent of dizygotic bovine twins, anastomosis of placental blood vessels occurs *in utero*, and, as a result, the erythrocytes of these animals become indiscriminately mixed. Mixing of hematopoietic stem cells also occurs, and, consequently, each calf will carry erythrocytes of its twin's phenotype for the rest of its life. A calf carrying this cell mixture is known as a chimera (see Chapter 7). Although no adverse consequences arise from this cell mixing and subsequent tolerance, problems may occur if the calves are of different sexes. In particular, the transfusion of male hormones to the female calf *in utero* may result in dysgenesis of the female reproductive tract. Externally, these female calves appear to be quite normal; on reaching reproductive age they are found to be infertile, however, and are known as freemartins. It is obviously desirable for a farmer to be able to identify a freemartin as early as possible in life so that it does not have to be maintained for over a year before its infertility is recognized. For this reason, tests have been developed in order to identify chimeras. One way this can be done is to test the erythrocytes of an animal in order to determine whether they are homogeneous or composed of a mixture of cells of different blood groups. The technique is known as differential hemolysis. Thus, antibodies and complement acting against blood group antigens present on only a portion of the red cell population will never be able to cause more than partial hemolysis of the blood, whereas if the antigens are present on all cells, total hemolysis will result. By using a battery of different antisera for testing, it is possible to determine whether the red cell population is homogeneous or comprises two antigenically different populations. If the latter is the case, then the animal is a chimera, and if it is also a female calf born with a male twin, then it is also likely to be a freemartin.

PARENTAGE TESTING

Under some circumstances it is necessary to establish the parentage of an animal. This may be accomplished by examining the erythrocyte antigens of an animal

---

Example 2. The use of blood groups in the identification of paternity. In this case this technique was used to identify the father of a litter of pups. (Courtesy of Mr. D. Colling.)

	Erythrocyte Groups				
	A_1	A_2	J	N	O
Putative father 1	+	+	−	+	−
Putative father 2	+	+	−	−	+
Mother	−	−	+	+	−
Puppy 1	+	+	−	−	−
2	+	+	−	+	−
3*	−	−	−	+	+
4	−	−	+	+	−

*Since Puppy No. 3 possesses O antigen, it cannot be derived from Father No. 1.

(Example 2), a method based on the principle that since blood group factors are inherited, they must be present on the erythrocytes of one or both parents. If a blood group factor is present in a tested animal but absent from both its putative parents, then parentage must be reassigned. Similarly, if one parent is known to be homozygous for a particular blood group factor, then this factor must of necessity appear in the offspring. It must be recognized, however, that blood tests can only exclude parentage, never prove parentage.

TYPE II HYPERSENSITIVITY REACTIONS AS A RESULT OF IMMUNE RESPONSES TO DRUGS

Some drugs may bind firmly to cells, especially those in the blood. For example, penicillin, quinine, L-dopa, aminosalicylic acid and phenacetin may adsorb onto the surface of erythrocytes. Since these cells are then modified, they may be recognized as foreign and eliminated by an immune response, resulting in the occurrence of hemolytic anemia. Sulfonamides, phenylbutazone, aminopyrine, phenathiazine and possibly chloramphenicol may cause agranulocytosis by binding to granulocytes, and phenylbutazone, quinine, apronalide (Sedormid), chloramphenicol and sulfonamides may provoke thrombocytopenia. If the cells from animals suffering from these conditions are examined by means of a direct antiglobulin test, antibody may be demonstrated on their surface. If these antibodies are eluted, they can be shown to be directed not against the blood cells but against the offending drug.

TYPE II HYPERSENSITIVITY IN INFECTIOUS DISEASES

Just as drugs can adsorb to erythrocytes and render them immunologically foreign, so also can bacterial antigens such as the salmonella lipopolysaccharides, viruses such as equine infectious anemia virus and Aleutian disease virus, rickettsia such as the anaplasma, and protozoa such as the trypanosomes and babesia. These altered red cells, being regarded as foreign, are either lysed by antibody and hemolytic complement or phagocytosed by mononuclear phagocytes. Clinically severe anemia is, therefore, characteristic of all these infections.

ADDITIONAL SOURCES OF INFORMATION

Animal Blood Groups and Biochemical Genetics is a journal that covers the most recent developments in the areas of animal blood groups and histocompatibility antigens.
Dimmock CK, Clark IA, and Hill MWM. 1976. The experimental production of hemolytic disease of the newborn in calves. Res Vet Sci 20 244–248.
Colling DT, and Saison R. 1980. Canine blood groups. I. Description of new erythrocyte specificities. Anim Blood Groups Biochem Genet 11 1–12.
Kallfelz FA, Whitlock RH, and Schultz RD. 1978. Survival of ^{59}Fe-labeled erythrocytes in cross-transfused equine blood. Am J Vet Res 39 617–620.
Linklater K. 1977. Post-transfusion purpura in a pig. Res Vet Sci 22 257–258.
Saison R, and Bull RW. 1976. Animal blood groups and biochemical polymorphisms. Handbook of laboratory animal science (Melby, E.C. and N.H. Altman Eds.) 3 463–478. C.R.C. Press, Cleveland, Ohio.
Scott AM, and Jeffcott LB. 1978. Hemolytic disease of the newborn foal. Vet Rec 103 71–74.
Stormont C. 1977. The etiology of bovine neonatal isoerythrolysis. Bovine Pract 12 22–27.
Tucker EM. 1971. Genetic variation in the sheep red blood cell. Biol Rev 46 341–386.

19

Type III Hypersensitivity: Pathological Consequences of Immune Complex Deposition

The formation of immune complexes through the combination of antibody with antigen is the initiating step in a number of biological processes. One of the most significant of these processes is the complement cascade. When complement-fixing immune complexes are deposited in tissues, the subsequent generation of chemotactic factors leads to a local accumulation of neutrophils. These neutrophils release hydrolytic enzymes normally contained within lysosomes, and these enzymes in turn cause local tissue destruction. Lesions generated in this fashion are classified as type III or immune complex–mediated hypersensitivity reactions.

CLASSIFICATION OF TYPE III HYPERSENSITIVITY REACTIONS

The site, severity and significance of type III hypersensitivity reactions depends, as might be expected, upon the amount and site of deposition of immune complexes. In general, two major types of reaction are recognized. One is known as the Arthus reaction, named after the biologist who first described it. The Arthus reaction occurs when antigen and, hence, immune complexes are deposited locally within tissues. Arthus reactions may be induced in any tissue into which antigen can be injected.

A second form of type III hypersensitivity reaction results from the formation of large quantities of immune complexes within the circulation, as may occur when antigen is administered intravenously to a hyperimmune recipient. Complexes generated in this way tend to be deposited in the walls of blood vessels. Local activation of

286

complement then leads to neutrophil accumulation and the development of a vasculitis. Circulating immune complexes are also deposited within glomeruli, and the occurrence of a glomerulonephritis is also, therefore, characteristic of this type of hypersensitivity. If the complexes bind to the formed elements of the blood, anemia, agranulocytosis or thrombocytopenia may also occur.

It might reasonably be pointed out that the combination of antigen with antibody inevitably results in the generation of immune complexes. It seems, however, that the occurrence of clinically significant type III hypersensitivity reactions is related to the formation of very large amounts of immune complexes. For instance, several grams of antigen are needed to sensitize an animal such as a rabbit in order to produce experimental Arthus reactions or generalized immune complex disease. In addition, it is becoming apparent that minor immune complex–mediated lesions arise relatively frequently following the normal immune responses to many antigens, without giving rise to clinically significant disease.

LOCAL TYPE III HYPERSENSITIVITY REACTIONS

The Arthus Reaction. If antigen is injected subcutaneously into an animal that possesses circulating antibody capable of precipitating that antigen, then an acute inflammatory reaction will develop within several hours at the site of injection. The reaction starts as an erythematous, edematous swelling; eventually local hemorrhage and thrombosis occur and, if severe, culminate in necrosis.

Histologically, the first changes observed following antigen injection are neutrophil adherence to vascular endothelium followed by emigration through the walls of small blood vessels, particularly venules. By six to eight hours, when the reaction has reached maximal intensity, the injection site is densely infiltrated by very large numbers of these cells (Fig. 19–1). As the reaction progresses, severe destruction of blood vessel walls occurs, resulting in hemorrhage and edema. Platelet aggregation and thrombosis are also associated with this vascular destruction. By eight hours, mononuclear cells may be observed within the lesion, and by 24 hours or later, depending on the amount of antigen injected, they become the predominant cell type. Eosinophil infiltration is not a significant feature of this type of hypersensitivity.

The fate of the injected antigen may be determined by means of a technique such as the direct fluorescent antibody test. It can be shown that antigen diffuses away from the injection site through tissue spaces. When small blood vessels are encountered, the antigen will diffuse into the vessel walls, where it comes into contact with circulating antibody. Consequently, immune complexes are generated and deposited between and beneath endothelial cells. If these immune complexes fix complement, a number of events follow, the most important of which is neutrophil chemotaxis and accumulation (Fig. 19–2).

Neutrophils are attracted by C3a, C5a and C567, all products of the complement cascade. In addition, the neutrophils of some species have a C3 receptor and so will adhere to immune complexes containing this component. Neutrophils that encounter immune complexes in this way promptly phagocytose them, and eventually the immune complexes are eliminated. However, during this process, large quantities of active hydrolytic enzymes are released into the tissues. These enzymes mediate the tissue damage seen in the Arthus reaction.

Neutrophil hydrolytic enzymes are normally stored within lysosomes. They may

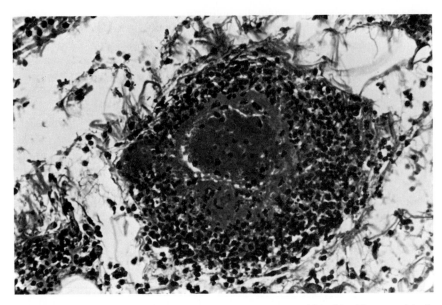

Figure 19–1 Histological section of an Arthus reaction in rabbit skin. The vessel is thrombosed, and fibrinoid material is deposited in the wall. Neutrophil accumulation is extensive. (From Thomson RG., 1978. General Veterinary Pathology. WB Saunders Company, Philadelphia. Courtesy of Dr. Thomson.)

be released into tissues through a number of processes, the most obvious of which is cell death; however, other release mechanisms are probably of greater importance in the Arthus reaction. For example, when neutrophils attempt to phagocytose immune complexes attached to a nonphagocytosable structure, such as a basement membrane, they secrete their lysosomal contents directly into the surrounding medium. Similarly, they may release lysosomal enzymes into the phagosome before immune complexes are completely enclosed, so that the enzymes escape into the surrounding tissues.

The lysosomal enzymes released in this way are primarily hydrolytic (see Table 2–1). They include collagenases that disrupt collagen fibers, neutral proteases that destroy ground substances and basement membranes, and elastases that destroy elastic tissue. Other enzymes released by neutrophils may degranulate mast cells or generate kinins. As a result of this enzyme release, destruction of tissues, especially blood vessel walls, occurs, resulting in the development of the edema, vasculitis and hemorrhage characteristic of the Arthus reaction.

In addition to causing neutrophil accumulation, complement activated by immune complexes may also cause platelets to clump and release procoagulants (Chapter 8). This, in conjunction with the severe vascular damage, may result in extensive thrombosis. Finally, the production of anaphylatoxins (C3a and C5a) and of the C2 kinin and the release of kininogens from neutrophils and vasoactive amines from neutrophils, platelets and mast cells all contribute to the development of a severe local inflammatory response.

The antibodies involved in the Arthus reaction must be both precipitating and complement-fixing and are therefore usually of the IgG class. Some studies have suggested that horse antibodies are relatively poor in provoking this reaction and give

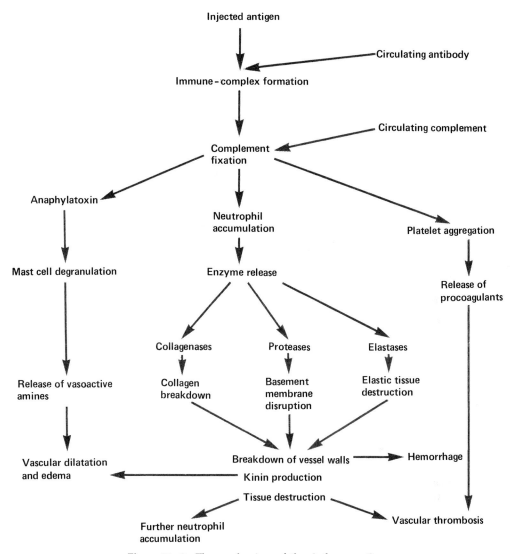

Figure 19–2 The mechanism of the Arthus reaction.

a considerably less severe response than an equivalent amount of rabbit antibodies.

Although the "classical" direct Arthus reaction is produced by local administration of antigen to hyperimmunized animals, any technique that permits immune complexes to be deposited in tissues will stimulate a similar response. A "reversed" Arthus reaction can therefore be produced if antibody is administered intradermally to an animal with a high level of circulating antigen. Injected preformed immune complexes, particularly those containing a moderate excess of antigen, will provoke a similar reaction, although, as might be anticipated, there is less involvement of blood vessel walls and the reaction is less severe. A "passive" Arthus reaction can be produced by giving antibody intravenously to a nonsensitized animal followed by an intradermal injection of antigen, and real enthusiasts can produce a "reversed passive" Arthus reaction by giving antibody intradermally followed by intravenous antigen.

NATURALLY OCCURRING LOCAL TYPE III
HYPERSENSITIVITY REACTIONS

As mentioned previously, it is unusual for hypersensitivity reactions of only a single type to occur under natural conditions. Nevertheless, there exist a number of relatively common hypersensitivities in the domestic animals in which type III hypersensitivity plays a major role.

Blue Eye.   The classical Arthus reaction is usually produced in the skin, since that is the most convenient site in which to administer the antigen. Local reactions of this type can, however, occur in many locations, the precise site depending upon the location of antigen. An example of this is "blue eye," a condition seen in a proportion of dogs either infected or vaccinated with live canine adenovirus type 1 (see Figs. 14–5 and 14–6). The lesion in blue eye consists of a transient anterior uveitis, corneal edema and opacity. The cornea is infiltrated by neutrophils, and, by means of immunofluorescence, virus-antibody complexes may be detected in the lesion. This reaction occurs around one to three weeks after the onset of infection and resolves spontaneously as virus is eliminated.

Hypersensitivity Pneumonitis.   Local type III hypersensitivity reactions occur in the lungs when highly sensitized animals inhale antigen. For example, cattle housed during the winter are usually exposed to dust arising from hay. Normally, these dust particles are relatively large and become deposited in the upper respiratory tract where they are trapped in mucus and eliminated. If, however, hay is stored when damp, the growth of microorganisms will result in heating. This heating may permit thermophilic actinomycetes to grow. One of the most important of these thermophilic actinomycetes is *Micropolyspora faeni*, which produces very large quantities of extremely small spores (1 μm in diameter) and which on inhalation can penetrate as far as the alveoli. If cattle are fed moldy hay during the winter months, constant inhalation of *M. faeni* spores will result in sensitization and in the development of high titered precipitating antibodies to *M. faeni* antigens in serum. In late winter, therefore, inhaled spore antigen may encounter antibody within the alveolar walls, and the resulting generation of immune complexes and complement fixation may result in the development of an interstitial pneumonia, the basis of which is a type III hypersensitivity reaction.

The lesion of this "hypersensitivity pneumonitis" consists of an acute alveolitis together with some vasculitis and exudation of fluid into the alveolar spaces (Fig. 19–3). The alveolar septa may be thickened, and the entire lesion is infiltrated with inflammatory cells. Since many of these cells are eosinophils and lymphocytes, it is obvious that the reaction is not a "pure" type III reaction. Nevertheless, immunofluorescent studies on the lungs of affected cattle show deposits of immunoglobulin, complement and antigen. In animals exposed to low levels of antigen over a long period of time, a proliferative bronchiolitis and fibrosis may be observed. Clinically, hypersensitivity pneumonitis presents as a pneumonitis occurring between 5 and 10 hours after exposure to grossly moldy hay. The animal may be severely dyspneic and may cough repeatedly. In chronically affected animals, dyspnea may be continuous. The most important method of treating this condition is by removing the source of antigen. The administration of steroids may also be beneficial.

A hypersensitivity pneumonitis due to exposure to *M. faeni* spores also occurs in farmers chronically exposed to dust from moldy hay and is known as "farmer's lung." Many other syndromes in man have an identical pathogenesis and are usually named

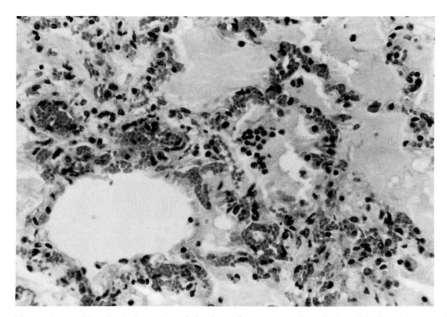

Figure 19–3 Histological section of the lung from a cow that died suddenly 24 hours after being fed moldy hay. The acute alveolitis is probably due to a hypersensitivity reaction to inhaled actinomycete spores. × 400. (Courtesy of Dr. B. N. Wilkie).

after the source of the offending antigen. Thus "pigeon breeder's lung" arises following exposure to the dust from pigeon feces, "mushroom grower's disease" is due to hypersensitivity to inhaled spores from actinomycetes in the soil used for growing mushrooms and "librarian's lung" results from inhalation of dusts from old books! Heaves in horses (chronic obstructive pulmonary disease) is a hypersensitivity pneumonitis of complex origin involving both type I and type III hypersensitivities (see page 272). The offending antigens in this case are probably derived from molds in dusty hay.

Although hypersensitivity pneumonitis as an entity occurs in response to inhaled antigens, it should be remembered that the immune response to pneumonia-causing microorganisms such as pasteurella may also contribute to the development of pathological lesions through a similar mechanism.

Staphylococcal Hypersensitivity in Dogs. Staphylococcal hypersensitivity is a chronic dermatitis of dogs generally presenting as a seborrheic dermatitis and deep or interdigital furunculosis, folliculitis and impetigo. Skin testing with staphylococcal antigens suggests that type III hypersensitivity may be involved, as do the histological findings of neutrophilic dermal vasculitis.

GENERALIZED TYPE III HYPERSENSITIVITY REACTIONS

If antigen is adminstered intravenously to animals with a high level of circulating antibodies, then immune complexes form within the circulation. Most of these complexes, especially the large ones, are removed by the cells of the mononuclear-phagocytic system. However, some complexes, particularly those formed with excess antigen, are soluble and hence poorly phagocytosed. In addition, alternate pathway complement components are capable of inserting themselves into and solubilizing large immune complexes. These soluble complexes may fix complement and stimulate platelet aggregation and the release of vasoactive amines, thus affecting the properties of the vascular endothelium. Consequently, immune complexes may be deposited in the walls of blood vessels, particularly medium-sized arteries and in vessels where there is physiological effusion of fluid — for example, glomeruli, synovia and the choroid plexus (Fig. 19–4).

Acute Serum Sickness. Many years ago, when the use of antisera for passive immunization was in its infancy, it was observed that individuals who had received a very large single dose of foreign (horse) serum showed a characteristic series of side effects about 10 days later. These side effects consisted of a generalized vasculitis with erythema, edema and urticaria of the skin, neutropenia, lymph node enlargement, joint swelling and proteinuria. The reaction was usually of short duration, subsiding within a few days, and was known as serum sickness.

A similar reaction can be produced experimentally in rabbits by a single high dose of antigen given intravenously. Its occurrence can be shown to coincide with the presence of large quantities of immune complexes in the circulation as a result of the immune response to circulating antigen (Fig. 19–5). Histologically, two types of lesion

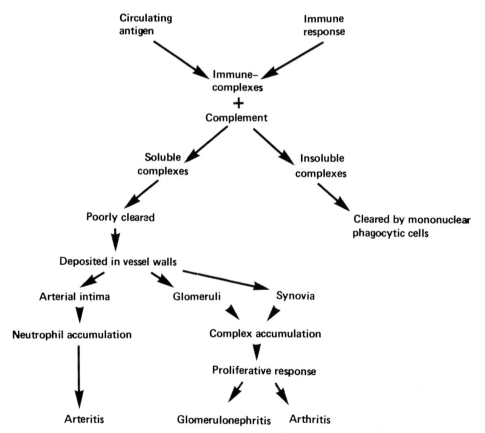

Figure 19–4 The pathogenesis of serum sickness.

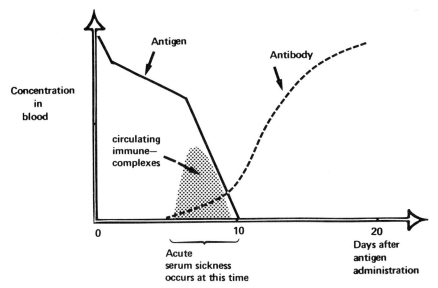

Figure 19–5   The time course of acute serum sickness.

may be seen. First, there is a transient glomerulonephritis, the nature of which tends to vary with the size of immune complexes involved. Thus, relatively large complexes in slight antigen excess appear to penetrate the vascular endothelium but not the basement membrane, and so become deposited in the subendothelial region, where they stimulate endothelial swelling and proliferation (Fig. 19–6). In contrast, if very small complexes are formed, as occurs in gross antigen excess, then these can penetrate both the vascular endothelium and the basement membrane and stimulate epithelial swelling and proliferation. Neutrophils do not normally accumulate within these glomeruli; nevertheless, damage does occur and results in the development of proteinuria. The precise mechanism of this damage is not clear, but it is probably due largely to the vasoactive properties of fixed complement.

Second, widespread arterial lesions develop. The most important of these is an Arthus-type lesion — neutrophil infiltration, disruption of the internal elastic membrane and medial necrosis that occurs in medium-sized muscular arteries. This is presumably due to local deposition of immune complexes. Although the mechanisms of this deposition are not clear, it is probable that a transient type I hypersensitivity reaction may be required to initiate the arteritis.

Chronic Serum Sickness.   If, instead of a single high dose of antigen, an animal is given repeated injections of small doses of antigen, then two other types of glomerular lesion may develop (Fig. 19–6). Continued deposition of subepithelial immune complexes may lead to an apparent increase in the thickness of the glomerular basement membrane, forming the so-called wire loop lesion and causing a membranous glomerulopathy. Alternatively, these immune complexes may be deposited in the mesangial region of glomeruli. Mesangial cells are probably a form of mononuclear phagocyte; as such they possess receptors for immune complexes and complement as well as being phagocytic. They respond to these immune complexes by proliferation (Fig. 19–7). Normally, such proliferation scarcely affects glomerular function unless the mesangial cells expand to completely surround the glomerular

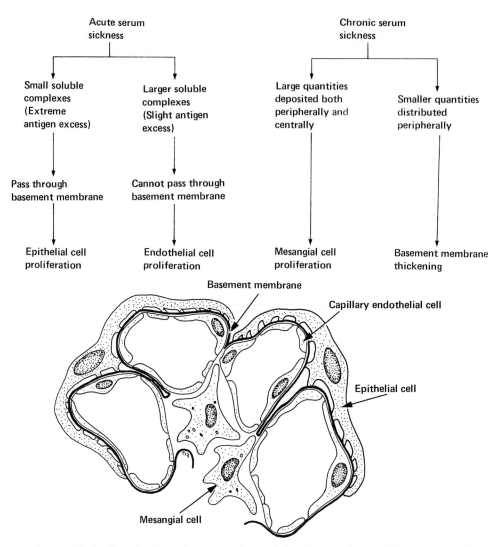

Figure 19–6 The structure of a glomerulus and the different forms of immune complex–induced glomerulopathy.

capillaries. By immunofluorescence it can be shown that "lumpy-bumpy" aggregates of immune complexes are deposited in capillary walls and on the epithelial side of the glomerular basement membrane (Fig. 19–8). Arteritis is not a significant feature of experimental chronic serum sickness.

CLINICAL ASPECTS OF IMMUNE COMPLEX–MEDIATED GLOMERULAR DISEASE

In general, immune complex-mediated lesions occur when prolonged antigenemia persists in the presence of antibodies. Glomerulonephritis is, therefore, characteristic of such chronic virus diseases as equine infectious anemia, Aleutian disease of mink

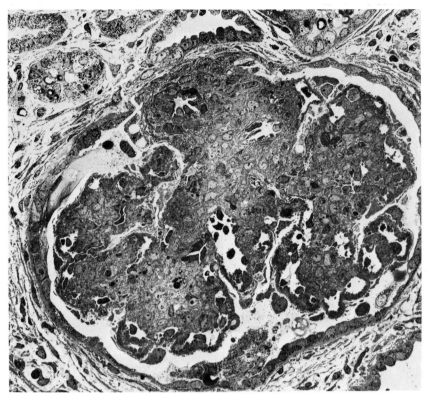

Figure 19–7 A thin section of a glomerulus from a Finnish-Landrace lamb suffering from mesangiocapillary glomerulonephritis, showing dramatic mesangial cell proliferation and basement membrane thickening. (From Angus KW et al. 1974. J Comp Pathol *84* 319–330. Used with permission.)

and African swine fever (Table 19–1). Immune complex glomerulopathy has also been reported to occur in dogs suffering from pyometra, chronic pneumonias, distemper encephalitis, acute pancreatic necrosis, bacterial endocarditis, systemic lupus erythematosus (Chapter 21) and certain malignant tumors, particularly lymphosarcomas and mastocytomas. It may also arise in the absence of an obvious predisposing cause. The most common pathological lesion is mesangial proliferation, but diffuse membranous thickening is also occasionally seen.

The presence of immune complexes within glomeruli leads to an increase in their permeability to protein, and as a result plasma proteins are lost in the urine. The major protein lost is albumin, since it is a relatively small molecule. This loss of protein, if severe, may exceed the capacity of the body to replace it. As a consequence, the animal becomes hypoalbuminemic, the plasma colloid osmotic pressure falls, fluid passes into tissue spaces and the animal may become edematous and ascitic. The loss of fluid into tissue spaces results in a reduction of blood volume, a compensatory increase in secretion of antidiuretic hormone, increased sodium retention and accentuation of the edema. The decreased blood volume will also result in a drop in renal blood flow, reduction in glomerular filtration, retention of urea and creatinine, azotemia and hypercholesterolemia. Although all these may occur as a result of

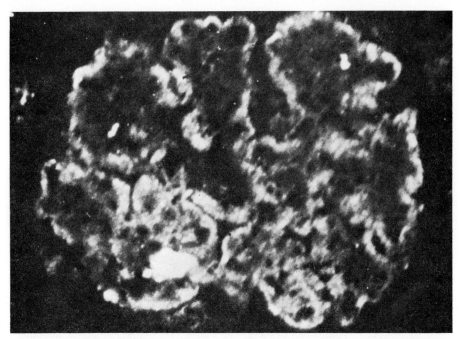

Figure 19-8 Fluorescent micrograph of a section of a glomerulus from a Finnish-Landrace lamb suffering from mesangiocapillary glomerulonephritis. The labeled antisheep globulin reveals "lumpy-bumpy" deposits characteristic of immune-complex deposition. (From Angus KW et al. 1974. J Comp Pathol *84* 319–330. Used with permission.)

Table 19-1 INFECTIOUS DISEASES WITH A SIGNIFICANT TYPE III
HYPERSENSITIVITY COMPONENT

ORGANISM OR DISEASE	*MAJOR LESION*
Erysipelothrix insidiosa *(E. rhusiopathiae)*	Arthritis
Mycobacterium johnei	Enteritis
Leptospira interrogans	*Opthalmia*
Streptococcus equi	Purpura
Staphylococcus aureus	Dermatitis
Canine adenovirus I	Uveitis, glomerulonephritis
Feline leukemia	Glomerulonephritis
Feline infectious peritonitis	Peritonitis, glomerulonephritis
Aleutian disease	Glomerulonephritis, anemia, arteritis
Hog cholera	Glomerulonephritis
Bovine virus diarrhea	Glomerulonephritis
Equine viral arteritis	Arteritis
Equine infectious anemia	Anemia, glomerulonephritis
Dirofilaria immitis	Glomerulonephritis

immune complex deposition within glomeruli, the development of this nephrotic syndrome is not inevitable. In fact, the clinical course of these conditions is extremely unpredictable, some animals showing a progressive decline in renal function while others show spontaneous remissions. Many animals may be clinically normal in spite of the presence of immunoglobulin deposits within their glomeruli, and immune complex deposits are not uncommonly observed in apparently healthy old dogs, horses and sheep. Because of the unpredictable occurrence of spontaneous remissions, it is difficult to judge the effects of treatment on this condition. It is usual to treat affected animals with corticosteroids and immunosuppressive drugs, but the rationale of this treatment is open to question. The glomerular lesion is not inflammatory, and although the lesion in primary immune complex glomerulopathy contains immunoglobulin, there is no evidence to suggest that the condition occurs as a result of hyperactivity of the immune system. In addition, steroid treatment of rabbits with experimental immune complex disease has been shown to exacerbate the condition.

Finnish-Landrace Glomerulopathy. Some lambs of the Finnish-Landrace breed die when about 6½ weeks of age as a result of a glomerulopathy. The glomerular lesions are similar to those seen in chronic serum sickness, with mesangial cell proliferation and basement membrane thickening (Fig. 19–7). In extreme cases epithelial cell proliferation may result in Bowman's capsule being filled by an epithelial crescent. Neutrophils may be present in small numbers within glomeruli, and the rest of the kidney may exhibit diffuse interstitial lymphoid infiltration and necrotizing vasculitis. Deposits containing IgM, IgG and C3 are found within the glomeruli (Fig. 19–8) and in the choroid plexus, and serum C3 levels are low. The lesions are, therefore, probably produced as a result of immune complex deposition within these organs, although the nature of the inducing antigen is unknown.

OTHER IMMUNE COMPLEX−MEDIATED LESIONS

Polyarteritis Nodosa. This is a condition seen in man, swine, dogs and cats. It is characterized by a widespread but focal arteriolar necrosis in which there is extensive neutrophil infiltration of the arterial media. Renal arteries are most commonly involved. The origin of polyarteritis nodosa is unknown, but because of the similarity of the lesion to that seen in acute serum sickness of humans, it is possible that it represents a type III hypersensitivity reaction to an unidentified antigen. Polyarteritis nodosa is usually detected as an incidental finding on autopsy, although ocular defects may present clinically if the arteries of the eye are involved.

Drug Hypersensitivities. In the previous chapter, it was pointed out that if a drug attached itself to a cell such as an erythrocyte, then the immune response against the cell could lead to its elimination. A similar reaction may occur through type III hypersensitivity reactions if immune complexes bind directly to host cells. In this case, the cells are recognized as being opsonized and are removed by phagocytosis. There are obviously only minor differences in mechanism between antibody binding to antigen-coated cells and antibody-antigen complexes coating cells directly, and it is therefore usually very difficult to distinguish between the two. As might be predicted, if immune complexes bind to erythrocytes, anemia results; if they bind to platelets, thrombocytopenia and purpura result; and binding to granulocytes leads to agranulocytosis and, consequently, recurrent infection. In many cases, however, it is difficult to distinguish between the toxic effects of a drug and type III hypersensitivity unless specific antibodies can be eluted from affected cells.

Dirofilariasis. Some dogs heavily infected with the heartworm *Dirofilaria immitis* develop glomerular lesions and proteinuria. The lesions involve thickening of the glomerular basement membrane with minimal endothelial or mesangial proliferation. Since "lumpy-bumpy," IgG1-containing deposits may be found on the epithelial side of the basement membrane, it has been suggested that immune complexes formed by antibodies to helminth antigens provoke these lesions. Other investigators dispute the immune complex nature of these lesions, however, and claim that the lesions develop in response to the physical presence of microfilariae within glomerular blood vessels. The fact that infected dogs may develop amyloidosis (Chapter 22) suggests strongly that they mount a significant immune response to the worms.

ADDITIONAL SOURCES OF INFORMATION

Angus KW, and Gardiner AC. 1979. Mesangio-capillary glomerulonephritis in Dorset-Finnish–Landrance cross lambs. Vet Rec *105* 471.

Cochrane CG, and Koffler D. 1973. Immune-complex disease in experimental animals and man. Adv Immunol *16* 186–224.

Drazner FH. 1978. Renal amyloidosis and glomerulonephritis secondary to dirofilariasis. Canine Pract *5* 66–68.

Germuth FG, and Rodriguez E. 1973. Immunopathology of the renal glomerulus. Immune complex deposition and anti-basement membrane disease. Little, Brown & Co, Boston.

Krakowka S. 1978. Glomerulonephritis in dogs and cats. Vet Clin North Am (Small Animal Practice) *8* 629–639.

Littlejohn A. 1979. Chronic obstructive pulmonary disease in horses. Vet Bull *49* 907–917.

Morrison WI, and Wright NG. 1976. Immunopathological aspects of canine renal disease. J. Small Anim Pract *17* 139–148.

Murray M, and Wright NG. 1974. A morphological study of canine glomerulonephritis. Lab Invest *30* 213–221.

Schatz M, Patterson R, and Fink J. 1979. Immunologic lung disease. N Engl J Med *300* 1310–1320.

Scott DW, Macdonald JM, and Schultz RD, 1978. Staphylococcal hypersensitivity in the dog. J Am Anim Hosp Assn *14* 766–779.

Slauson DO, and Lewis RM. 1979. Comparative pathology of glomerulonephritis in animals. Vet Pathol *16* 135–164.

Theofilopoulos AN, and Dixon FJ. 1979. The biology and detection of immune complexes. Adv Immunol *28* 89–220.

Weissman G, Smolen JE, and Korchak HM. 1980. Release of inflammatory mediators from stimulated neutrophils. N Engl J Med *303* 27–34.

20

Cell-Mediated (Type IV) Hypersensitivity

When certain antigens are injected into the skin of sensitized animals, an inflammatory response, taking many hours to develop, may occur at the injection site. Since this "delayed hypersensitivity" reaction cannot be transferred from sensitized to normal animals by serum, but only through lymphocytes, it is apparently cell-mediated. Delayed hypersensitivity reactions of this sort are classified as type IV hypersensitivity and occur as a result of the interaction between the injected antigen and sensitized T lymphocytes. An important example of a delayed hypersensitivity reaction is the tuberculin response, the reaction mediated in a tuberculous animal as a result of an intradermal injection of tuberculin — an antigenic extract derived from the tubercle bacillus.

TUBERCULIN REACTION — A CLASSICAL TYPE IV REACTION

Tuberculin is the name given to extracts of *Mycobacterium tuberculosis, Mycobacterium bovis* or *Mycobacterium avium*, which are employed as antigens when skin testing animals in an effort to identify those suffering from tuberculosis. Several types of tuberculin have been employed for this purpose. These include old tuberculin (OT), which is the supernatant fluid from a broth culture of the organism concentrated by boiling; heat concentrated synthetic medium (HCSM) tuberculin, which is similar to OT but grown on synthetic medium; and purified protein derivative (PPD) tuberculin, which is prepared by growing organisms in synthetic medium, killing them with steam and filtering. The PPD tuberculin is precipitated from this filtrate with trichloracetic acid, washed and finally resuspended in buffer ready for use.

When PPD tuberculin is injected intradermally into a normal animal, there is no significant local inflammatory response. On the other hand, if it is injected into an animal sensitized by infection with the tubercle bacillus, a delayed hypersensitivity response will occur. Following injection of tuberculin into such an animal, no changes are detectable either grossly or histologically for several hours. Later, however, vasodilation and increased vascular permeability occur, as a result of which erythema and swelling are observed. This swelling is characteristically indurated (hard). On histological examination, the lesion is observed to differ from the classical acute inflammatory response in that the infiltrating cell population consists largely of mononuclear cells (macrophages and lymphocytes) (Fig. 20–1), although a transient neutrophil accumulation also occurs in the early stages of the reaction. The reaction reaches its greatest intensity by 24 to 72 hours after injection and may persist for several weeks before gradually fading. In very severe reactions, necrosis may occur at the injection site.

The tuberculin reaction is an immunologically specific reaction mediated by T cells. It is believed that circulating antigen-sensitive T cells encounter the injected antigen and respond both by recruiting other lymphocytes and by dividing, differentiating and releasing lymphokines (Fig. 20–2). The lymphokines involved and the order in which they act are unclear, but it is thought that macrophages accumulate at the site through the release of macrophage chemotactic factors and that their emigration from this site is then inhibited by migration inhibitory factors. The vascular changes are probably mediated through the release of "skin-reactive factors" and lysosomal en-

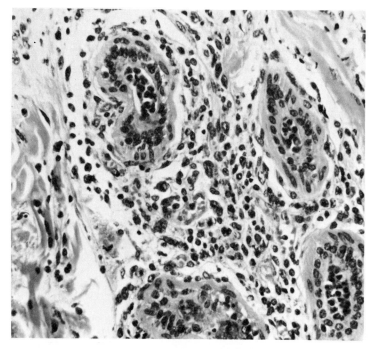

Figure 20–1 Histological section of a positive tuberculin reaction in bovine skin. Note the perivascular mononuclear cell infiltration. (From Thomson RG 1978. General Veterinary Pathology, WB Saunders Company, Philadelphia. Courtesy of Dr. Thomson.)

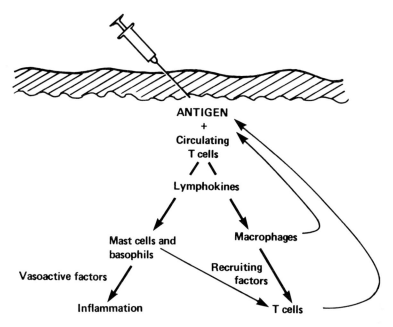

ANTIGEN
+
Circulating
T cells

Lymphokines

Mast cells and
basophils

Macrophages

Vasoactive factors

Recruiting
factors

Inflammation

T cells

Figure 20—2 Schematic diagram depicting the pathogenesis of the delayed hypersensitivity reaction. It is essentially an inflammatory reaction in which both macrophages and T cells participate in order to eliminate the inducing antigen.

zymes from macrophages. The macrophages ingest and eventually destroy the injected antigen, so that its elimination removes the stimulus for further lymphokine production, permitting the tissues to return to normal.

The initial T-cell response also generates a lymphokine that attracts basophils and causes local mast cells to degranulate. Serotonin from these cells enhances the migration of mononuclear cells into the lesion.

Cutaneous Basophil Hypersensitivity. Some antigens may elicit a different form of delayed inflammatory response in skin. In these cases, the lesion is infiltrated with large numbers of basophils as well as mononuclear cells. This reaction, called cutaneous basophil hypersensitivity (CBH), can be transferred between animals with antibody, with purified B cells or with T cells. It is, therefore, a very heterogeneous phenomenon that probably arises through a number of different mechanisms. CBH is observed in chickens in response to intradermal Rous sarcoma virus, in rabbits in response to schistosomes, and in humans in allergic contact dermatitis and renal allograft rejection.

Tuberculin Reaction as a Diagnostic Test in Cattle. Because the tuberculin reaction occurs only in animals that have, or have had, tuberculosis, it may be employed to identify animals affected by this disease. Indeed, this test has provided the basis for all tuberculosis eradication schemes that involve the detection and subsequent elimination of infected animals.

Tuberculin testing of cattle may be performed in several ways. The simplest of these is the single intradermal (SID) test. In this test, 0.05 ml of PPD tuberculin derived from either *M. tuberculosis* or *M. bovis* is injected into one anal fold and the injection site is examined 72 to 96 hours later. A comparison is easily made between the injected and the uninjected folds, and a positive reaction consisting of a diffuse indurated swelling at the injection site is readily detected.

In the United States two injections are made, one into the mucocutaneous junction of the vulva and the other into an anal fold; in other countries the injection is normally made into the skin on the side of the neck. The neck site is more sensitive than the anal folds, but restraint of the animal may be more difficult and good injection technique is critical.

The advantage of the SID test is its simplicity; its disadvantage is that by using this test it is not possible to distinguish between infection with the different species of mycobacteria that include *M. avium*, *Mycobacterium paratuberculosis* and the related *Nocardia* group of organisms. A second disadvantage is the relatively high prevalence of animals that react positively to the test but on necropsy do not have detectable lesions of tuberculosis. The reasons for this are not clear but may involve inapparent infection with nonpathogenic mycobacteria.

False negative SID tests may occur in animals with advanced tuberculosis, in animals with very early infection, in animals that have calved within the preceding four to six weeks, in very old cows and in animals tested within the preceding 1 to 10 weeks. The anergy seen in advanced cases of tuberculosis is also observed in clinical Johne's disease and appears to be due to the presence of a blocking factor in the serum of these animals—perhaps an antibody, which prevents T cells from reacting with antigen; there is also, however, evidence for the development of suppressor cells in this condition. Because of these defects in the SID, several modifications of this test have been developed (Table 20–1). The comparative test, for example, employs both avian and bovine tuberculins. Each of these is injected into the side of the neck at separate sites, and these sites are examined 72 hours later. In general, if the avian tuberculin site shows the greatest reaction, the animal is considered to be infected with *M. avium* or *M. paratuberculosis*. On the other hand, if the *M. bovis* site shows the greatest reaction, then it is felt that the animal is infected with either *M. tuberculosis* or *M. bovis*. Therefore, this test is useful when a high prevalence of avian tuberculosis or Johne's disease is anticipated, and it has been used with success in the United Kingdom. PPD from *M. bovis* is more specific in cattle than *M. tuberculosis*, giving less cross-reaction with *M. avium* as well as being more appropriate for use in cattle, and is therefore preferred.

Other modified tuberculin tests include the short thermal test, in which a large volume of tuberculin solution is given subcutaneously and the animal examined for a rise in temperature between four and eight hours later. (Antigen-stimulated T cells release a lymphokine pyrogen.) The Stormont test relies on the increased sensitivity of a test site, which occurs after a single injection; it is performed by giving two doses of tuberculin at the same injection site seven days apart. Both these tests are relatively sensitive and may be used in postpartum cows as well as for the testing of heavily infected animals.

TUBERCULIN TESTING IN ANIMALS OTHER THAN CATTLE.   Tuberculin testing has never been a widely employed procedure in domestic animals other than cattle, so information on these is scanty. Nevertheless, it appears that the capacity of different species to mount a classical tuberculin reaction varies greatly. In the pig and cat, for example, the tuberculin test is unreliable, being positive for only a short period following infection. In the pig and dog, the best test is a SID test given behind the ear, whereas in the cat the short thermal test is probably the best. In sheep, goats and horses the antigen is usually given in the caudal fold, but the results also tend to be

Table 20–1 SOME TUBERCULIN TESTS USED IN CATTLE

TEST	*USAGE*	*ADVANTAGES*	*DISADVANTAGES*
Single intradermal (SID)	Routine testing	Simple	False positives; poor sensitivity
Comparative	When much avian T.B. or Johne's disease is present	More specific than SID	More complex than SID
Short thermal	Use in post-partum animals and in advanced cases	High efficiency	Time consuming; potential risk of anaphylaxis
Stormont	Use in post-partrum animals and in advanced cases	Very sensitive and accurate	Three visits required; leads to a long de-sensitization period

highly erratic in these species. In birds, good reactions may be obtained by inoculating tuberculin into the wattle or wing web.

Johnin Reaction. Animals infected with *M. paratuberculosis* may exhibit a delayed hypersensitivity to an antigenic extract of this organism known as johnin. Johnin can be used in a single intradermal test but, like tuberculin, generally gives a negative result in animals with clinical disease. As an alternative to the SID test, an intravenous johnin test may be preferable. In this test the antigen is administered intravenously and the animal's temperature noted at intervals thereafter. A rise in temperature of 1.5°F or a neutrophilia after six hours is considered a positive result. These tests are probably of limited usefulness in individual animals but may be used for the identification of infected herds.

Other Diagnostic Skin Tests Involving Delayed Hypersensitivity. Positive delayed hypersensitivity reactions may be obtained in any infectious disease in which cell-mediated immunity plays a significant role. Thus, various extracts of *Brucella abortus* have been used from time to time in attempts to diagnose brucellosis. These include "brucellin," a filtrate of a 20-day broth culture, and "brucellergen," a nucleoprotein extract. Because these preparations may stimulate production of antibody to brucella, they must not be employed in areas where eradication is monitored by serologic tests. In glanders of horses, a culture filtrate of the organism *Pseudomonas mallei*, termed "mallein," is used for skin testing. Mallein can be used in either a short thermal test or an ophthalmic test. An ophthalmic test, also occasionally employed in tuberculosis, is performed by dropping the antigen solution into an eye. A transient conjunctivitis develops if the test is positive. Another and perhaps preferable hypersensitivity test for glanders is the intrapalpebral test, in which mallein is injected into the skin of the lower eyelid, where a positive reaction causes swelling and ophthalmia.

Skin tests are also employed in the diagnosis of many fungal diseases; thus, "histoplasmin" is used for histoplasmosis, "coccidioidin" in coccidioidomycosis and so on. In these cases, the tests are not particularly specific, and the test procedure may effectively sensitize the tested animal, causing it to become serologically positive. This problem also arises when "toxoplasmin" is used in attempts to diagnose toxoplasmosis (Chapter 15).

PATHOLOGICAL CONSEQUENCES OF TYPE IV
HYPERSENSITIVITY

Tubercle Formation.   Although the intradermal tuberculin reaction is artificial in that antigen is administered by injection, a similar host response occurs if living tubercle bacilli lodge in tissues. However, *M. tuberculosis* is resistant to intracellular destruction until a cell-mediated immune response has developed (Chapter 6), and dead organisms are very slowly removed because they contain large quantities of poorly metabolized waxes. As a result of this, the delayed hypersensitivity reaction to whole organisms tends to be prolonged, and, consequently, macrophages accumulate in very large numbers. Many of these macrophages attempt to ingest the bacteria and die in the process, whereas others fuse to form multinucleated giant cells. The lesion that develops around invading tubercle bacilli therefore consists of a mass of necrotic material containing both living and dead organisms and is surrounded by a layer of macrophages, which in this location are known as epithelioid cells (Chapter 2). The entire lesion is known as a tubercle (Fig. 20–3). Persistent tubercles may become relatively well organized and develop fibrous tissue resulting in the formation of a granuloma. (Some lymphokines may stimulate collagen production by fibroblasts and hence contribute to this process.) Granuloma formation is a frequent consequence of local chronic inflammation. This inflammation may be of immunological origin, as in tuberculosis or brucellosis in some species, but it may also occur as a result of the presence in tissues of other chronic irritants. For example, granulomas may arise in response to the prolonged irritation caused by talc or asbestos particles.

In chronic interstitial nephritis (CIN) of dogs associated with leptospiral infection, it has been suggested that the organisms persisting in the kidney may induce a chronic inflammatory reaction in which delayed hypersensitivity as well as local antibody

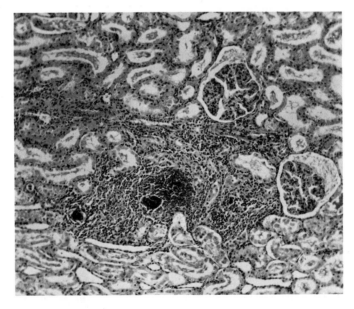

Figure 20–3 Histological section from the kidney of a black buck showing a small tubercle. × 250. (From a specimen kindly provided by Dr. R. G. Thomson.)

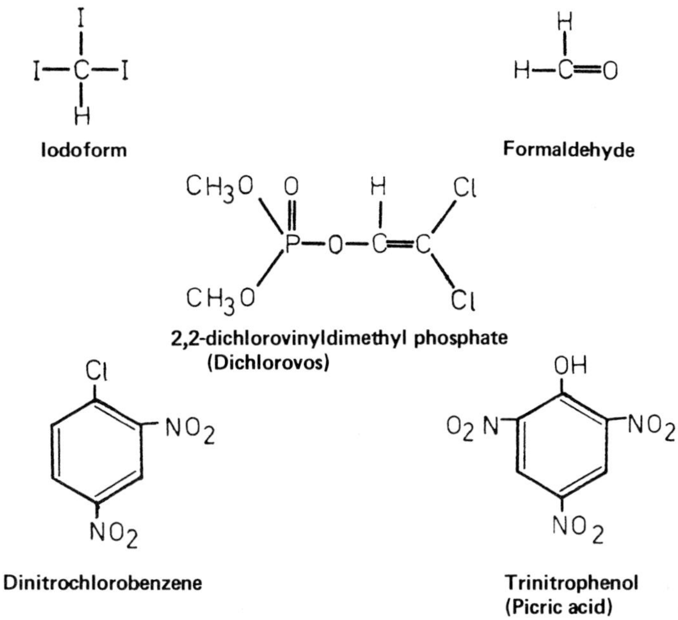

Figure 20–4 Some of the simple chemicals that may cause allergic contact dermatitis.

production plays a role. Certainly, the histology of CIN shows remarkable resemblances to that of chronic renal allograft rejection in the dog.

Allergic Contact Dermatitis. Under some circumstances, exposure of tissue cells to reactive chemicals leads to the formation of protein-chemical complexes. If these complexes are regarded as foreign, affected cells may be "rejected" through a cell-mediated immune response. If this reaction occurs in the skin, it gives rise to a condition known as allergic contact dermatitis.

The chemicals that induce allergic contact dermatitis are usually relatively simple; they include such compounds as formaldehyde, picric acid, aniline dyes, plant resins, organophosphates and salts of metals such as nickel and beryllium (Fig. 20–4). Thus, allergic contact dermatitis can occur on pathologists' fingers as a result of exposure to formaldehyde, on the foot pads and ventral abdomen of dogs on exposure to some carpet dyes, on parts of the body exposed to the resins (urushiol) of the poison ivy plant (*Rhus radicans*) and around the neck of animals as a result of exposure to dichlorovos (2,2-dichlorovinyldimethyl phosphate) in flea collars. Allergic contact dermatitis involving the muzzle of dogs has been reported to occur as a result of sensitivity to components of plastic food bowls. Some dogs, instead of developing the more usual type I hypersensitivity to pollen proteins, suffer from allergic contact dermatitis as a result of a type IV hypersensitivity to pollen resins. It is unusual for allergic contact dermatitis to severely affect the haired areas of the skin unless the allergen is a liquid.

The lesions of allergic contact dermatitis generally vary greatly in severity, ranging from a mild erythema to severe erythematous vesiculation. Because of the intense pruritus, however, self-trauma, excoriation, ulceration and secondary pyoderma often mask the true nature of the lesion. In chronic lesions, hyperkeratosis, acanthosis and dermal fibrosis may be produced. Histologically, the lesion is marked by a

Table 20-2 COMPARISON OF THE TWO MAJOR FORMS OF
ALLERGIC DERMATITIS

	ATOPIC DERMATITIS	*ALLERGIC CONTACT DERMATITIS*
Pathogenesis	Type I hypersensitivity	Type IV hypersensitivity
Clinical signs	Hyperemia, urticaria, intense pruritus leading to self-mutilation	Spotty hyperemia, occasional vesiculation, erythematous alopecia, pruritis
Distribution	Face, nose, eyes, feet, perineum	Hairless areas, usually ventral abdomen, feet, nose
Major allergen	Foods and pollens, commonly seasonal; occasionally arthropod-associated	Reactive chemicals only after prolonged contact with skin
Diagnosis	Rapid erythematous response to intradermal and patch testing; commonly, other signs of allergy; eosinophilia or eosinophilic infiltration of lesions	Delayed (24 to 48 hr) response to patch test; mononuclear infiltration of the lesions
Treatment	Antihistamines, steroids, hyposensitization therapy	Steroids

mononuclear cell infiltration and vacuolation of skin cells under attack by cytotoxic T cells (Table 20-2).

Diagnosis is made by removal of the suspected antigen and by patch testing. In patch tests, a small area of skin is shaved and covered with a patch of tissue or cloth impregnated with the suspected "allergen." After 24 to 48 hours the patch may be removed, a positive reaction is indicated by local erythema and vesiculation. Treatment makes use of steroids as well as antibiotics to control secondary infections.

Arthropod Hypersensitivity. Although most of the arthropod hypersensitivities in the domestic animals have a strong type I component (Chapter 17), the role of type IV reactions should not be ignored.

DEMODECTIC MANGE. The mange mite *Demodex folliculorum* appears to be a normal symbiont commonly present in hair follicles and only occasionally causing disease. When demodectic mange does occur, the reaction around mites and mite fragments tends to be infiltrated by mononuclear cells together with a few plasma cells. Granuloma formation may occasionally occur. Although it has been suggested that this lesion is a type IV hypersensitivity reaction, perhaps a form of allergic contact dermatitis, it is more likely to be a chronic foreign-body reaction. The absence of eosinophils and edema in the lesion suggests that type I hypersensitivity is relatively unimportant in this condition. Animals suffering from generalized demodecosis appear to be immunosuppressed in that their lymphocytes are unreactive to plant mitogens such as phytohemagglutinin. Serum from these animals is also capable of suppressing the reactivity of lymphocytes from normal animals. It is of interest to note that immunosuppressive agents such as antilymphocyte serum tend to predispose animals to the development of demodectic mange.

FLEA BITE DERMATITIS. Biting fleas secrete saliva into the skin wound. Some of the components of flea saliva are of relatively low molecular weight but can act as haptens by binding to dermal collagen. As a consequence of this, a local type IV hypersensitivity reaction characterized by a mononuclear cell infiltration occurs. In sensitized animals, this type IV reaction is gradually replaced over a period of months by a type I reaction, and so the mononuclear cell infiltration gradually changes to an eosinophil infiltration as infestation persists.

TICK INFESTATION. It has been observed that ticks on nonimmune animals are larger than those on immune animals. Although the nature of this resistance is unclear, it has been suggested that local cell-mediated and immune complex hypersensitivities to tick saliva may act together to restrict the blood flow to the tick thus reducing its food supply and stunting its growth.

THE MEASUREMENT OF CELL-MEDIATED IMMUNITY

Although diagnostic immunology is based largely upon the detection of antibodies, measurement of cell-mediated immune responsiveness in animals may be desirable under some circumstances. Currently, three major groups of techniques are widely used.

The simplest is the intradermal skin test described earlier in this chapter. The resulting inflammatory response may be considered cell-mediated, provided that it has the characteristic time-course and histology of a type IV reaction. Intradermal skin tests are not always convenient, and injection of antigen into an animal may effectively sensitize it. In addition, there is good evidence to suggest that tuberculin testing may promote the spread of infections such as bovine leukosis between animals. For these reasons, *in vitro* tests may be more appropriate. The *in vitro* tests are designed to measure either the proliferation of T lymphocytes in response to antigen or their production of lymphokines.

In order to measure T-cell proliferation in response to antigen, a suspension of purified peripheral blood lymphocytes from the animal to be tested is mixed with antigen and cultured for 48 to 96 hours. Twelve hours before harvesting, thymidine labeled with the radioactive isotope tritium is added to the cultures. Normal, nondividing lymphocytes do not take up thymidine but dividing cells do, because they are actively synthesizing DNA. Thus, if the T cells are proliferating, they will take up the tritiated thymidine and the radioactivity of the washed cells will provide a measure of the degree of proliferation. The greater the response of the cells to antigen, the greater the radioactivity. The ratio of the radioactivity in the stimulated cultures to the radioactivity in the controls is the stimulation index.

The measurement of lymphokine release by T cells is a much more complicated procedure. One of the commonest techniques involves incubating a purified lymphocyte suspension with antigen. After 24 to 48 hours, the supernatant fluid of the culture is removed and assayed for MIF (migration inhibitory factor) activity. This may be done by measuring the ability of the supernatant to inhibit the migration of macrophages out of a capillary tube (see Fig. 6–10).

It is sometimes useful to measure the ability of an animal to mount cell-mediated immune responses in general. One way to do this is to surgically graft the animal with allogeneic skin and measure its survival time. A much simpler technique is to paint the animal's skin with a sensitizing chemical such as dinitrochlorobenzene. The intensity of the resulting contact dermatitis provides a rough estimate of the animal's ability to mount a cell-mediated immune response.

An alternative *in vitro* technique is to measure the response of lymphocytes to mitogenic lectins such as phytohemagglutinin, concanavalin A or pokeweed mitogen (Chapter 6). The intensity of the lymphocyte proliferative response, as measured by tritiated thymidine uptake, provides an estimate of the reactivity of an animal's lymphocytes (see Fig. 22–4). In addition, if phytohemagglutinin is injected intradermally, it provokes a reaction with many of the features of a delayed hypersensitivity response. This is a very convenient and rapid method of assessing an animal's ability to mount a cell-mediated response without the need for first sensitizing the animal to an antigen.

None of the currently available techniques to measure cell-mediated immunity, with the possible exception of intradermal testing, lends itself readily to use by any but investigators in well-equipped laboratories. The measurement of cell-mediated immunity has become an increasingly important feature of the analysis of immune reactivity, however, and refined and much simpler techniques are expected to become available in future.

ADDITIONAL SOURCES OF INFORMATION

Adams DO. 1976. The granulomatous inflammatory response: a review. Am J Pathol *84* 164–191.

Angus K, and Young TJ. 1978. Lymphocyte response to phytohemagglutinin: temporal variation in normal dogs. J Immunol Methods *21* 261–269.

Dixon JB, Allan D, and West CR. 1979. Hematological correlates of phytohemagglutinin-induced lymphocyte transformation in horses. Res Vet Sci *26* 59–65.

Dvorak HF. 1974. Delayed hypersensitivity. *In* Zweifach BW, Grant L, and McCluskey RT (eds). The Inflammatory Process, Vol 3 Academic Press, New York, pp 292–335.

Gershon RK, Askenase PW, and Gershon MD. 1975. Requirement for vasoactive amines for production of delayed-type hypersensitivity skin reactions. J Exp Med *142* 732–747.

Grant DI, and Thoday KL. 1980. Canine allergic contact dermatitis: a clinical review. J Small Anim Pract *21* 17–27.

Hirsch DC, Baker BB, Wiger N, *et al*. 1975. Suppression of *in vitro* lymphocyte transformation by serum from dogs with generalized demodecosis. Am J Vet Res *36* 1591–1595.

Knox S, and Shifrine M. 1980. Cell-mediated immunity in the dog in relation to disease: a reveiw. Comp Immunol Microbiol Infect Dis *2* 405–514.

Legendre AM, Mallman VH, and Michel RL. 1977. Migration-inhibition response of peripheral leukocytes to tuberculin in cats sensitized with *Mycobacterium bovis* (BCG). Am J Vet Res *38* 819–822.

Scherba G, Gustafson DF, Kanitz CL, and Sun IL. 1978. Delayed hypersensitivity reaction to pseudorabies virus as a field diagnostic test in swine. JAVMA *173* 1490–1493.

Toews GB, Bergstresser PR, Streilein JW, and Sullivan S. 1980. Epidermal Langerhans cell density determines whether contact hypersensitivity or unresponsiveness follows skin painting with DNFB. J Immunol *124* 445–453.

21

Autoimmunity: Breakdown in Self-Tolerance

It was believed for many years that normal healthy animals lacked the ability to mount any immune response against self-antigens as a result of self-tolerance. It is now clear, however, that a degree of immune reactivity against normal body constituents is physiological. Thus, a small number of lymphocytes, reactive to normal tissue antigens, are always present in the spleen. Stimulation of these cells by nonspecific mitogens such as bacterial endotoxin will provoke a transient appearance of antibodies in serum; these antibodies can react with normal tissues but have no adverse effects. Normally, however, these self-reactive cells are suppressed and do not make significant quantities of autoantibody.

In other situations, some responses to self-antigens (autoimmune responses) play a physiological role. For example, naturally occurring anti-idiotype antibodies appear to serve as physiological regulators of the immune system (Chapter 7).

On occasion, the suppression of the autoreactive cells may break down. When this happens, clones of normally quiescent lymphocytes will grow and generate very large quantities of autoantibodies or autoreactive T cells. When this happens, the immune responses against normal cells or tissues will cause disease—autoimmune disease.

MECHANISMS OF BREAKDOWN IN SELF-TOLERANCE

Exposure of Previously Hidden Antigens.   There are a number of ways in which immunological unreactivity to normal body components may be overcome. For example, some antigens may exist in locations not normally "visited" by circulating lymphocytes. These locations, which include the central nervous tissue and testicular tissue, are usually not directly drained by the lymphatic circulation. If the brain or testes is injured, either by trauma or by infection, then the resulting breakdown in vascular barriers may permit antigens released by damaged cells to reach the general circulation, encounter antigen-sensitive cells and stimulate an immune response. Similar considerations apply to antigens that are normally found only within cells and to which tolerance may not be established. For example, after myocardial infarction, autoantibodies may be produced against intracellular components such as mitochondria, although myocardial infarction is manifestly not an autoimmune disease.

Development of New Antigenic Determinants.   The formation of autoantibodies may be provoked by the development of new antigenic determinants in normal body or tissue proteins. Two examples of autoantibodies generated in this fashion are rheumatoid factors and immunoconglutinins.

Rheumatoid factors (RF) are antibodies (largely IgM) that are directed against antigenic determinants on other immunoglobulins. When an immunoglobulin binds to antigen, the Fab regions of the molecule are stabilized in such a way that new antigenic determinants are exposed on the Fc region. These new determinants stimulate rheumatoid factor formation. Rheumatoid factors are consequently found in serum in diseases in which large quantities of immune complexes are generated, such as in the non–organ-specific immune disorders, rheumatoid arthritis (page 325) and systemic lupus erythematosus (page 322).

Immunoconglutinins (abbreviated to IK after the German spelling) are antibodies directed against antigenic determinants on the activated complement components C2, C4 and C3. The most important of these is the IK directed against C3. The antigenic determinants that stimulate IK formation are sites on the complement components newly revealed by complement activation. The level of IK in serum is a measure of the amount of complement activation occurring, and this, in turn, is a measure of the degree of antigenic stimulation to which an animal is subjected. IK levels may, therefore, be employed as nonspecific indicators of the prevalence of infectious disease within a population.

Minor antigenic changes in normal body components may also be generated artificially. For example, chemically modified thyroglobulin can be used to stimulate the production of autoantibodies against normal thyroglobulin. It is also possible to render normal tissues antigenic by incorporating them into Freund's complete adjuvant.

Cross-Reactivity with Microorganisms.   In porcine enzootic pneumonia, antibodies to *Mycoplasma hyopneumoniae* cross-react with pig lung, and in contagious bovine pleuropneumonia there is cross-reactivity between *Mycoplasma mycoides* antigens and normal bovine lung. It is not known to what extent autoantibodies of this type contribute to the pathogenesis of these diseases.

It has been suggested that the heart lesions that develop in rheumatic fever in children arise as a result of the production of antibodies to group A streptococci, which cross-react with myocardium. Recent evidence has, however, shown major flaws in the experimental evidence for this, and the myocardial lesions are very different from those associated with other autoimmune diseases.

Development of Previously Suppressed Immunologically Competent Cells. Most autoimmune disorders probably occur as a consequence of the development of cells that had previously been suppressed by the normal control mechanisms of the body. For example, it can be shown that the severity of autoimmune thyroiditis in the OS strain of chickens (page 313) is increased following neonatal thymectomy. It has been suggested that this may be due to the removal of suppressor T cells, which normally prevent the development of an immune response to normal thyroid antigens.

It is not uncommon to find autoimmune disease associated with lymphoid tumors. For example, myasthenia gravis (page 321) may be associated with the presence of a thymoma. In humans, there is a fourfold increase in the incidence of rheumatoid diseases in patients with malignant lymphoid tumors, and there is evidence for a similar association in animals. The reasons for this are poorly understood, but since many lymphoid tumors may arise as a consequence of a failure in immunological control mechanisms, a simultaneous failure in self-tolerance may also occur. Alternatively, some tumors may represent the development of a "forbidden clone" of cells producing autoantibodies. One other possibility that should be considered is that lymphoid tumors may arise as a consequence of the continued stimulation of the immune systems by autoantigens.

Viruses as Inducers of Autoimmunity. A growing body of evidence has served to link many diseases currently considered to be autoimmune to virus infections, and it has been suggested that viruses, particularly those that infect lymphoid tissues, may be capable of interfering with immunological control mechanisms and so permit autoimmunity to occur. Thus, in New Zealand Black (NZB) mice, persistent infection with a type C retrovirus leads to the development of autoantibodies against nucleic acids and erythrocytes. Systemic lupus erythematosus (SLE) of dogs and humans is a similar condition in which the presence of autoantibodies to many different organs is possibly associated with either a type C retrovirus or paramyxovirus infection (see page 324).

MECHANISMS OF TISSUE DAMAGE IN AUTOIMMUNE DISEASE

Autoimmune Reactions Involving Type I Hypersensitivity. Milk allergy in cattle is an autoimmune disorder in which milk α casein, normally found only in the udder, gains access to the general circulation and so stimulates an immune response. This happens when milking is delayed and intramammary pressure forces milk proteins into the circulation. For some reason the immune response stimulated by α casein is of the IgE type, and affected cows show clinical signs of acute systemic anaphylaxis (Chapter 17). A similar condition is seen occasionally in other domestic animals such as the mare. Although antibodies to milk proteins are commonly found in human serum after rapid weaning, type I hypersensitivity is not a usual sequel.

Autoimmune Reactions Involving Type II Hypersensitivity. Autoantibodies directed against cell-surface antigens may cause lysis with the assistance of either complement or cytotoxic cells. If the autoantibodies are directed against erythrocytes, then autoimmune hemolytic anemia may result. If directed against platelets, thrombocytopenia will occur; and if against thyroid cells, thyroiditis will result. In one form of this reaction in humans, autoantibodies directed against thyroid-stimulating-hormone receptors in the thyroid may stimulate thyroid activity rather than mediate its destruction. This antibody is known as long-acting thyroid stimulator (LATS).

Autoimmune Reactions Involving Type III Hypersensitivity. Autoantibodies will form immune complexes when bound to antigen, and these complexes may participate in type III hypersensitivity reactions. This occurs, for example, in systemic lupus erythematosus in the dog, a disease in which a wide variety of autoantibodies are produced, the most significant of which are those directed against nucleic acids. DNA-antibody complexes are formed in affected animals and are deposited in glomeruli to provoke the development of a membranous glomerulonephritis (Chapter 19). Similarly, in rheumatoid arthritis, immune complexes formed between rheumatoid factor (the antibody) and antigen-bound IgG (the antigen) are deposited in joint tissues and, by fixing complement, contribute to the local inflammatory response.

Autoimmune Reactions Involving Type IV Hypersensitivity. Many lesions in autoimmune conditions are heavily infiltrated with mononuclear cells, and it is probable, therefore, that autosensitized T lymphocytes may contribute to the pathogenesis of disease of this type. Examples of such diseases include autoimmune thyroiditis, in which thyroid antigens may be shown to cause macrophage migration inhibition; experimental allergic encephalitis, in which cytotoxic T cells can cause demyelination; and ulcerative colitis, in which cytotoxic T cells may destroy colon cells growing in culture. Another example of a disease that may in some cases be due to a cell-mediated autoimmune response is juvenile diabetes mellitus in humans. In some of these cases, lymphocytes from diabetics have been shown to be cytotoxic for pancreatic islet cells.

AUTOIMMUNE DISEASES OF ANIMALS

Autoimmune disorders may be divided into those affecting mainly one organ or tissue only and those in which a wide variety of organs or tissues are affected.

ORGAN-SPECIFIC AUTOIMMUNE DISEASES

Autoimmune Thyroiditis. Dogs and chickens suffer from a naturally occurring autoimmune thyroiditis, the occurrence of which is genetically determined.

The disease in dogs generally occurs in beagles and is associated with the presence of antibodies against thyroglobulin, against follicular cell microsomes, and against an unidentified colloid antigen. These dogs may also show a delayed hypersensitivity reaction to intradermally injected thyroid extract, suggesting that cell-mediated immune mechanisms may also particpate in the disease process. Histologically, the gland is infiltrated with plasma cells and with large and small lymphocytes to such an extent that germinal center formation may occur (Fig. 21–1).

The clinical signs of autoimmune thyroiditis are those of hypothyroidism — that is, the animals are fat and inactive, they show patchy hair loss, and they are relatively infertile. Tests of thyroid function such as plasma-bound–iodine levels tend to confirm the existence of hypothyroidism, but their usefulness depends upon the severity of the condition. In order to confirm the diagnosis of autoimmune thyroiditis, thyroid biopsy must show the characteristic lymphocytic infiltration, and antithyroid antibodies must be detected in serum. These antibodies may be detected by a number of techniques. For example, a passive hemagglutination test using erythrocytes sensitized with thyroglobulin will detect antibodies to this protein. A complement fixation test will detect

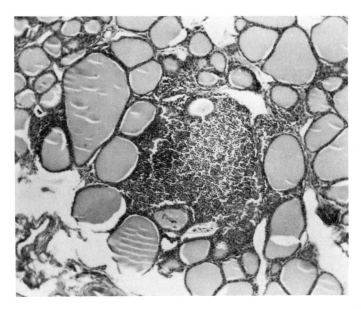

Figure 21-1 A lymphocytic nodule in the thyroid of a beagle suffering from an autoimmune thyroiditis. × 100. (From a specimen kindly provided by Dr. B. N. Wilkie.)

antibodies directed against cytoplasmic antigens in thyroid follicular cells, and an indirect fluorescent antibody test may detect antibodies to a thyroid colloid protein (not thyroglobulin). If none of these relatively sophisticated techniques are available to the clinician, an immunodiffusion test in agar-gel, in which the test serum is reacted against dog thyroid extract, may yield useful results. Appropriate negative controls should be incorporated in all these tests. Treatment of autoimmune thyroiditis involves replacement therapy with thyroxine or desiccated thyroid together with steroids to suppress the immune response.

Autoimmune thyroiditis occurs naturally in the OS (obese) strain of white Leghorn chickens. The normal thyroid tissue of these birds is heavily infiltrated by lymphocytes and plasma cells, which may organize to form germinal centers. Autoantibodies are directed against the thyroglobulin, and affected birds are hypothyroid.

This thyroiditis appears to be the result of several interacting genetic lesions. First, the B cells of these chickens make antithyroglobulin, a trait linked to the major histocompatibility complex. Second, these chickens possess a thymic abnormality that results in unusually early maturation of the T cell system. As a result, autoimmune responses are stimulated before they can be prevented by suppressor cells. Third, these chickens have defective thyroid function in that they are refractory to thyroid stimulating hormone. Neonatal thymectomy prevents the development of lesions, but adult thymectomy may increase its severity by removing suppressor T cells, which presumably moderate the disease.

Autoimmune Encephalitis and Neuritis. Because brain antigens are normally sequestered behind the "blood-brain" barrier, it is relatively easy to induce an experimental autoimmune encephalitis. Known as experimental allergic encephalomyelitis (EAE), this condition may be produced in animals by inoculating them with brain tissue emulsified in Freund's complete adjuvant. After a few weeks, dogs or cats treated in this way show erratic focal encephalitis and myelitis, possibly with paralysis, and the brain lesions consist of focal vasculitis, mononuclear (lymphocyte and macrophage) infiltration associated with perivascular demyelination, and some axon damage. It is possible to detect antibodies to brain tissue in the serum of these animals by means of a complement fixation test, although the lesion itself develops primarily as a result of a cell-mediated autoimmune response.

A clinically significant encephalitis, identical in many features to EAE, occurred following administration of older types of rabies vaccines containing phenolized brain tissue. The clinical signs of this postvaccinal encephalitis appeared between 4 and 15 days after vaccination. For this reason, suckling mouse brain tissue taken prior to myelination is now used in the production of rabies vaccines. It is possible that postdistemper demyelinating leukoencephalopathy is also of autoimmune origin (Chapter 14), although, as pointed out previously, the production of antimyelin antibodies appears to be a frequent sequel to central nervous tissue destruction, regardless of its cause.

If nerve tissue such as that of the sciatic nerve is used to immunize experimental animals, it may lead to the development of an experimental allergic neuritis (EAN) (Fig. 21–2). Like EAE, there is a latent period of 6 to 14 days before an ascending polyneuritis develops, which causes gradual paresis. EAN resembles idiopathic polyneuritis (Guillain-Barré syndrome) in humans, neuritis of the cauda equina in horses, and coonhound paralysis in dogs. It is possible, therefore, but not proved, that these conditions may also be autoimmune disorders. Treatment of this condition in humans involves the use of steroids.

Autoimmune Reproductive Disorders. Orchitis may be produced in animals such as bulls by administration of testicular extracts emulsified in Freund's complete adjuvant. Autoantibodies to sperm may also be detected in the serum of some animals, particularly following injury to the testes or long-standing obstruction of the seminiferous ducts. A typical example of this occurs in male dogs infected with *Brucella*

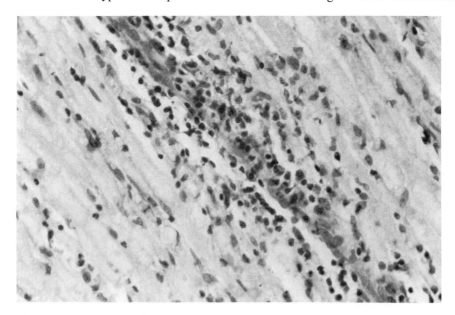

Figure 21–2   A section of rat sciatic nerve showing a mononuclear cell infiltration. This is the lesion of experimental allergic neuritis produced by inoculation of rat sciatic nerve in Freund's complete adjuvant. × 400. (Courtesy of Dr. B. N. Wilkie.)

canis. These animals suffer from a chronic epididymitis and become sensitized by sperm antigens carried to the circulation after phagocytosis by macrophages. These antigens stimulate the production of autoantibodies of the IgG or, less commonly, the IgA class. The autoantibodies agglutinate and immobilize sperm, and, as a consequence, affected animals may be infertile. In cows, antibodies to sperm have been reported to arise as a result of the absorption through the vagina, uterus, fallopian tubes or peritoneum. If these antibodies reach high levels, they may cause infertility.

If dogs are immunized with bovine or ovine luteinizing hormone (LH), then the antibodies produced may cross-react with canine LH and neutralize its activity. Similarly, it has proved possible to provoke autoantibodies that neutralize gonadotrophin-releasing hormone in several species. As a consequence of both these procedures, the reproductive cycle is abolished in females and testicular, epididymal and prostatic atrophy occurs in males, which leads to sterility. This technique shows promise of becoming an effective immunological contraceptive method for animals.

Autoimmune Skin Diseases (Fig. 21–3) Dermatologists, unlike immunologists, have a tendency to use complicated terminology to describe relatively simple conditions. This is especially apparent in the nomenclature of the major autoimmune skin diseases. These diseases usually involve blister or vesicle formation in the skin, and dermatologists use the terms pemphigus or pemphigoid to describe them, after the Greek word *pemphix* meaning "a blister."

PEMPHIGUS. The term pemphigus applies to two skin disorders that occur in humans, dogs, and cats. The more severe form is called pemphigus vulgaris. Bullae (vesicles or blisters) develop around the mucocutaneous junctions, especially the nose, lips, eyes, prepuce and anus, and also on the tongue and the inner surface of the ear. These bullae are fragile and rupture readily, leaving weeping, denuded areas that may become secondarily infected. Histological examination of intact bullae shows a separation of the skin cells (acantholysis) in the suprabasal region of the lower epidermis (Figs. 21–4 and 21–5). Pemphigus vegetans is a very rare and mild variant of pemphigus vulgaris in which either bullae or pustules form and papillomatous proliferation of the base of these occurs on healing.

Pemphigus foliaceous is a milder and much commoner disease than pemphigus vulgaris. It has been described in humans, dogs, cats and horses. It, too, is a vesicular disease, but it is not confined so definitely to the mucocutaneous junctions, and it tends, at least in dogs, to present as a scaling eruptive dermatitis. Histological examination of the bullae reveals that the acantholysis and hence the vesicle formation

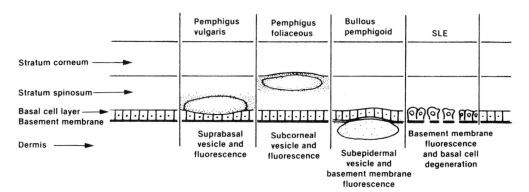

Figure 21–3 The differential histology of the autoimmune skin diseases.

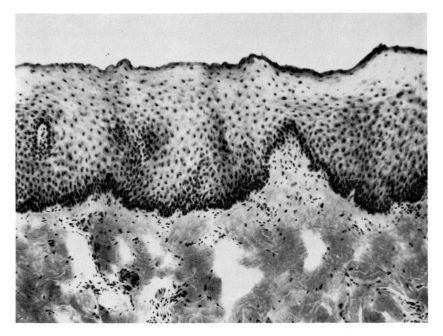

Figure 21–4 A section of normal canine mucous membrane. Note the absence of any cellular separation within the epithelium or between the epithelium and the underlying skin. (From Bennett D, *et al.* 1980. Vet Rec *106* 497. Used with permission.)

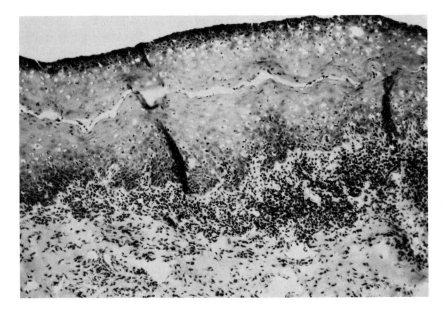

Figure 21–5 A section of an oral lesion of canine pemphigus vulgaris. Note the cleft formation within the epithelium. (From Bennett D, et al. 1980. Vet Rec *106* 497. Used with permission.)

occur superficially in the subcorneal region. The vesicles are very fragile and therefore rarely persist. A milder variant of pemphigus foliaceous is known as pemphigus erythematosus. It may merely be an early stage of pemphigus foliaceous. The lesions in this case tend to be confined to the head and neck and are very similar to those of systemic lupus erythematosus.

All cases of pemphigus arise as a result of the formation of autoantibodies directed against intercellular cement in the skin. The different location of the lesions of pemphigus vulgaris and pemphigus foliaceous is probably due to antigenic differences between intercellular cements in different regions of the skin. The autoantibodies, by binding to intercellular cement, induce nearby cells to release proteinases, which disrupt adhesion between cells to cause acantholysis and bulla formation. Direct immunofluorescent examination of skin lesions reveals immunoglobulins and possibly complement deposited on the intercellular cement (Fig. 21–6).

It is important to differentiate between the two major forms of pemphigus for prognostic reasons. Pemphigus vulgaris has a relatively poor prognosis: treatment tends to be unsatisfactory and the lesions are persistent. Owners of affected animals may become dissatisfied with the intractable disease and request euthanasia. In contrast, pemphigus foliaceous is milder and the results of treatment may be more satisfactory. Treatment of either disease involves the use of prednisolone (2 to 4 mg/kg daily in divided doses) with antibiotic cover. In refractory cases, cyclophosphamide, azathioprine or gold salts may be of assistance. It may be necessary to continue the steroid treatment for a very long time, since the disease often recurs when treatment is stopped.

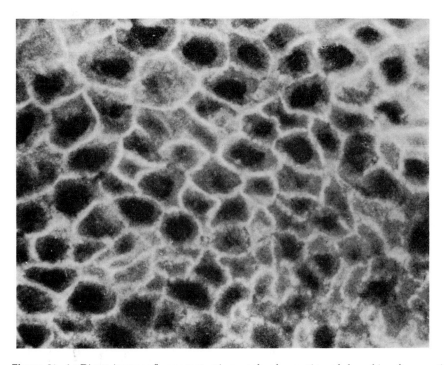

Figure 21–6 Direct immunofluorescent micrograph of a section of dog skin after reacting with serum from a dog suffering from pemphigus. Note staining of the intercellar space substance. (Courtesy of Dr. A. I. Hurvitz.)

BULLOUS PEMPHIGOID.   Bullous pemphigoid is the second most common bullous skin disease in dogs and clinically resembles pemphigus vulgaris. Multiple bullae develop around mucocutaneous junctions and in the groin and axillae. This disease differs from pemphigus vulgaris, however, in that the bullae arise in the subepidermis (Fig. 21–7) (and are therefore less likely to rupture), they tend to be filled with fibrin as well as mononuclear cells or eosinophils, and they heal spontaneously. Bullous pemphigoid is associated with the presence of autoantibodies directed against the basement membrane of the skin and mucous membranes. The deposition of IgG on the basement membrane may be demonstrated by immunofluorescent staining. The prognosis of bullous pemphigoid is good, but recovery may be hastened by the use of steroids.

DERMATITIS HERPETIFORMIS.   Another autoimmune skin disease that has been reported to occur in dogs is dermatitis herpetiformis. In this disease the autoantibodies are directed against antigens in dermal papillae and are usually of the IgA class. Clinically, the lesions are pustular and papular, resembling pyoderma, although there are also eosinophil-filled subepidermal vesicles. The lesions are intensely pruritic. The drug dapsone is the specific treatment for this condition.

Autoimmune Nephritis.   There   are   two   immunopathogenic   types   of glomerulonephritis. In the immune complex type, immune complexes containing complement are deposited in a lumpy, granular fashion on glomerular basement membranes (GBM) (see Fig. 19–7). In contrast, if autoantibodies are produced against GBM antigens, they become deposited in a smooth, linear fashion. These anti-GBM antibodies may be produced experimentally in animals; however, they may arise spontaneously in a condition known as Goodpasture's syndrome in humans. In this

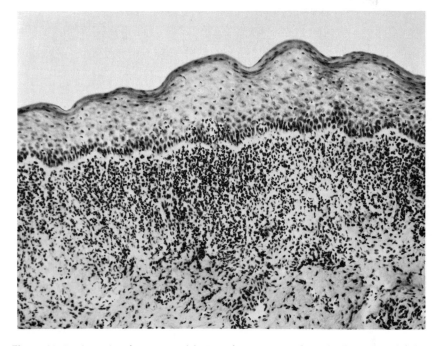

Figure 21–7 A section from an oral lesion of canine pemphigoid. There is a cleft between the epithelium and the underlying dermis. Inflammatory cells are present in the superficial connective tissue and to a lesser extent within the epithelium. (From Bennet D, et al. 1980. Vet Rec *106* 497. Used with permission.)

condition, the autoantibodies react not only with the GBM but also with the basement membrane of pulmonary alveolar septae and capillaries. No condition exactly parallel to Goodpasture's syndrome has been observed to arise spontaneously in animals. However, horses may develop antibodies to GBMs, which may provoke a glomerulonephritis. Clinically, the condition is characterized by signs of renal failure. Immunofluorescent studies of the kidneys of affected animals show the basement membrane to be evenly coated with a smooth, linear deposit of immunoglobulin. As discussed earlier (Chapter 19), these deposits provoke a proliferative response in the glomerular epithelial cells, which, if severe, may result in epithelial crescent formation.

Autoimmune Hemolytic Anemia (AIHA). Autoantibodies to erythrocytes will provoke erythrocyte destruction and thus cause an anemia. This destruction is due either to intravascular hemolysis mediated through complement or, much more commonly, to removal of antibody-coated erythrocytes by the macrophages of the spleen and liver. AIHA is not uncommon in dogs and cats and has been described in horses and cattle. It is commonly associated with other autoimmune disorders, such as systemic lupus erythematosus and autoimmune thrombocytopenia, and with lymphoid tumors such as feline leukemia. Usually, however, AIHA develops without any predisposing cause.

Autoimmune hemolytic anemias may be divided into two major groups depending upon whether the autoantibody is of the IgG or IgM class (Table 21–1).

AIHA MEDIATED BY IgG ANTIBODIES. Most cases of AIHA in dogs and cats are caused by IgG antibodies, which react optimally with red cells at 37°C. Since IgG antibodies are relatively small, they are usually unable to counteract the zeta potential of the red cells and therefore will usually not cause direct agglutination. In a very small proportion of cases, the IgG antibodies may cause direct agglutination, which may then be observed when the blood is withdrawn. Since IgG does not fix complement efficiently, intravascular hemolysis is not a feature of this form of AIHA. The red cells, however, are destroyed by phagocytosis largely in the spleen. In very severe cases, a blood smear may show extensive erythrophagocytosis.

Table 21–1 COMPARISON OF THE MAJOR FORMS OF AUTOIMMUNE HEMOLYTIC ANEMIA

	IgG-MEDIATED	*IgM-MEDIATED*
Optimal temperature	37°C	4° or 37°C
Action of antibody	Incomplete (rarely direct agglutination)	Direct agglutination (4°C) Incomplete antibody (4°C) Hemolysis (37°C)
Fate of erythrocytes	Splenic phagocytosis	Hepatic phagocytosis Intravascular hemolysis
Major clinical findings	Progressive anemia	Necrosis of extremities Progressive anemia
Treatment	Steroids, cytotoxic drugs, splenectomy	Steroids, cytotoxic drugs
Prognosis	Fair to good	Poor

reflecting erythrocyte destruction, although jaundice is uncommon. Most of these animals also have hepatosplenomegaly and lymphadenopathy. IgG-mediated AIHA is diagnosed by demonstrating the presence of nonagglutinating, or incomplete, antibodies on the animal's red cells. This is done by means of a direct antiglobulin or Coombs' test (Chapter 9). The erythrocytes of the affected animal are first washed to remove free serum and then exposed to an antiglobulin serum. Erythrocytes coated with autoantibody will be agglutinated. If the antiglobulin serum possesses anticomplement (anti-C3) activity, it may give a false positive reaction, since positive complement reactions of this type are not uncommon in canine internal diseases.

Treatment of AIHA involves specific management of the anemia and administration of corticosteroids both to cause immunosuppression and to reduce erythrophagocytosis. Steroid treatment may be supplemented with cyclophosphamide in acute cases. Splenectomy may be of assistance in refractory cases.

AIHA MEDIATED BY IgM ANTIBODIES. IgM autoantibodies mediate a different type of disease from that caused by IgG. Some IgM antibodies that act at 37°C activate complement and thus provoke intravascular hemolysis. Other IgM anti–red cell antibodies cannot agglutinate red cells at body temperature but agglutinate them when the blood is chilled. In animals with these "cold-agglutinins," erythrocyte destruction may occur *in vivo*. As blood circulates through an animal's extremities (tail, toes, ears, etc.) it may be cooled significantly; as a result, erythrocyte destruction may occur within capillaries. This can lead to vascular stasis, tissue ischemia and, eventually, necrosis. Affected animals may therefore present with necrotic lesions at the extremities of the body. Anemia may or may not be a significant feature. As might be anticipated, this form of AIHA is most severe during the winter.

Cold agglutinins can be detected by cooling a blood sample to below 20°C, at which point clumping will occur. The agglutination is reversed upon rewarming. Other cold-acting antibodies may combine with red cells when chilled but will not agglutinate them. These antibodies can only be identified by an antiglobulin test conducted at 4°C.

AIHA due to direct-acting agglutinins or to hemolysis is usually of acute onset, is rapidly progressive and has a poor prognosis. Steroids and cyclophosphamide may be used to treat the affected animal. Splenectomy is of little assistance in IgM-mediated AIHA, since the erythrocytes are largely trapped in the liver.

Similar acute anemias have been observed in horses following infection with *Streptococcus fecalis,* in sheep following leptospirosis and in pigs with eperythrozoonosis. In all these cases cold agglutinins are produced, which are capable of clumping erythrocytes from normal animals of the same species when chilled.

Hemoglobin itself may act as an autoantigen on occasion. Antihemoglobin antibodies are detectable in the serum of cattle severely infected with *Corynebacterium pyogenes,* perhaps as a consequence of bacterial hemolysis. The clinical significance of this is not clear.

Immune Suppression of Hematopoiesis. It has been demonstrated in humans, and surmised in dogs, that autoimmune responses may be directed against hematopoietic stem cells. For example, autoantibodies to erythroid precursors may give rise to red cell aplasia, and autoantibodies to myeloid precursors may provoke an immune neutropenia. These conditions can only be diagnosed by demonstrating these autoantibodies by immunofluorescence on bone marrow smears.

Autoimmune Thrombocytopenia. Thrombocytopenia may be induced by the development of antiplatelet autoantibodies. This condition has been reported in horses, dogs and cats. It is observed clinically as a purpura of relatively sudden onset, and it results in the development of petechiae and ecchymoses in the skin and mucous membranes. If severe, epistaxis, hematuria and melena may be seen. The condition is very commonly observed in conjunction with AIHA, systemic lupus erythematosus or lymphoproliferative disorders.

Antibodies to platelets may be measured by a number of techniques, including agglutination, complement fixation, immunofluorescence on megakaryocytes, and antiglobulin tests. However, the best test for this purpose is one that measures the release of factor 3 from platelets as a result of exposure to antibodies directed against the platelet membrane. This may be done by incubating platelets with a globulin fraction of the serum under test and then estimating the amount of procoagulant activity released into the supernatant fluid.

Steroids are used to treat this condition, since they lower the titer of antiplatelet antibody and reduce platelet sequestration by mononuclear phagocytes. As with AIHA, splenectomy or azathioprine treatment or both may be of assistance in the control of patients who do not respond to steroid therapy.

Sjögren's Syndrome. In this disease, which has been described in both humans and dogs, autoimmunity develops against exocrine glands, most notably the lacrimal and salivary glands. As a result, the secretion of these glands is greatly reduced and affected animals suffer from corneal dryness resulting in keratoconjunctivitis sicca and xerostomia (mouth dryness). These animals subsequently develop gingivitis, dental caries and excessive thirst.

Sjögren's syndrome is often associated with rheumatoid arthritis, systemic lupus erythematosus, polymyositis and autoimmune thyroiditis. The first two cases described in dogs were found in a colony maintained for investigations into canine systemic lupus erythematosus.

The condition may be treated by palliative dentistry and artificial tears. It would be logical to use immunosuppressive agents in refractory cases.

Myasthenia Gravis. Myasthenia gravis, a disease of humans, dogs and cats, is a disorder of skeletal muscle characterized by the occurrence of abnormal fatigue and weakness after relatively mild exercise. For example, a dog with myasthenia gravis will collapse exhausted after trotting for only a few yards. Myasthenia gravis occurs as a result of a blockage or deficiency of acetylcholine receptors on the motor end plate of striated muscle. In Jack Russell terriers, Springer spaniels and fox terriers, a congenital form of the disease occurs as a result of an inherited deficiency of receptors. It is, therefore, a disease of young dogs. In adult dogs, however, an effective receptor deficiency occurs as a result of the production of autoantibodies to the acetylcholine receptors. Not only do these antibodies block the receptors, they also accelerate their degradation. As a result, the number of effective acetylcholine receptors is drastically reduced. Consequently, the end-plate potentials induced at the neuromuscular junctions fall below threshold levels and fail to trigger the muscle to contract. Repeating the stimulus is ineffective, since all available receptors are saturated with acetylcholine.

In some animals with myasthenia gravis, the thymus may show medullary hyperplasia, germinal center formation or even a thymoma. Since normal thymus tissue contains a population of "myoid" cells, which are striated muscle cells that possess acetylcholine receptors of their own, it is possible that the thymic changes result from immunological attack on myoid cells. Alternatively, since the thymic hormone thymopoietin is capable of neuromuscular blocking activity, thymoma-associated myasthenia may be due to excessive thymopoietin production. This is supported by the observation in humans that thymectomy usually, but not always, leads to significant remission of the disease.

Myasthenia gravis is a clinically obvious disease, and it is normally not necessary to resort to laboratory tests. Administration of a short-acting anticholinesterase such as edrophonium (1 to 2 mg intravenously) will lead to dramatic clinical improvement within seconds. The anticholinesterase, by permitting the acetylcholine to persist, enables it to stimulate the remaining receptors more effectively. It is possible to demonstrate the presence of antireceptor antibodies by means of a radioimmunoassay. In humans, but not in dogs, antimuscle antibodies may be detected by immunofluorescence. Their significance is unknown.

Myasthenia gravis is treated by means of long-acting anticholinesterase drugs such as pyridostigmine or neostigmine. In humans with myasthenia gravis, immunosuppressive therapy with corticosteroids, plasmapheresis and cyclophosphamide has been used with success.

DISEASES OF WIDE ORGAN SPECIFICITY ASSOCIATED WITH AUTOIMMUNE COMPONENTS

In addition to the organ-specific autoimmune conditions discussed so far, there exist a number of diseases that involve many organs throughout the body and that are, at least in part, autoimmune.

Systemic Lupus Erythematosus. Systemic lupus erythematosus (SLE) is a generalized immunologic disorder, that has been described in humans, dogs and cats. About 75 per cent of the reported canine cases have occurred in females.

SLE occurs as a result of a loss of overall control of the specificity of the B-cell system. In some, but not all, cases this has been associated with defective suppressor cell function. As a result of this loss of control, affected animals make autoantibodies against a great range of normal organs and tissues. These multiple autoantibodies in turn give rise to a wide spectrum of pathological lesions and clinical manifestations.

One consistent feature of SLE is the development of autoantibodies against nucleic acids. Several different antinuclear antibody systems have been described in the disease, the most important of which are antibodies to DNA. These autoantibodies can cause damage by several mechanisms. They can combine with free DNA to form DNA–anti-DNA immune complexes. These immune complexes may be deposited in glomeruli (Chapter 19), causing a membranous glomerulonephritis and giving rise to a "wire-loop" lesion in the glomerular tufts. The complexes may also be deposited in arteriolar walls, where they result in local fibrinoid necrosis and fibrosis, or in synovia, where they provoke arthritis. Antinuclear antibodies also bind to the nuclei of degenerating cells. In tissues this results in the presence of round or oval masses of DNA bound to antibody, known as hematoxylin bodies; these are found in the skin, kidney, lung, lymph nodes, spleen and heart. Within the blood vascular system these "opsonized" nuclei may be phagocytosed, giving rise to the structures known as lupus erythematosus (LE) cells (Fig. 21–8). LE cells are found mainly in bone marrow and, less commonly, in blood.

Although antibodies to nucleic acids are important features of SLE, a great variety of other autoantibodies are also produced. Autoantibodies to red cells, for example, commonly give rise to an antiglobulin-positive hemolytic anemia. Antibodies

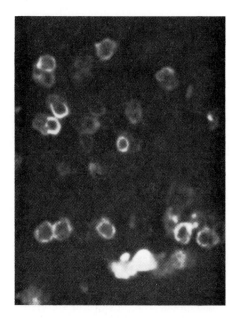

Figure 21–8 A positive ANA reaction (titer 1:160) showing rim fluorescence, from a dog with SLE. × 450. (From Quimby FW, et al. 1980. Am J Vet Res *41* 1662. Used with permission.)

to platelets give rise to an immunologically mediated thrombocytopenia. Antilymphocyte antibodies may be present, and it is suggested that they may selectively destroy suppressor cells, thus enhancing the excessive immune reactivity. Antimuscle antibodies may provoke myositis, and antimyocardial antibodies may provoke myocarditis or endocarditis. Antibodies to skin components give rise to a characteristic bilaterally symmetrical dermatitis characterized by changes in the thickness of the epidermis, focal mononuclear cell infiltration, collagen degeneration and immunoglobulin deposits at the dermo-epidermal junction. (see Fig. 21–3). The lesions are commonly restricted to the bridge of the nose and the area around the eyes. The results of this grossly excessive immune reactivity are also reflected in a polyclonal hypergammaglobulinemia, enlargement of lymph nodes with medullary disruption, and thymic enlargement with germinal center formation.

The great variety of autoantibodies produced in SLE can give rise to an equally great variety of clinical manifestations. A simple diagnostic rule could, therefore, be stated as follows: Suspect SLE in an animal with multiple autoimmune disorders and either a positive test for antinuclear antibodies or a positive test for LE cells (Table 21–2).

Table 21–2 THE DIAGNOSTIC CRITERIA FOR SYSTEMIC LUPUS
ERYTHEMATOSUS

Any two of the following:
    Characteristic skin lesions
    Polyarthritis
    Antiglobulin-positive hemolytic anemia
    Thrombocytopenia
    Proteinuria

and either
    A positive ANA test or a positive LE cell test

Antinuclear antibodies are generally demonstrated by immunofluorescence. The target may be either cultured cells or frozen sections of mouse or rat liver. Dilutions of a patient's serum are applied to this, and the material is incubated and then washed off. The binding of antinuclear antibodies to the cell nuclei is revealed by incubating the tissue in a fluorescent labeled antiserum to canine or feline immunoglobulins and then re-washing. A variety of different nuclear staining patterns have been described for humans, and their clinical correlations have been analyzed. In animals, staining patterns have been less thoroughly investigated, and their significance is currently unclear. Some authorities believe that a granular or rim fluorescence pattern is most significant (Fig. 21–8).

LE cells, as previously described, are polymorphonuclear neutrophils (PMNs) that have phagocytosed nuclei from effete cells. They therefore look somewhat like binucleated cells (Fig. 21–9). Their presence may be detected in the bone marrow and occasionally in buffy coat preparations from animals with SLE. It is usually necessary, however, to attempt to produce them *in vitro*. This can be accomplished by allowing the blood of an affected animal to clot and incubating it at 37° C for two hours. During this time, normal PMNs will phagocytose the nuclei of any effete or damaged cells. The clot is then disrupted by pressing it through a fine mesh, the resulting cell suspension is centrifuged, and the buffy coat is examined. The presence of LE cells is essentially pathognomonic for SLE, but their absence is not, since only 60 per cent of affected animals are positive in any one sample. Some normal dogs and some dogs with liver disease or lymphosarcoma may have detectable antinuclear antibodies, so both of these tests must be interpreted only in close conjunction with the clinical picture.

PATHOGENESIS OF SLE (Fig. 21–10).   Although it is clear that SLE involves a loss of control of the specificity of the B-cell response with resulting multiple autoimmune disorders, the initiating cause remains obscure. There is good evidence for a genetic predisposition in humans, since SLE is associated with an increased familial incidence and the presence of certain histocompatibility antigens. The bulk of the present evidence suggests that a virus infection is responsible for initiation of the condition. Various viruses have been implicated. Thus, individuals with SLE commonly have high titered antibodies to parainfluenza 1 and measles. Myxovirus-like

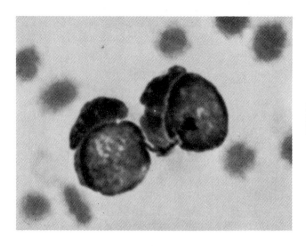

Figure 21–9 Two LE cells from a dog with SLE. × 1000. (From Quimby FW, et al. Am J Vet Res *41* 1662. With permission.)

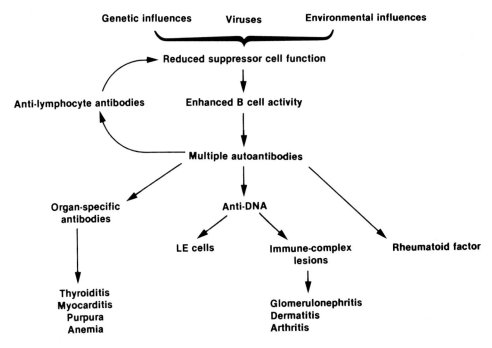

Figure 21–10   A speculative scheme for the pathogenesis of SLE.

structures have been observed within renal endothelial cells from SLE patients. Similarly, certain type C retroviruses have been isolated from SLE patients and associated with the disease.

When dogs affected by SLE are bred, the number of affected offspring is higher than can be accounted for genetically, suggesting that the condition can be vertically transmitted. Cell-free filtrates from asymptomatic but LE cell–positive dogs, when administered to newborn mice, have been reported to provoke the appearance of antinuclear antibodies and the development of some lymphoid tumors. Type C viruses have been isolated from these tumors, and antisera to these viruses may be used to demonstrate viral antigen on the lymphocytes and in the glomeruli of humans with SLE. Cell-free filtrates of these mouse tumors have also been reported to induce the formation of antinuclear antibodies and the production of LE cells in newborn puppies.

TREATMENT OF SLE.   SLE usually responds well to corticosteroids (prednisolone).

Discoid Lupus Erythematosus.   Discoid lupus erythematosus is a mild variant of SLE characterized by the occurrence of subepidermal deposits of immunoglobulin in skin lesions and the absence of other pathological lesions as well as negative ANA and LE tests. The distribution of the skin lesions, as in SLE, may be restricted to the bridge of the nose and the area around the eyes. Discoid LE has been described in dogs, especially Shetland sheep dogs.

Rheumatoid Arthritis.   Rheumatoid arthritis is a common, crippling disease in humans that is also seen in domestic animals, especially dogs. Although, as its name suggests, it typically involves the joints, other body systems are commonly affected. Dogs with rheumatoid arthritis may present with depression, anorexia and pyrexia in addition to lameness, which tends to be most severe after inactivity (for example, immediately after awakening in the morning) and mainly affects peripheral joints, which show swelling and stiffness. The joint swelling is often symmetrical. Rheumatoid arthritis tends to pursue a progressive course and eventually leads to severe joint destruction and deformities. In advanced cases the joints may even fuse as the result of the formation of bony ankyloses. Radiological findings are variable, but the swelling is generally seen to involve soft tissues only, and there may be subchondral rarefaction, cartilage erosion and narrowing of the joint space.

Histologically, the disease commences as synovitis characterized by extensive infiltration by neutrophils. As the disease progresses, the synovia swell and begin to proliferate. Outgrowths of this proliferating synovia extend into the joint cavities, where they are known as pannus. Pannus consists of fibrous, vascular tissue, that, as it invades the joint cavity, releases proteolytic enzymes that erode the articular cartilage and the neighbouring bony structures. As the arthritis progresses, the infiltrating neutrophils may be partially replaced by lymphocytes, which can form lymphoid nodules and germinal centers. Another feature of rheumatoid arthritis that is commonly encountered is the development of subcutaneous nodules — necrotic foci surrounded by fibrous connective tissue containing lymphocytes and plasma cells. In addition, amyloidosis, disseminated arteritis, glomerulonephritis and lymphatic hyperplasia are occasional complications.

The immediate cause of rheumatoid arthritis is unknown. It is probably due to the chronic deposition of immune complexes in synovia. The offending antigen has not been identified, but development of autoantibodies to IgG is characteristic of the disease. These autoantibodies, called rheumatoid factors, are of the IgM class and are directed against determinants in the C_H2 regions of antigen-bound IgG. Rheumatoid factors are found not only in rheumatoid arthritis but also in SLE and other conditions in which extensive immune-complex formation occurs.

Rheumatoid factors may be detected by allowing them to agglutinate antibody-coated particles. In humans, latex coated with IgG is used for this purpose. In dogs, it is easier to make a canine antisheep erythrocyte serum and to coat sheep erythrocytes with this in a subagglutinating dose. After washing, these erythrocytes will agglutinate when mixed with positive dog serum. In humans this technique is known as the Rose-Waaler test.

Although rheumatoid factors are of great diagnostic importance, their clinical significance is unclear. Rheumatoid factors can be found in joint fluid, where their titer tends to correlate with the severity of the lesions, and the lesions themselves may be exacerbated by intra-articular inoculation of autologous immunoglobulins. Nevertheless, some individuals with rheumatoid arthritis may not have detectable rheumatoid factors, and it is not uncommon to find humans who have no arthritis despite the presence of rheumatoid factor in their serum.

Over many years, attempts have been made to associate rheumatoid arthritis with infectious agents. Thus, mycoplasmas such as *Mycoplasma hyorhinis* and bacteria such as *Erysipelothrix insidiosa* (*E. rhusiopathiae*) produce a chronic nonsuppurative arthritis in pigs with a histological picture very similar to that seen in rheumatoid arthritis in humans. In spite of this and occasional reports of the isolation of bacteria or mycoplasmas from rheumatoid joints, no definite evidence is yet available to substantiate an infectious basis for this condition.

Diagnosis of rheumatoid arthritis in animals (Table 21–3) is generally based on the criteria established for human rheumatoid arthritis. At least five of the clinical features should be present and any one of the first five shown in Table 21–3 should

Table 21-3 THE DIAGNOSTIC CRITERIA FOR CANINE RHEUMATOID
ARTHRITIS

---

*Any five of the following signs must be present. One of the first five features on the list
must be present for at least six weeks, and ANA or LE tests must be negative.*
  Morning stiffness
  Pain on moving a joint
  Soft tissue swelling
  Swelling of at least one other joint within a three-month period
  Symmetrical joint swelling

  Subcutaneous nodules
  Consistent radiographic findings
  Presence of rheumatoid factor
  Characteristic synovial histology
  Characteristic nodule histology
  Poor mucin production in synovial fluid*

---

*This diagnostic test involves treating a synovial fluid sample with glacial acetic acid. This causes
the protein in the sample to clot. The clot from normal joint fluid forms a solid mass. The clot from
rheumatoid joints tends to be loose and friable.

have been present for at least six weeks. In addition, steps should be taken to exclude
SLE (by testing for antinuclear antibody) and to exclude an infectious cause for the
arthritis.

Salicylates such as acetylsalicylic acid are the drugs of first choice in treating
early, uncomplicated cases. Steroids such as prednisolone should be reserved for late,
severe cases in which salicylates have proved inadequate. This is because steroids,
although they produce dramatic clinical remissions, permit articular damage to proceed
unabated.

Feline Chronic Progressive Polyarthritis. This disease of male cats is characterized by polyarthritis with either osteopenia and periosteal new bone formation,
periarticular erosions and eventual collapse or subchondral erosions, joint instabilities
and deformities closely resembling those of rheumatoid arthritis. Affected cats may be
infected with feline syncytia-forming virus or feline leukemia virus, or both. It is
described here because of suggestions that it is of immunological origin. These
suggestions are based on the massive mononuclear cell infiltration of affected joints
and the presence of an immune complex type of glomerulonephritis. However, affected cats are rheumatoid factor– and ANA-negative, and their serum immunoglobulin levels tend to be close to normal.

Other Conditions Involving Autoimmunity. Although, theoretically, autoimmune disorders may involve any tissue in the body and in practice many can be
experimentally induced, the range of naturally occurring autoimmune disorders in
animals is not wide. As has been pointed out, the presence of autoantibodies is
insufficient by itself to identify a disease as autoimmune. For example, autoantibodies
commonly arise following tissue damage. Thus, antibodies directed against mitochon-
drial antigens develop in animals suffering from liver or heart damage. In diseases
such as trypanosomiasis or tuberculosis in which widespread tissue disturbances occur,
autoantibodies to a wide range of tissue antigens may be detected at low titers in
serum.

In order for a disease to be identified as autoimmune, the disease process must,
therefore, be demonstrated to occur as a consequence of the autoimmune response.
Thus, the autoantibodies should be detectable in all cases of the disease. The disease

should be experimentally reproducible by some form of immunization with the anti-gen, and the disease should be transferable from an affected animal to a normal animal by means of either serum or living lymphoid cells.

ADDITIONAL SOURCES OF INFORMATION

Alexander JW. 1978. Rhematoid arthritis in the dog. Canine Practice 5 41–45.

Banks KL. 1979. Antiglomerular basement membrane antibody in horses. Am J Path 94 443–446.

Drachman DB. 1978. Myasthenia gravis. N Engl J Med 298 136–142, 186–193.

Dumonde DC (ed). 1976. Infections and Immunology in the Rheumatic Diseases. Blackwell, Oxford.

Fauci AS. 1980. Immunoregulation in autoimmunity. J Allergy Clin Immunol 66 5–17.

Halliwell REW. 1978. Autoimmune disease in the dog. Adv Vet Sci Comp Med 22 221–263.

Kae I, and Drachman DB. 1977. Thymic muscle cells bear acetylcholine receptors: possible relation to myasthenia gravis. Science 195 74–75.

Pedersen NC, Pool RR, and O'Brien T. 1980. Feline chronic progressive polyarthritis. Am J Vet Res 41 522–535.

Quimby FW, Jensen C, Nawrocki D, and Scollin P. 1978. Selected autoimmune diseases in the dog. Vet Clin North Am (Small Animal Practice) 8 665–682.

Quimby FW, Smith C, Brushwein M, and Lewis RW. 1980. Efficacy of immunodiagnostic procedures in the recognition of canine immunologic disease. Am J Vet Res 41 1662–1666.

Schwartz RS. 1975. Viruses and systemic lupus erythematosus. N Engl J Med 293 132–136.

Wick G, Sundick RS, and Albini B. 1974. A review. The obese strain (OS) of chickens: and animal model with spontaneous autoimmune thyroiditis. Clin Immunol Immunopathol 3 272–300.

Wilkins RJ, Hurvitz AI, and Dodds-Laffin WJ. 1973. Immunologically mediated thrombocytopenia in the dog. JAVMA 163 277–282.

22

Defects in the Immune System: Immunological Deficiencies, Neoplasia and Hyperactivity

This chapter considers disorders of the immune system that are reflected in either immunological deficiency or hyperactivity. The former group includes deficiencies that may arise in animals as a result of either inherited defects in the development of the immune system or tumors of that system.

The diseases that produce, or are a consequence of, hyperactivity of cells of the immune system include some tumors such as the myelomas, which consist of plasma cells that secrete excessive quantities of a uniform immunoglobulin product; the autoimmune disorders discussed in the previous chapter; certain infectious diseases such as Aleutian disease of mink (discussed in Chapter 14); and amyloidosis, a condition that probably arises, at least in some instances, as a result of an attempt on the part of the body to control immunological hyperactivity. The two classes of generalized disorders, deficiency and hyperactivity, are also linked in that the commitment to production of neoplastic lymphoid tumor cells generally renders an animal immunodeficient by default.

IMMUNODEFICIENCIES

Any failure of the immune system and its associated systems, such as the mononuclear-phagocytic system, usually becomes apparent as a result of the increased susceptibility of affected animals to infectious diseases. Because of the nature of medical care, these conditions have been investigated primarily in humans, as infants, who would otherwise die, are kept alive by intensive efforts and the nature of their veterinary medicine, individual animals are unlikely to either receive this amount of attention or be so thoroughly investigated. Nevertheless, on the basis of the immunodeficiency syndromes studied so far, it is apparent that the same types of inherited deficiencies occur in both man and domestic animals.

INHERITED DEFECTS IN ANTIGEN PROCESSING

Two major classes of congenital deficiency syndromes associated with phagocytic failure have been reported in humans. In one there is a failure in opsonization; in the other there is a failure in intracellular killing.

Failures in opsonization have so far not been recorded as occurring in the domestic animals. If such a deficiency is suspected, it is possible to measure the opsonic activity of a serum by a simple test in which bacteria, phagocytic cells (such as buffy coat cells) and serum are mixed and incubated. After a standard period the cells may be fixed, stained and examined for the presence of phagocytosed bacteria. By comparing the phagocytic activity of cells from a normal animal in the presence of normal and suspect serum, a rough indication of the opsonic activity of the serum may be obtained.

The most important phagocytic deficiency syndrome to occur in humans is known as chronic granulomatous disease. This has not yet been reported as occurring in domestic animals. Children affected with chronic granulomatous disease suffer from recurrent infections characterized by the development of septic granulomata in lymph nodes, lungs, bones and skin. Analysis of the defect reveals that the neutrophils of these children are less capable than normal cells of destroying organisms such as staphylococci and coliforms. It is probable that the specific defect is an absence of the lysosomal enzyme superoxide dismutase. As a consequence of this, the generation of oxidizing radicals by the respiratory burst fails to occur (Chapter 2), and the bactericidal efficiency of the neutrophils is grossly impaired. This impairment may be detected by incubating the neutrophils of an affected individual in nitro-blue tetrazolium. Normal cells degrade this to produce a black formazan deposit, whereas defective cells do not.

Although chronic granulomatous disease has not yet been reported to occur in animals, three other phagocytic deficiency syndromes have. One, the Chédiak-Higashi syndrome, is an inherited disease of cattle (particularly Herefords), Aleutian mink, Persian cats, white tigers, killer whales and humans. It is associated with a defect in cell structure that results in the production of abnormally large primary granules in neutrophils and eosinophils and in enlarged melanin granules (Fig. 22–1). The abnormal melanin granules give rise to a very pale coat color and light-colored irises (pseudoalbinism). Cats with this condition have a red fundic light reflection rather than the normal yellow-green. The primary granules of affected animals are more fragile than those of normal animals, rupturing spontaneously and causing tissue damage, such as cataracts. The leukocytes of these animals have defective chemotactic responsiveness and a reduced capacity for intracellular killing. The Chédiak-Higashi gene also regulates the development of natural killer cells, which may be reflected in an increased susceptibility to tumors and to some viruses such as the Aleutian disease agent. Affected animals commonly succumb to recurrent pyogenic bacterial infections or lymphoid tumors. The Chédiak-Higashi syndrome may be diagnosed either by examining a stained blood smear for the presence of grossly enlarged primary granules within leukocytes or by examining hair shafts for enlarged melanin granules.

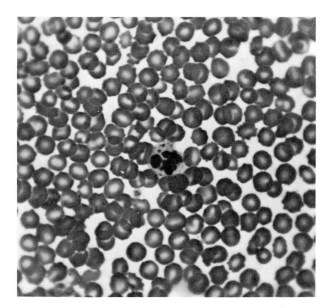

Figure 22–1 A neutrophil from an Aleutian mink. The large dark granules in this cell are abnormal primary granules and are characteristic of the Chédiak-Higashi syndrome. × 750. (From a specimen kindly provided by Dr. S. H. An.)

The canine granulocytopathy syndrome is an autosomal recessive condition observed in Irish setters. These dogs suffer from recurrent severe bacterial infections, especially suppurative skin lesions, gingivitis and lymphadenopathy. Affected dogs may have a pronounced leukocytosis, and their neutrophils are morphologically normal. In spite of this, these cells are unable to kill opsonized *E. coli* or *Staph. aureus* organisms. Closer examination of the neutrophils of these dogs has shown that their respiratory burst is depressed, as reflected by a decrease in glucose oxidation. Nevertheless, they are more effective than normal cells at reducing nitro-blue tetrazolium, implying that O_2^- is produced in greater quantities than normal. Further studies are clearly needed to clarify the precise nature of the defect of these cells in microbial killing.

The third genetically determined neutrophil defect reported to occur in animals is the Gray collie syndrome. This is a disease seen in collie dogs. It is associated with abnormal skin pigmentation, eye lesions and cyclical neutropenia. The loss of neutrophils occurs about every 11 days, and in their absence the animals become severely infected. They suffer from severe enteric disease, respiratory infections, bone disease and lymphadenitis. Immunoglobulin levels are somewhat elevated as a result of the recurrent antigenic stimulation. If affected animals are kept alive by aggressive antibiotic therapy, the continued stimulation of their lymphoid tissues may lead to the development of amyloidosis. The nature of the defect is not clear but appears to be due to the presence of a block in neutrophil maturation within the bone marrow and to a myeloperoxidase deficiency.

INHERITED DEFICIENCIES IN THE IMMUNE SYSTEM

The consequences of inherited immunological defects have served as excellent indicators of the site of the genetic lesion and have confirmed the overall arrangement

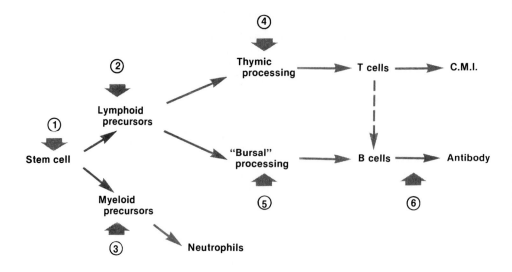

1 Reticular dysgenesis
2 Severe combined immunodeficiency
3 Neutrophil defects
4 Thymic aplasia
5 Agammaglobulinemia
6 Deficiencies in individual immunoglobulins

Figure 22–2 The points in the immune system at which development blocks may lead to immune deficiencies.

of the immune system, as outlined in Figure 22–2. For example, if both the cell- and antibody-mediated immune responses are deficient, it may be assumed that the genetic lesion operates at a point prior to the points of both thymic and bursal cell processing — that is, it is a stem-cell lesion. A defect that occurs only in thymic development will be reflected in an inability to mount a cell-mediated immune response, although antibody production will be normal. Similarly, a lesion restricted to the B cell system will be reflected in an absence of antibody-mediated immune responses.

Immunodeficiencies of Horses (Fig. 22–3). Horses are among the few domestic animals whose economic worth has permitted a thorough analysis of neonatal mortality. As a result, a significant number of primary immunodeficiency syndromes have been identified.

COMBINED IMMUNODEFICIENCY. Probably the most important equine immunodeficiency is the combined immunodeficiency syndrome (CID) of Arabian foals. Affected foals fail to produce functional T or B cells. As a result, they are born with very few circulating lymphocytes. If they suckle successfully they will acquire maternal immunoglobulins. Once these have been catabolized, however, the foal is unable to produce its own antibodies and eventually becomes totally agammaglobulinemic. Affected foals are, therefore, born healthy, but they sicken by two months of age. All are usually dead by 4 to 6 months as a result of overwhelming infection by a variety of low-grade pathogens. Organisms that have been implicated in these deaths include adenovirus, *Pneumocystis carinii* (an ill-defined protozoan-like organism), *Cryptosporidium* (a coccidian) and many different bacteria.

On necropsy, the spleen of affected animals is found to be devoid of both germinal centers and periarteriolar lymphoid sheaths. The lymph nodes lack lymphoid

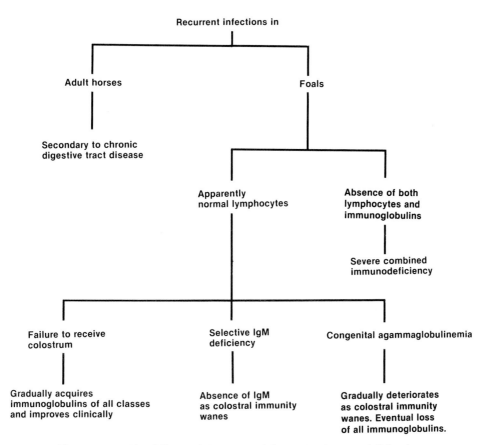

Figure 22—3 The differential diagnosis of the equine immunodeficiencies.

follicles and germinal centers and are depleted of cells in the paracortical zone, and the thymus is severely hypoplastic. Effective treatment is not possible, although several unsuccessful attempts have been made to reconstitute these animals with grafts of fetal equine liver, thymus or bone marrow.

CID is inherited in an autosomal recessive manner, and its occurrence indicates that both parents carry the offending gene. Accurate diagnosis is therefore of great importance, since it significantly reduces the economic value of the parent animals. The diagnosis of CID requires that at least two of the following three criteria be established: (1) Very low (consistently below 1000/cu mm) or no circulating lymphocytes; (2) histology typical of CID, that is, gross hypoplasia of the primary and secondary lymphoid organs; and (3) an absence of serum IgM. (Maternal antibody provides serum IgG, whereas IgM is the first immunoglobulin synthesized by the newborn foal.) If at all possible it should be shown that the foal is unable to mount both cellular and humoral immune responses.

The presence of humoral immunity may be demonstrated by injecting an antigen, such as sheep erythrocytes, antibodies to which are not present in equine colostrum. Antibodies appear in normal foals two to three weeks after a single inoculation of sheep erythrocytes.

By using large quantities of blood it is possible to obtain sufficient lymphocytes and demonstrate that they are unreactive to mitogens such as phytohemagglutinin

(Chapter 7). It may also be possible to attempt to provoke a type IV hypersensitivity reaction by painting the skin with a contact allergen such as dinitrochlorobenzene or by inoculating the T-cell mitogen phytohemagglutinin intradermally.

AGAMMAGLOBULINEMIA.   At least two cases of primary agammaglobulinemia have been described in foals. The animals were devoid of identifiable B cells (cells with surface immunoglobulin) and were almost totally devoid of all immunoglobulins. Their lymphoid tissues had no primary follicles, germinal centers or plasma cells. Nevertheless, they possessed circulating blood lymphocytes that could respond to phytohemagglutinin and produce migration inhibitory factor. Intradermal inoculation of phytohemagglutinin caused a type IV delayed hypersensitivity reaction. Both animals suffered from recurrent bacterial infections but survived for 17 to 18 months.

SELECTIVE IgM DEFICIENCY.   Several cases of equine IgM deficiency have been described. The foals suffered from recurrent respiratory tract infections often involving *Klebsiella pneumoniae*. Their immune functions appeared to be normal in all respects except for very low or absent IgM.

SELECTIVE IgG DEFICIENCY.   A single case of putative IgG deficiency has been described in a 3-month-old foal with salmonellosis. The animal had normal IgA and IgM but no germinal centers, lymphoid follicles, splenic follicles or periarteriolar lymphoid sheaths. Serum IgG was extremely low.

TRANSIENT HYPOGAMMAGLOBULINEMIA.   Between two and three months of age, some foals experience a transient episode of hypogammaglobulinemia as a result of a delayed onset of immunoglobulin synthesis. These animals may suffer from recurrent infections during the period when immunoglobulin levels are low.

The most important immunological defect in foals is not inherited but results from a failure to absorb sufficient colostral antibody from the mare (see Chapter 11). This may affect up to 10 per cent of all foals. Combined immunodeficiency occurs in 2 to 3 per cent of Arab foals (the gene is carried by 28 to 30 per cent of these horses) and is 10 times more common than selective IgM deficiency. Selective IgM deficiency is, in turn, 10 times more common than agammaglobulinemia.

Immunodeficiencies of Cattle. TRAIT A-46.   Certain Black Pied Danish cattle carry an autosomal recessive trait (trait A-46) of thymic and lymphocytic hypoplasia. Affected calves are born healthy, but by four to eight weeks they begin to suffer from severe skin infections. If untreated, they die a few weeks later, and none survive for longer than four months. Affected calves have exanthema, hair loss on the legs, and parakeratosis around the mouth and eyes. It can be shown that these animals are deficient in T cells and have depressed cell-mediated immunity but normal antibody responses. Thus they have a normal response to tetanus toxoid but respond poorly to dinitrochlorobenzene or tuberculin. If these calves are treated by oral zinc oxide, they recover fully and acquire the ability to mount normal cell-mediated responses. The precise mechanisms are unknown, but it is probable that these animals inefficiently absorb zinc from the intestine. T cells require zinc in order to respond to antigen.

SELECTIVE IgG2 DEFICIENCY.   IgG2 deficiency has been reported in Red Danish cattle. About 1 to 2 per cent of this breed are completely deficient in this immu-noglobulin subclass and as a result suffer from an increased susceptibility to pneu-monias and gangrenous mastitis. In addition, up to 15 per cent of this breed have subnormal IgG2 levels, although they do not appear to suffer any ill effects in consequence.

Immunodeficiencies of Dogs.   Some lines of inbred Weimaraners show a wasting disease as a result of thymic atrophy. These animals have normal γ globulin levels, but their response to T-cell mitogens is depressed. A selective IgM deficiency has been reported in Doberman pinschers; it was associated with only a chronic nasal discharge, so its significance is in doubt. The death of six male miniature dachshunds from *P. carinii* pneumonia has led to the suggestion that they were suffering from an immunodeficiency. This was not proven, although *P. carinii* is usually found only in immunosuppressed or immunodeficient animals.

Immunodeficiencies of Chickens. Birds of the hypothyroid OS strain have a selective IgA deficiency. Birds of the UCD 140 line have a selective IgG deficiency known as hereditary dysgammaglobulinemia. These birds have normal immunoglobulin levels for about 50 days after hatching; then their IgG drops and their IgM rises. This is probably because of the development of specific suppressor cells. In addition to the hypogammaglobulinemia, these birds show evidence of immune complex lesions; it has been suggested that this condition is mediated by a vertically transmitted virus.

Immunodeficiencies of Humans. A large number of well-characterized immunodeficiency syndromes have been reported in humans. It is anticipated that, in the future, investigators will succeed in identifying most of these syndromes in domestic animals as well.

The most severe immunodeficiency state in humans results from a defect in the development of primordial stem cells, as a result of which neither myeloid nor lymphoid cells develop. This condition, known as reticular dysgenesis, results in the very early death of affected individuals. An only slightly less severe disease occurs as a result of failure of the lymphoid stem cells to develop. The resulting lesion gives rise to combined immunodeficiency disease. In humans, some of these cases are due to a congenital deficiency of the enzymes adenine deaminase or purine nucleoside phosphorylase. Deficiency of adenine deaminase results in the accumulation of excessive adenosine, which suppresses T-cell function by stimulating cyclic AMP production. A deficiency of purine nucleoside phosphorylase results in accumulation of lymphotoxic deoxyribonucleotides.

Humans may be born with congenital defects in thymic function. The most severe of these conditions, DiGeorge's syndrome, results from a failure of the third and fourth thymic pouches to develop. In consequence, little or no thymic epithelial tissue develops and few, if any, cells populate the T-dependent areas of the secondary lymphoid tissues. Since these individuals have no functional T cells, they can neither mount a delayed hypersensitivity reaction nor reject allogeneic tissue grafts. The importance of the T-cell system in providing protection against virus diseases is emphasized by the observation that individuals with DiGeorge's syndrome generally die from virus infections but remain resistant to bacterial invasion.

A variety of other congenital T-cell lesions have been described in man. They are generally associated with a poorly developed thymus, lymphopenia and deficient cell-mediated immune responses. They may also be associated with hypogammaglobulinemia. They are differentiated on the basis of their mode of inheritance.

B-cell deficiencies also occur in humans. The most severe of these, known as "Bruton-type" agammaglobulinemia, is an X-linked recessive condition; affected infants are devoid of all immunoglobulin classes and subclasses. They suffer from recurrent infections due to organisms such as pneumococci, staphylococci and streptococci but are usually resistant to viral, fungal and protozoan infections. Inherited deficiencies of individual immunoglobulin classes have also been recorded in humans. As might be anticipated, there are many possible combinations of deficiencies in IgG, IgM, IgA and IgE and a tendency to give each a specific name leads to confusion.

One of the most important of these is the Wiscott-Aldrich syndrome. In this disease, a selective IgM deficiency is associated with multiple infections, eczema and thrombocytopenia. Another such syndrome is ataxia-telangiectasia, in which serum IgA and IgE levels are extremely low or absent and cerebellar and cutaneous abnormalities exist. Affected children, lacking an effective surface immune system, suffer from recurrent bacterial respiratory tract infections.

SECONDARY IMMUNOLOGICAL DEFECTS

Although immunodeficiencies may occur as a result of a congenital defect in an animal's immune system, it is more common for a defect to be secondary to an identifiable provocation. Perhaps the most important cause of secondary immunological defects are virus infections. Equine herpes virus 1, canine distemper, feline leukemia, and bovine virus diarrhea are all capable of causing widespread and severe lymphoid tissue destruction. Thymic atrophy and lymphopenia are common manifestations of many virus infections, and before a congenital immunodeficiency syndrome is identified, rigorous steps must be taken to exclude the possibility that it is secondary to a virus infection. In addition, immunosuppression generally accompanies infestation with *Demodex, Toxoplasma* or trypanosomes, helminths such as *Trichinella spiralis* and bacteria such as *Pasteurella haemolytica*. Many environmental toxins such as polychlorinated biphenyls, polybrominated biphenyls, iodine, lead, cadmium, methyl mercury and DDT have a suppressive effect on the immune system, as do deficiencies of zinc and selenium.

Immunoglobulin synthesis is generally very much reduced in animals suffering from absolute protein deficiencies. Thus, immunosuppression occurs in the nephrotic syndrome, in malnutrition, in heavily parasitized or tumor-bearing animals and following severe burns or trauma. Adult horses with chronic diarrhea are immunosuppressed, as reflected by a hypogammaglobulinemia A and reduced lymphocyte responses to phytohemagglutinin. It is debatable whether the immunosuppression is due to a protein-losing enteropathy or the immunosuppression causes the diarrhea.

By chilling newborn puppies for five to ten days, it is possible to provoke an immunodeficiency syndrome very similar in appearance to CID.

Destruction of lymphoid tissue leading to immunosuppression may occur in tumor-bearing animals, especially if the tumors themselves are lymphoid in origin (Table 22–1). Some endocrine disorders such as thyrotoxicosis and diabetes may also cause immunosuppression.

NEOPLASMS OF LYMPHOID CELLS

The immune response requires that antigen-sensitive cells stimulated by appropriate exposure to antigen respond in a controlled fashion by division and differentiation. Much of the complexity of the immune system outlined in earlier chapters is presumably due to the need for rigid control of this cellular response; consequently, a failure in this control system may result in uncontrolled lymphoid cell proliferation. Surveillance was orginally proposed as a function of the immune system when it was observed that immunosuppressed animals and humans suffered from an increased prevalence of tumors. Analysis of the types of tumors seen in these individuals, however, shows that an unusually high proportion of them are of lymphoid origin. It is not unlikely, therefore, that at least some of these lymphoid tumors in immunosuppressed indivduals arise as a result of a failure in the immunological control systems rather than from a failure in surveillance.

Neoplastic transformation may occur in lymphoid cells of both branches of the immune system at almost any stage in their maturation process. Providing that the tumor cells have not dedifferentiated as a result of very rapid growth (as in acute lymphatic leukemia of calves), it is possible to identify the cells present in a lymphoid tumor by means of surface markers. The presence of cell-surface immunoglobulin is considered characteristic of B cells, and the capacity to form rosettes with sheep erythrocytes is an identifying feature of T cells.

Lymphoid tumors usually cause immunosuppression (Fig. 22–4); as a broad generalization, it may be claimed that T-cell tumors interfere with the cell-mediated immune system and B-cell tumors interfere with the antibody-mediated immune system (Table 22–1). Most cases of canine lymphosarcoma, Marek's disease, calf leukosis and feline leukemia are of T-cell origin. In Marek's disease, affected birds are immunosuppressed as a result of the activities of suppressor macrophages. These macrophages act

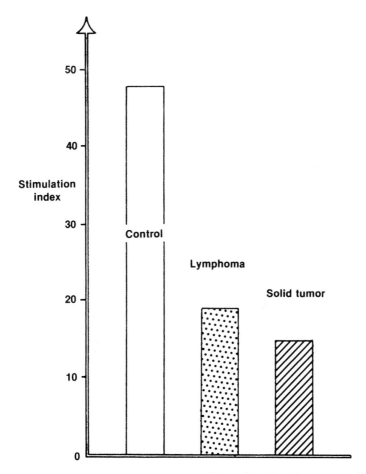

Figure 22–4 Immunosuppression in dogs suffering from lymphomas or solid tumors as compared to normal control dogs. The stimulation index is a measure of the response of lymphocytes to the mitogenic lectin phytohemagglutinin (see page 307). (Data taken from Weiden PL, et al. 1974. J Natl Cancer Inst 53 1053. Used with permission.)

Table 22–1　THE IMMUNOSUPPRESSIVE EFFECTS OF LYMPHOID TUMORS

TUMOR	CELL TYPE	EVIDENCE FOR IMMUNOSUPPRESSION	MECHANISMS
Feline leukemia	T cell	Lymphopenia Prolonged skin grafts Increased susceptibility to infection Lack of response to mitogens	Suppressive viral protein Suppressor cells
Marek's disease	T cell	Lack of response to mitogens Depressed cell-mediated cytotoxicity Depressed IgG production	Suppressor macrophages
Avian lymphoid leukosis	B cell	Increased susceptibility to infection	Suppressor lymphocytes
Bovine leukosis	B cell	Depressed serum IgM	Soluble serum factor
Myeloma	B cell	Increased susceptibility to infection	Soluble tumor-cell factor
Canine malignant lymphoma	B cell	Predisposition to infection associated with autoimmune disorders	Unknown

to restrict the replication of the tumor cells but in doing so suppress the resistance of birds to other infections.

The adult forms of bovine and ovine leukosis, the alimentary forms of feline leukemia, and avian leukosis are usually of B-cell origin, as reflected by the presence of immunoglobulin on the tumor cell surface. Animals with advanced bovine leukosis

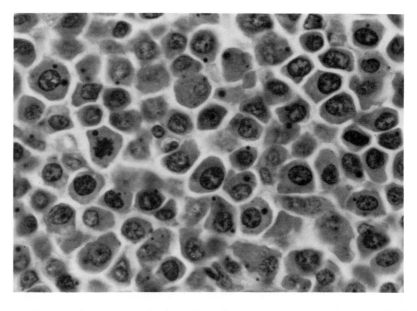

Figure 22–5　A photomicrograph of a section of a myeloma nodule in a dog. × 900. (From a specimen kindly provided by Dr. R. G. Thomson.)

are usually immunosuppressed as a result of the presence in their serum of an ill-defined suppressor factor. This suppression is commonly associated with lowered serum IgM levels. Occasionally the neoplastic cell in bovine leukosis may be sufficiently differentiated to secrete immunoglobulin, and excess immunoglobulin may be produced in a manner similar to that in myelomas. Similarly, although birds with avian lymphoid leukosis and cats with leukemia are normally severely immunosuppressed, some cases of these diseases may present with a hypergammaglobulinemia.

Myelomas. Malignant transformation of a single B cell may give rise to the development of a clone of immunoglobulin-producing tumor cells. The morphological features of these cells may vary, but they are usually recognizable as plasma cells (Fig. 22–5). Plasma cell tumors are known as myelomas or plasmacytomas. Because myelomas apparently arise from a single precursor cell, they produce a homogeneous immunoglobulin product known as a myeloma protein or M protein.

TERMINOLOGY

Myeloma proteins are also known as *paraproteins* and their presence in serum is termed *paraproteinemia*. The term *gammopathy* or *hypergammaglobulinemia* is used to denote any condition in which a pathological increase in immunoglobulin levels occurs. In general, the gammopathies are of two types. *Monoclonal gammopathies*, as are found in the myelomas, are characterized by a great rise in a single molecular type of immunoglobulin. This is readily seen as a very narrow, sharp peak on an electrophoretic scan. *Polyclonal gammopathies* (see page 341) are characterized by an overall rise in gammaglobulin levels, which may be readily identified on electrophoresis, since there is a rise in all the proteins in the globulin region, thus producing a broad peak on the electrophoretic scan (Fig. 22–6).

Myeloma proteins may belong to any immunoglobulin class. For example, IgG, IgA and IgM myelomas have been reported in the dog (Fig. 22–7). In humans, in addition to myelomas of the major immunoglobulin classes, rare cases of IgD and IgE myelomas have also been described. In general, the prevalence of the various immunoglobulin classes in myeloma proteins correlates well with their relative quantities in normal serum, suggesting that the condition arises as a consequence of a random mutation of a single plasma-cell clone. Light chain disease is a condition in which light chains alone are produced or the production of light chains is greatly in excess of the production of heavy chains. Similarly, there is a very rare variant of this condition in which Fc fragments alone are produced. This condition is erroneously termed heavy chain disease.

Myelomas have been reported to occur in humans, mice, dogs, cats, horses, cows, pigs and rabbits. The most common clinical manifestation in dogs is a bleeding problem that occurs as a result of a hyperviscosity syndrome as well as an effective loss of clotting components due to their binding to myeloma proteins. The hyper-

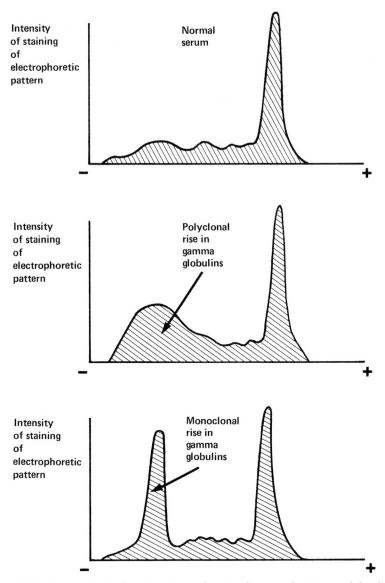

Figure 22−6 Serum electrophoretic patterns showing the normal pattern and the differences observed in monoclonal and polyclonal gammopathies.

viscosity syndrome results from the presence in serum of abnormally large quantities of immunoglobulins and is particularly severe in animals suffering from an IgM myeloma (macroglobulinemia). As a result of the increase in blood viscosity, the heart must work harder and congestive heart failure, retinopathy and neurologic signs may ensue. Because myeloma cells are also osteolytic, the presence of tumor masses in bone may lead to bone pain and to the development of multiple radiolucent osteolytic lesions and diffuse osteoporosis, both of which are readily observed by radiography. It may also lead to the occurrence of pathological fractures. Light chains, being relatively small (22,000 daltons), pass through the glomerulus and are excreted in the

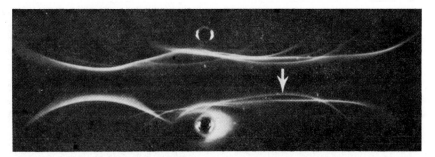

Figure 22−7   Immunoelectrophoresis of serum from a dog suffering from an IgM myeloma. The arrow points to the myeloma component band. The cathode is on the right and the developing reagent is rabbit anticanine whole serum. Note that both the IgG and IgA precipitin bands (first and second from right in the normal serum tracing) are diminished in the myeloma serum tracing. Furthermore, the IgM precipitin band is sharper and has moved closer to the center well in the myeloma sample, indicating an elevated concentration of IgM. (From Quimby FW, et al. 1980. Am J Vet Res *41* 1662. Used with permission.)

urine. Unfortunately, these molecules appear to be toxic for renal tubular cells, and as a result myelomas may be associated with renal failure. These light chains may also be detected in urine by electrophoresis of concentrated urine or, in some cases, by heating the urine. Light chains may precipitate when heated to 60°C but redissolve as the temperature is raised to 80°C. Proteins possessing this curious property are known as Bence-Jones proteins, and their presence in urine is suggestive of a myeloma.

Because of the overwhelming commitment of the body's immune resources to the production of neoplastic plasma cells as well as to the replacement of normal marrow tissue by tumor cells and to the negative feedback induced by elevated serum immunoglobulins, animals with myelomas are profoundly immunosuppressed. As a consequence of this, they commonly suffer from pyogenic bacterial infections. In humans, in fact, renal failure and overwhelming infection are the commonest causes of death in this disease. On occasion, old dogs and humans may show monoclonal gammopathy in the absence of myeloma. The cause is unknown, but the prognosis is good.

Polyclonal Gammopathies.   In contrast to monoclonal gammopathies, which are generally associated with myelomas, polyclonal gammopathies are observed in a wide variety of pathological conditions. The condition that might most resemble myeloma is Aleutian disease of mink (Chapter 14). Animals infected by the Aleutian disease virus show, in the progressive form of the disease, marked plasmacytosis and lymphocyte infiltration of many organs and tissues (Fig. 22–8) as well as polyclonal (occasionally monoclonal) gammopathy (Fig. 22–9). As a result of the elevated immunoglobulin levels, affected mink suffer from blood hyperviscosity and are severely immunosuppressed.

Other causes of polyclonal gammopathy include autoimmune disease such as systemic lupus erythematosus, rheumatoid arthritis and myasthenia gravis (Chapter 21); certain infections such as tropical pancytopenia of dogs (*Ehrlichia canis*) and African trypanosomiasis, in which B cells are polyclonally stimulated; and chronic bacterial infections such as pyometra and pyoderma, in which the prolonged antigenic stimulus leads to a hypergammaglobulinemia G. In horses heavily parasitized with *Strongylus vulgaris*, IgG(T) levels rise significantly. Polyclonal gammopathy also occurs in virus infections such as feline infectious peritonitis and African swine fever and in conditions in which there is extensive liver damage.

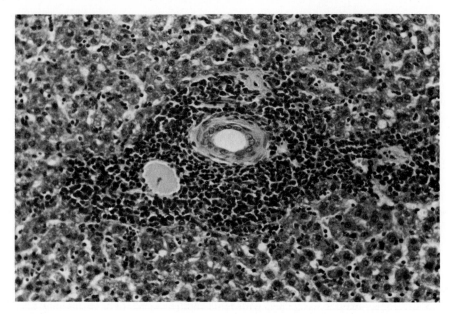

Figure 22–8 A section from the liver of an Aleutian disease–infected mink showing the marked plasma cell and lymphocyte infiltration. × 250. (From a specimen kindly provided by Dr. S. H. An.)

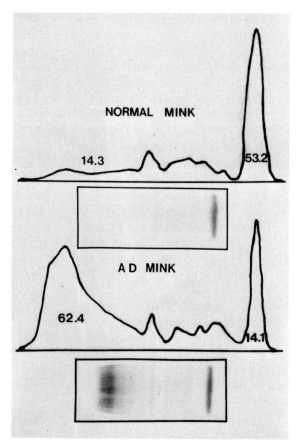

Figure 22–9 A comparison of the serum electrophoretic patterns seen in normal and Aleutian disease–infected mink. The serum of the infected animal shows a polyclonal gammopathy so that the gamma globulins account for 62.4 per cent of the serum proteins in contrast to the normal level of 14.3 per cent. (Courtesy of Dr. S. An.)

HYPERACTIVITY OF THE IMMUNE SYSTEM

Amyloidosis. Amyloid is the name given to an amorphous, eosinophilic, hyaline, extracellular substance that infiltrates tissues in certain pathological conditions. It is found in all domestic animals, particularly cattle, horses and dogs. It may be classified either as "immunocytic," if it is associated with a myeloma or other lymphoid tumor, or as "reactive," if it is associated with chronic suppurative conditions such as mastitis, osteomyelitis, abscesses, traumatic pericarditis or tuberculosis. Reactive amyloidosis is a major cause of death in animals repeatedly immunized for commercial antiserum production. It is also commonly associated with autoimmune disorders. Several other well-defined forms of amyloidosis are seen in domestic animals; for example, old dogs may suffer from vascular amyloidosis in which amyloid is deposited in the media of leptomeningeal and cortical arteries. Tumor-like amyloid nodules and subcutaneous amyloid have been reported in horses, but in general, amyloid deposits are usually found in the liver, spleen (Figs. 22–10 and 22–11) and kidneys, particularly within glomeruli. Amyloidosis may be produced in laboratory mice by feeding them a diet rich in casein or by injecting large or repeated doses of bacterial endotoxin or Freund's complete adjuvant.

On electron microscopy all forms of amyloid can be shown to consist of a felt-like mass of protein fibrils. By x-ray crystallography it can be further shown that all amyloid proteins have their polypeptide chains arranged in the form known as β-pleated sheets. This is a uniquely stable molecular conformation that renders the fibrils both extremely insoluble and almost totally resistant to normal proteolytic enzymes. Consequently, once deposited in tissues, they are almost impossible to remove. The accumulation of amyloid in tissues is, therefore, essentially irreversible, leading to gradual cell loss and tissue destruction.

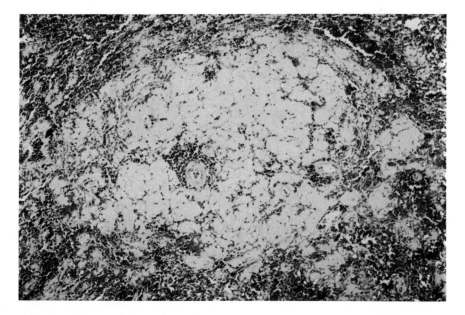

Figure 22–10 Amyloidosis in the spleen of a dog suffering from visceral leishmaniasis. × 25. (From Corbeil LB, et al. 1976. Clin Immunol Immunopathol 6 165–173. Used with permission.)

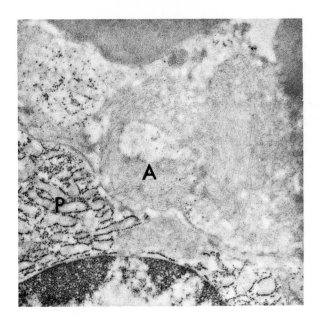

Figure 22–11 An electron micrograph of splenic amyloid from a dog suffering from visceral leishmaniasis. Note the close association between the amyloid fibrils (A) and a plasma cell (P). × 16,750. (From Corbeil LB, et al. 1976. Clin Immunol Immunopathol 6 165–173. Used with permission.)

The β-pleated sheet configuration of amyloid also gives it unique staining properties; for example, it stains metachromatically with toluidine-blue and binds specifically to congo-red.

Although all amyloid proteins have the β-pleated sheet configuration, biochemical analysis has shown that most are composed of one of two basic proteins (Fig. 22–12). In immunogenic amyloid and a few cases of reactive amyloid, this protein is known as AL. AL protein is a proteolytic digestion product of immunoglobulin light chains. In myeloma, light chains (Bence-Jones proteins) are usually generated in excess, and limited proteolytic digestion of these permits the V_L region to assume a β-pleated configuration. It has been suggested that immunogenic amyloid deposits consist of light chains modified by proteolytic enzymes from cells such as macrophages and deposited in tissues in excessive amounts.

The major protein component of reactive amyloid is known as AA. AA is not immunoglobulin derived but may be deposited in close association with plasma cells. It is probably derived from proteolytic digestion of an α globulin found in serum called SAA. SAA is found in high concentrations in the serum of humans and animals with experimental or natural amyloidosis and in the serum of patients undergoing chronic antigenic stimulation, as in tuberculosis or rheumatoid arthritis. It is found in low levels in normal serum and is produced by hepatocytes and fibroblasts. Since SAA has been shown to be strongly immunosuppressive in mice, it has been suggested that SAA normally serves to control the immune response and that, under conditions of chronic antigenic stimulation, excessive production of SAA and its subsequent digestion can lead to the deposition of AA as amyloid in tissues.

Reactive amyloid also contains, in addition to AA, a small quantity of a basement membrane protein known as AP component, which is related to C-reactive protein (Chapter 7). Although AP is probably unimportant in the pathogenesis of amyloidosis, C-reactive protein is known to be immunosuppressive, and the presence of AP, like that of AA, might be a reflection of an attempt by the body to control excessive immune reactivity.

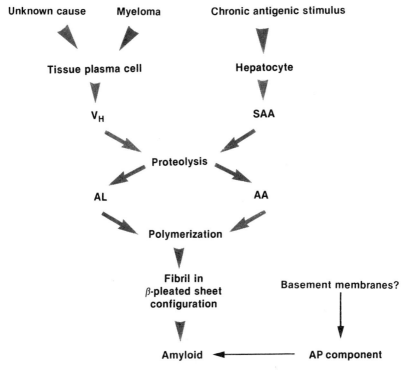

Figure 22–12   The pathogenesis of immunogenic and reactive amyloidosis.

Although AL and AA are associated with the two major forms of amyloid, it must be emphasized that any protein that can form extensive β-pleated sheets will give rise to amyloid if deposited in tissues. Many of the less common manifestations of amyloidosis may, therefore, be caused by proteins distinct from AL or AA. It has been suggested that a more appropriate collective term for the amyloidoses is β fibrilloses, since the β-1 pleated conformational structure is the common feature of all these conditions.

ADDITIONAL SOURCES OF INFORMATION

Buntain B. 1981. IgG immunodeficiency in a half-Arabian foal with salmonellosis. Vet Med Small Anim Clin 76 231–234.

Chusid MJ, Bujak JS, and Dale DC. 1975. Defective polymorphonuclear leukocyte metabolism and function in canine cyclic neutropenia. Blood 46 921–930.

Cockerell GL. 1978. Naturally occurring acquired immunodeficiency diseases of the dog and cat. Vet Clin North Am (Small Animal Practice) 8 613–628.

Glenner GG. 1980. Amyloid deposits and amyloidosis. The β-fibrilloses. N Engl J Med 302 1283–1292, 1333–1343.

Holmberg CA, Manning JS, and Osburn BI. 1976. Feline malignant lymphomas: comparison of morphologic and immunologic characteristics. Am J Vet Res 37 1455–1460.

Kennard J, and Zolla-Pazner S. 1980. Origin and function of suppressor macrophages in myeloma. J Immunol 124 268–273.

Koller LD. 1979. Effects of environmental contaminants on the immune system. Adv Vet Sci Comp Med 23 267–295.

Kulkarni PE. 1971. IgG2 deficiency in gangrenous mastitis in cows. Acta Vet Scand 12 611–614.

McGuire TC, Poppie MJ, and Banks KL. 1974. Combined (B- and T-lymphocyte) immunodeficiency: a fatal genetic disease in Arabian foals. JAVMA 164 70–76.

Perryman LE. 1979. Primary and secondary immune deficiencies of domestic animals. Adv Vet Sci Comp Med *23* 23–52.

Perryman LE, Buening GM, McGuire TC, *et al*. 1979. Fetal tissue transplantation for immunotherapy of combined immunodeficiency in horses. Clin Immunol Immunopathol *12* 238–251.

Perryman LE, and McGuire TC. 1980. Evaluation for immune system failures in horses and ponies. JAVMA *176* 1374–1377.

Weiden PL, and Blaese RM. 1971. Hemolytic anemia in agammaglobulinemic chickens — a model of autoimmune disease in immune deficiency. J Immunol *107* 1004–1013.

Index

Note: Page numbers in *italic* indicate an illustration.
Page numbers followed by t indicate a table.